Psychiatric Diagnosis:
Challenges and Prospects

Psychiatric Diagnosis
Challenges and Prospects

Editors

Ihsan M. Salloum

*Professor of Psychiatry and Director, Division of Alcohol and Substance Abuse:
Treatment and Research, University of Miami Miller School of Medicine, FL, USA
Section on Classification, Diagnostic Assessment and Nomenclature,
World Psychiatric Association*

Juan E. Mezzich

*Professor of Psychiatry and Director, International Center for Mental Health and
Division of Psychiatric Epidemiology, Mount Sinai School of Medicine,
New York University, NY, USA
Past President, World Psychiatric Association*

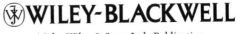
WILEY-BLACKWELL

A John Wiley & Sons, Ltd., Publication

This edition first published 2009
© 2009 John Wiley & Sons Ltd.

Wiley-Blackwell is an imprint of John Wiley & Sons, formed by the merger of Wiley's global Scientific, Technical and Medical business with Blackwell Publishing.

Registered office
John Wiley & Sons Ltd, The Atrium, Southern Gate, Chichester, West Sussex, PO19 8SQ, UK

Other Editorial Offices
9600 Garsington Road, Oxford, OX4 2DQ, UK
111 River Street, Hoboken, NJ 07030-5774, USA

For details of our global editorial offices, for customer services and for information about how to apply for permission to reuse the copyright material in this book please see our website at www.wiley.com/wiley-blackwell

The right of the author to be identified as the author of this work has been asserted in accordance with the Copyright, Designs and Patents Act 1988.

Wiley also publishes its books in a variety of electronic formats. Some content that appears in print may not be available in electronic books.

Designations used by companies to distinguish their products are often claimed as trademarks. All brand names and product names used in this book are trade names, service marks, trademarks or registered trademarks of their respective owners. The publisher is not associated with any product or vendor mentioned in this book. This publication is designed to provide accurate and authoritative information in regard to the subject matter covered. It is sold on the understanding that the publisher is not engaged in rendering professional services. If professional advice or other expert assistance is required, the services of a competent professional should be sought.

The contents of this work are intended to further general scientific research, understanding, and discussion only and are not intended and should not be relied upon as recommending or promoting a specific method, diagnosis, or treatment by physicians for any particular patient. The publisher and the author make no representations or warranties with respect to the accuracy or completeness of the contents of this work and specifically disclaim all warranties, including without limitation any implied warranties of fitness for a particular purpose. In view of ongoing research, equipment modifications, changes in governmental regulations, and the constant flow of information relating to the use of medicines, equipment, and devices, the reader is urged to review and evaluate the information provided in the package insert or instructions for each medicine, equipment, or device for, among other things, any changes in the instructions or indication of usage and for added warnings and precautions. Readers should consult with a specialist where appropriate. The fact that an organization or Website is referred to in this work as a citation and/or a potential source of further information does not mean that the author or the publisher endorses the information the organization or Website may provide or recommendations it may make. Further, readers should be aware that Internet Websites listed in this work may have changed or disappeared between when this work was written and when it is read. No warranty may be created or extended by any promotional statements for this work. Neither the publisher nor the author shall be liable for any damages arising herefrom.

Library of Congress Cataloguing-in-Publication Data

Psychiatric diagnosis : challenges and prospects / editors, Ihsan M. Salloum, Juan E. Mezzich.
    p.   ;   cm.
  Includes bibliographical references and index.
  ISBN 978-0-470-72569-6
  1. Mental illness—Classification.   2. Psychodiagnostics.
  I. Salloum, Ihsan M.   II. Mezzich, Juan E.
  [DNLM: 1. Mental Disorders—classification.   2. Mental Disorders—diagnosis.
  3. Comorbidity.   4. Models, Psychological. WM 141 P97357 2009]
  RC455.2.C4.P78 2009
  616.89′075—dc22

                                                                         2008051201

ISBN: 978-0-470-72569-6 (H/B)

A catalogue record for this book is available from the British Library.

Set in 10/12pt Times by Integra Software Services Pvt. Ltd, Pondicherry, India.
Printed in Great Britain by Antony Rowe Ltd, Chippenham, Wiltshire.

First Impression   2009

Contents

List of contributors

Michaela Amering
Professor, Department of Psychiatry and Psychotherapy, Division of Social Psychiatry, Medical University of Vienna, Vienna, Austria

Gisèle Apter-Denon
Responsible Unite Ppumma (Unite de Psychiatric Périnatale d' Urgence Mobile en Maternité), Université Denis Diderot, Paris 7, France

Said Abdel Azim
Emeritus Professor of Psychiatry, Cairo University, Egypt

Olusegun Baiyewu
Professor of Psychiatry, College of Medicine, University of Ibadan, Nigeria

Claudio E. M. Banzato
Associate Professor of Psychiatry, University of Campinas – UNICAMP, Brazil

Marna S. Barrett
Department of Psychiatry, University of Pennsylvania School of Medicine, Philadelphia, PA, USA

Carlos E. Berganza
Professor of Child Psychiatry, San Carlos University School of Medicine, Guatemala; Past President, Executive Committee on the Latin American Guide for Psychiatric Diagnosis

Dinesh Bhugra
Professor of Social & Cultural Psychiatry, Institute of Psychiatry, London, UK; President, Royal College of Psychiatrists, UK

Michel Botbol
World Psychiatric Association Zonal Representative for Western Europe; Member of the steering committee of the Institutional Program on Psychiatry for the Person; Section on Psychoanalysis in Psychiatry, World Psychiatric Association

Ian Brockington
Professor Emeritus, University of Birmingham, Birmingham, UK

Yanfang Chen
Professor, Beijing Huilongguang Hospital, Teaching Hospital of Peking University, Beijing, China

Zhong Chen
Professor, Shandong Mental Health Center, Teaching Hospital of Shandong University, Jinan, China

George Christodoulou
Professor of Psychiatry, Athens University, Greece; Standing Committee on Ethics, World Psychiatric Association; European Division, Royal College of Psychiatry; Honorary President, Hellenic Psychiatric Association; President, Hellenic Center for Mental Health & Research, Athens, Greece

C. Robert Cloninger
Wallace Renard Professor of Psychiatry, Genetics & Psychology, Washington University School of Medicine, Department of Psychiatry, St Louis, MO, USA

Sally-Ann Cooper
Professor of Learning Disabilities, Section of Psychological Medicine, Division of Community Based Sciences, Faculty of Medicine, University of Glasgow, Gartnavel Royal Hospital, Glasgow, UK

Sandra E. Cordoba
International Center for Mental Health, Mount Sinai School of Medicine, New York University, NY, USA

John Cox
Professor Emeritus, Keele University, Staffordshire, UK

Felipe Navarro Cremades
Universidad Miguel Hernandez, Alicante, Spain

Michael B. First
Professor of Clinical Psychiatry, Columbia University, NY, USA; Research Psychiatrist, New York State Psychiatric Institute, New York, NY, USA

KWM (Bill) Fulford
Professor of Philosophy and Mental Health, University of Warwick, UK; Fellow of St Cross College and Member of the Philosophy Faculty, University of Oxford; Honorary Consultant Psychiatrist, University of Oxford, UK; Co-Director, Institute for Philosophy, Diversity and Mental Health, University of Central Lancashire, UK; National Fellow for Values-Based Practice, Department of Health, London, UK

Wolfgang Gaebel
Professor & Chair, Department of Psychiatry and Psychotherapy, Heinrich-Heine-University, Rhineland State Clinics, Düsseldorf, Germany; Chair, Section on Schizophrenia, World Psychiatric Association

Nicole Garret-Gloanec
Chef de Service de Psychiatric Infanto-Juvenile, Nantes, France

Linda Gask
Divisions of Psychiatry and Primary Care, University of Manchester, UK

Nady el-Guebaly
Addiction Division, University of Calgary, Canada; Chair, Section on Addiction Psychiatry, World Psychiatric Association

Christian Haasen
Professor, Zentrum für interdisziplinäre Suchtforschung, Hamburg, Germany

Paul Hoff
Professor, Department of General and Social Psychiatry, University of Zurich, Zurich, Switzerland

Robert Jakob
Office of Classifications, Terminologies, and Standards, World Health Organization, Geneva, Switzerland

Miguel Roberto Jorge
Professor, Department of Psychiatry, Federal University of São Paulo, Brazil; Secretary for Sections, World Psychiatric Association

Marianne Kastrup
Head, Centre Transcultural Psychiatry Psychiatric Clinic, Rigshospitalet, Copenhagen, Denmark

Heinz Katschnig
Professor, Ludwig Boltzmann Institute for Social Psychiatry, Vienna, Austria

Laurence J. Kirmayer
Professor & Director, Division of Social & Transcultural Psychiatry, McGill University, Culture & Mental Health Research Unit, Sir Mortimer B Davis–Jewish General Hospital, Montreal, Quebec, Canada

Michael S. Klinkman
Professor, Departments of Family Medicine and Psychiatry, University of Michigan, MI, USA

Juan J. López-Ibor, Jr
Chairman, Institute of Psychiatry and Mental Health, San Carlos Hospital, Complutense University, Madrid, Spain

María Inés López-Ibor
Professor of Psychiatry, Department of Psychiatry and Medical Psychology, Complutense University, Madrid, Spain

Juan E. Mezzich
Professor of Psychiatry and Director, International Center for Mental Health and Division of Psychiatric Epidemiology, Mount Sinai School of Medicine, New York University, NY, USA; Past President of the World Psychiatric Association

Giles Newton-Howes
Division of Neurosciences and Mental Health, Imperial College London, London, UK

Ángel Otero-Ojeda
Professor, Havana University School of Medicine, Cuba; Section on Diagnosis and
Classification, Latin American Psychiatric Association; Executive Committee on the
Latin America Guide for Psychiatric Diagnosis; Cuban Glossary of Psychiatry

Antonio Pacheco Palha
Hospital San Joao, University of Porto, Portugal

Aminta Parra
Universidad Central de Venezuela, Caracas, Venezuela

Zoltán Rihmer
Professor, Department of Clinical and Theoretical Mental Health, and Department of
Psychiatry and Psychotherapy, Semmelweis Medical University, Budapest, Hungary

Wolfgang Rutz
Professor, University Hospital, Uppsala, Sweden; University for Applied Sciences,
Coburg, Germany

Ihsan M. Salloum
Professor of Psychiatry and Director, Division of Alcohol and Substance Abuse: Treatment
and Research, University of Miami Miller School of Medicine, FL, USA; Section on
Classification, Diagnostic Assessment and Nomenclature, World Psychiatric Association

Luis Salvador-Carulla
Professor of Psychiatry, University of Cadiz (Spain); Section on Psychiatry of Intellectual
Disability, World Psychiatric Association

Benedetto Saraceno
Director, Department of Mental Health and Substance Abuse, World Health Organization,
Geneva, Switzerland

Norman Sartorius
Professor, University of Geneva, Switzerland

Shekhar Saxena
Programme Manager, Department of Mental Health and Substance Abuse, World Health
Organization, Geneva, Switzerland

Kenneth F. Schaffner
University Professor of History and Philosophy of Science, Professor of Psychiatry,
University of Pittsburgh, PA, USA

Lior Schapir
GEHA Mental Health Center, Tel Aviv University School of Medicine, Israel

Margit Schmolke
German Academy for Psychoanalysis, Munich, Germany; Co-Chair, World Psychiatric
Association Section on Preventive Psychiatry

Rubén Hernández Serrano
Universidad Central de Venezuela, Caracas, Venezuela

Raluca Sfetcu
Professor, Babes-Bolyai University, Cluj-Napoca, Romania

Chiara Simonelli
Professor, Institute of Sessuologia Clinica, University of La Sapienza, Rome, Italy

Michael E. Thase
Professor of Psychiatry, University of Pennsylvania School of Medicine, Philadelphia, PA, USA

Tim Thornton
Professor of Philosophy and Mental Health and Director of Philosophy, University of Central Lancashire, UK

Sam Tyano
Professor Emeritus in Psychiatry, Tel Aviv University School of Medicine, Israel

Peter Tyrer
Division of Neurosciences and Mental Health, Imperial College London, London, UK

T. Bedirhan Üstün
Head, Office of Classifications, Terminologies, and Standards, World Health Organization, Geneva, Switzerland

Jürgen Zielasek
Department of Psychiatry and Psychotherapy, Heinrich-Heine-University, Rhineland State Clinics, Düsseldorf, Germany

Preface

Diagnosis occupies a pivotal role in clinical care and public health. As it was cogently stated by Feinstein almost half a century ago, "*diagnostic categories provide the locations where clinicians store the observations of clinical experience*" and "*the diagnostic taxonomy establishes the patterns according to which clinicians observe, think, remember and act*" [1]. Diagnosis is the basic unit in the process of medical care. It is essential for communication among clinicians, for the identification and treatment of disorders, for education and training, for prevention and health promotion efforts, and for performing vital administrative and quality monitoring tasks.

Major developments in psychiatric diagnosis and classification were introduced into a standardized nosology with the publication of the Diagnostic and Statistical Manual of Mental Disorders, Third Edition (DSM-III) over a quarter of a century ago. These concepts emphasizing descriptive psychopathology have transformed the practice of psychiatry and contributed greatly to the extraordinary expansion in psychiatric research over this period. Improved reliability has been the most notable benefit of applying standardized descriptive criteria for psychiatric disorders. This approach, however, did not lead to similar advances in the validity of current nosological entities, and while the provision of diagnostic criteria for psychiatric disorder has enhanced research in general, empirical work on the classification system itself has been remarkably limited.

This book addresses current challenges and future prospects for psychiatric diagnosis, a central topic in clinical care and public health. This theme is especially timely as two major psychiatric diagnostic systems, the WHO International Classification of Diseases, Mental Disorders Chapter, and the APA Diagnostic and Statistical Manual of Mental Disorders, have started their revision processes. Additionally, new perspectives are emerging, such as the Person-centered Integrative Diagnosis model developed by the WPA Classification Section and Person-centered Psychiatry Program and those involving regional adaptations and annotations (such as the APAL Latin American Guide for Psychiatric Diagnosis). In line with the above, a number of conceptual, methodological and contextual issues as well as innovative prospects are arising, such as the distinction between *nosological diagnosis* and *full diagnosis* as discussed by Lain Entralgo [2], and that between *aetiopathogenic* and *clinical* validities of psychiatric diagnosis as outlined by Schaffner [3]. A range of these major issues and prospects are addressed in this volume by some of the most authoritative experts in the world.

The present monograph presents a systematic review of key concepts, the structure and context of psychiatric diagnosis along innovative emerging lines, including diagnostic systems that have been developed recently or are in the process of being developed. Leaders in the field offer a pointed look at fundamental areas concerning the future of psychiatric diagnosis.

A critical feature of this book is its broad consideration of psychiatry and mental health. From a conceptual perspective, Section I addresses mental health and illness across the world from historical, philosophical, ethical and cultural perspectives, as well as a broad notion of health, including its positive aspects such as resilience, resources and quality of life. Major specific psychopathology topics are covered in Section II, including new categorizations and dimensional approaches. Broad illness categories include dementia, psychotic disorders, mood disorders, anxiety disorders, substance-related disorders, sexual disorders, sleep disorders, personality disorders, intellectual disabilities, child and adolescent psychiatric disorders and perinatal mental disorders, as well as a key chapter on suicide. Section III broadly addresses the complex problem of comorbidity regarding conceptual and methodological issues with a special focus on comorbidity in mental and general health in persons presenting in primary care, and on comorbidity, positive aspects of health and integration of care.

Finally, Section IV focuses on diagnostic models, with a chapter addressing the crucial topic of validity of psychiatric diagnosis. Two chapters delineate the processes involved in the upcoming revision of the International Classification of Diseases, one focused on the overall development of ICD-11, and the second on the revision of the ICD-10 Chapter on Mental and Behavioral Disorders (Chapter V). Experience with the development of DSM-V is presented next, followed by experience with other national and regional classification and diagnostic systems, most prominently the Latin American Guide for Psychiatric Diagnosis and the Chinese Classification of Mental Disorders. The multiaxial schema for psychiatric diagnosis is heuristically discussed next. Finally, the WPA Person-centered Integrative Diagnosis, a novel model for comprehensive diagnosis with focus on both ill and positive aspects of health, concludes this volume.

Our purpose has been to include the broadest international perspectives given the importance and global impact of the topic for the whole community involved with mental health and general health, including clinicians, researchers, educators, trainees and policy makers. Practising mental and general health professionals, both young and experienced, may find it of interest as it presents challenging issues and innovative proposals for improved evaluation and care.

Ihsan M. Salloum and Juan E. Mezzich

REFERENCES

[1] Feinstein AR. *Clinical judgment*. Huntington, NY, USA: Robert E. Krieger, 1967.
[2] Lain-Entralgo, P: *Medical Diagnosis*. Barcelona, Spain, Salvat, 1982.
[3] Schaffner, KF: An Alternative Approach to Clarifying Kinds. In: K. S. Kendler and J. Parnas (eds) *Philosophical Issues in Psychiatry: Explanation, Phenomenology, and Nosology*, Baltimore, MD, USA: Johns Hopkins University Press, 2008.

World Psychiatric Association Evidence and Experience in Psychiatry Series

Series Editor: Helen Herrman (2005 -) WPA Secretary for Publications, University of Melbourne, Australia

The *Evidence & Experience in Psychiatry* series, launched in 1999, offers unique insights into both investigation and practice in mental health. Developed and commissioned by the World Psychiatric Association, the books address controversial issues in clinical psychiatry and integrate research evidence and clinical experience to provide a stimulating overview of the field.

Focused on common psychiatric disorders, each volume follows the same format: systematic review of the available research evidence followed by multiple commentaries written by clinicians of different orientations and from different countries. Each includes coverage of diagnosis, management, pharma and psycho-therapies, and social and economic issues. The series provides insights that will prove invaluable to psychiatrists, psychologists, mental health nurses and policy makers.

Depressive Disorders, 3e
Edited by Helen Herrman, Mario Maj and Norman Sartorius
ISBN: 978-0-470-98720-9

Substance Abuse
Edited by Hamid Ghodse, Helen Herrman, Mario Maj and Norman Sartorius
ISBN: 978-0-470-74510-6

Schizophrenia 2e
Edited by Mario Maj, Norman Sartorius
ISBN: 978-0-470-84964-4

Dementia 2e
Edited by Mario Maj, Norman Sartorius
ISBN: 978-0-470-84963-7

Obsessive-Compulsive Disorders 2e
Edited by Mario Maj, Norman Sartorius, Ahmed Okasha, Joseph Zohar
ISBN: 978-0-470-84966-8

Bipolar Disorders
Edited by Mario Maj, Hagop S Akiskal, Juan José López-Ibor, Norman Sartorius
ISBN: 978-0-471-56037-1

Eating Disorders
Edited by Mario Maj, Kathrine Halmi, Juan José López-Ibor, Norman Sartorius
ISBN: 978-0-470-84865-4

Phobias
Edited by Mario Maj, Hagop S Akiskal, Juan José López-Ibor, Ahmed Okasha
ISBN: 978-0-470-85833-2

Personality Disorders
Edited by Mario Maj, Hagop S Akiskal, Juan E Mezzich
ISBN: 978-0-470-09036-7

Somatoform Disorders
Edited by Mario Maj, Hagop S Akiskal, Juan E Mezzich, Ahmed Okasha
ISBN: 978-0-470-01612-1

Other World Psychiatric Association titles

Series Editor (2005 -): Helen Herrman, WPA Secretary for Publications, University of Melbourne, Australia

Special Populations

The Mental Health of Children and Adolescents: an area of global neglect
Edited by Helmut Remschmidt, Barry Nurcombe, Myron L. Belfer, Norman Sartorius and Ahmed Okasha
ISBN: 978-0-470-51245-6

Contemporary Topics in Women's Mental Health: global perspectives in a changing society
Edited by Prabha S. Chandra, Helen Herrman, Marianne Kastrup, Marta Rondon, Unaiza Niaz, Ahmed Okasha, Jane Fisher
ISBN: 978-0-470-75411-5

Families and Mental Disorders
Edited by Norman Sartorius, Julian Leff, Juan José López-Ibor, Mario Maj, Ahmed Okasha
ISBN: 978-0-470-02382-2

Disasters and Mental Health
Edited by Juan José López-Ibor, George Christodoulou, Mario Maj, Norman Sartorius, Ahmed Okasha
ISBN: 978-0-470-02123-1

Approaches to Practice and Research

Recovery in Mental Health: reshaping scientific and clinical responsibilities
By Michaela Amering and Margit Schmolke
ISBN: 978-0-470-99796-3

Handbook of Service User Involvement in Mental Health Research
Edited by Jan Wallcraft, Beate Schrank and Michaela Amering
ISBN: 978-0-470-99795-6

Psychiatry and Religion: beyond boundaries
Edited by Peter J Verhagen, Herman M van Praag, Juan José López-Ibor, John Cox, Driss Moussaoui
ISBN: 978-0-470-69471-8

Psychiatrists and Traditional Healers: unwitting partners in global mental health
Edited by Mario Incayawar, Ronald Wintrob and Lise Bouchard
ISBN: 978-0-470-51683-6

Psychiatric Diagnosis and Classification
Edited by Mario Maj, Wolfgang Gaebel, Juan José López-Ibor, Norman Sartorius
ISBN: 978-0-471-49681-6

Psychiatry in Society
Edited by Norman Sartorius, Wolfgang Gaebel, Juan José López-Ibor, Mario Maj
ISBN: 978-0-471-49682-3

Psychiatry as a Neuroscience
Edited by Juan José López-Ibor, Mario Maj, Norman Sartorius
ISBN: 978-0-471-49656-4

Early Detection and Management of Mental Disorders
Edited by Mario Maj, Juan José López-Ibor, Norman Sartorius, Mitsumoto Sato, Ahmed Okasha
ISBN: 978-0-470-01083-9

CONCEPTS OF MENTAL ILLNESS AND HEALTH ACROSS THE WORLD

CHAPTER 1

Historical Roots of the Concept of Mental Illness

Paul Hoff

Professor, Department of General and Social Psychiatry,
University of Zurich, Zurich, Switzerland

1.1 INTRODUCTION

Of all medical specialities, psychiatry and psychotherapy are probably the ones that are most intensively connected with political, historical and social developments taking place in society [1]. However, the relationship between psychiatry and society is typically an ambivalent one. On the one hand, society puts psychiatry in charge of mentally ill people, especially in order to develop efficient therapeutical tools and carry out research. On the other hand, there are often sceptical or even suspicious under currents when psychiatric issues are debated publicly. The complex reasons for this cannot be discussed here, but a historical perspective, especially the history of psychiatric ideas, might help to bring more clarity and scientific argument to the debate. Of course, any such overview shortens and, by this, simplifies the field. One of the main intentions of this chapter is to exemplify the practical significance of the historical perspective for present-day psychiatry.

1.2 ANCIENT GREECE TO THE ENLIGHTENMENT

The exponent of ancient Greek medicine, Hippokrates von Kos (460–377 BC), postulated – in a very modern way – that empirical data and not (only) theoretical speculation should guide our practical behaviour towards health and illness, explicitly including mental health and illness. He favoured a 'somatic' etiology of mental illness, but did not regard the brain as the central factor. His suggestion was that different types of illnesses ('humoral pathology') were caused when the equilibrium of body fluencies was disturbed. Therapeutic ideas included not only diatetic or somatic methods but also differentiated suggestions for how to

Psychiatric Diagnosis: Challenges and Prospects   Edited by I.M. Salloum and J.E. Mezzich
© 2009 John Wiley & Sons, Ltd

deal with disturbed people, which we might well call precursors of modern psycho- and sociotherapeutic techniques.

The Middle Ages and Renaissance saw more setbacks than positive developments in terms of the understanding of 'madness'. Although hospitals were beginning to accept mentally ill people as patients (e.g. 1409 in Valencia, Spain), at the same time there was discrimination against psychotic individuals, who were described as 'possessed' or 'witches', and even killed. Nevertheless, there were already critical voices. For example, in the writings of Paracelsus (1491–1541)[1] and Johann Weyer (1515–1588), we find a remarkable combination of highly speculative *and* empirical, 'pre-modern' arguments. Before and even during the Enlightenment, however, rationalistic and person-oriented behaviour towards mentally ill people was far from widespread. In their early days, the large mental asylums of Paris, such as Bicêtre and Salpêtrière, were a peculiar mixture of homes for orphans, poor and homeless people; prisons; and, finally, mental hospitals.

1.3   THE EMERGENCE OF PSYCHIATRY

It was not until the 18th century – in the context of enlightenment – that psychiatry began to emerge and define itself as a medical discipline, rooted in scientific research and debate, and dedicated to the treatment of the individual mentally ill person. The number of psychiatric hospitals increased and, all over Europe, there were initiatives to free especially severely psychotic persons from the many and often cruel mechanical and other restraints that had previously regularly been imposed upon them. Prominent figures in this context are Philippe Pinel in Paris, William Tuke in York and Johann Gottfried Langermann in Bayreuth. John Conolly (1794–1866) later became known as the leader of the 'non-restraint' movement.

From this time on, psychiatrists also began to be regarded as experts by the courts in civil law and issues regarding penal code. This development, in turn, partly influenced clinical psychiatry and especially the nosological debate. By creating the new diagnostic entity of 'moral insanity', the English psychiatrist James Cowles Prichard (1785–1848) initiated a controversy that has continued to the present day. He used the term to describe people who ignored the commonly accepted values, behaved egoistically and would not recognize their own behaviour as unjustified or even a problem at all. The controversy arises from that very question, of whether such individuals simply do not *want* to respect other people's rights (although they could) or they really *cannot* do so (due do their 'moral insanity'). Nowadays, precisely this issue is discussed with regard to the forensic relevance of personality disorders, especially antisocial personality disorder or 'psychopathy'.

1.4   THE NINETEENTH CENTURY

1.4.1   Romanticism

The first decades of the 19th century saw an influential group of psychiatric authors, mainly in German speaking countries, who were part of the romanticism movement. Philosophically, romanticism was strongly oriented to Schelling's philosophy of nature, and its emphasis was on affectivity, irrationality and vagueness, in contrast to the

Enlightenment's strong focus on rationality and measurement. Nowadays, this period is known mainly for the 'romantic' style of its art and literature, but there was also a strong interest in and influence on psychiatric issues. What is central, for our present context, is the interest that was taken by 'romantic psychiatry' in the subjective perspective of the individual person and his or her 'idiographic' development before becoming mentally disturbed. This, in a way, was opposed to the more or less 'nomothetic' approach of the Enlightenment some decades earlier. 'Romantic psychiatry' explicitly recognized the relevance of affects and emotions (*Leidenschaften*, to use the strong German expression) for normal and disturbed mental phenomena [2, 3, 4]. Prominent authors of this time were, for example, J.C.A. Heinroth (1773–1843) and K. Ideler (1795–1860) [5].

1.4.2   Griesinger

One of the most remarkable figures in the history of modern psychiatry, Wilhelm Griesinger (1817–1868), marked the turning point from romanticism in psychiatry to what may be called the rise of modern empirical, and especially neurobiological, research into mental illness. Griesinger postulated that psychiatry should deal with the mind-body relationship empirically (i.e. by clinical and psychophysiological research) and not metaphysically. But – and this is often underestimated – he also criticized any simple materialistic attitude towards mental phenomena, voting for a *methodological*, not a *metaphysical* materialism. This is important in order not to misinterpret his often quoted thesis, that 'mental illness is an illness of the brain' (in 19th century German: '*Geisteskrankheiten sind Gehirnkrankheiten*').

Griesinger's work also strongly influenced two other areas of psychiatric practice and research. Nosologically, he postulated the existence of only one psychotic illness, which can appear clinically in different stages ('unitary psychosis', or '*Einheitspsychose*') from affective syndromes to paranoid-hallucinatory and catatonic syndromes and, finally, to chronic states with severe cognitive deficits, nowadays called dementia (1845; 2nd ed. 1861 [6]).

Griesinger also gave strong impulses to develop community-based care models for mentally ill people ('*Stadtasyl*') and is therefore one of the forerunners of modern social psychiatry [7, 8]. So, Wilhelm Griesinger, although often regarded as *the* symbolic figure of neurobiologically oriented psychiatry, is in fact a very good example for the basic idea of person-centredness with all its perspectives.

1.4.3   Neuroanatomical and Biological Research

In the second half of the 19th century, neuroanatomical and biological research brought many new insights about the structure and the function of the brain. Many authors regarded mental illness predominantly as a biological disorder of the brain, e.g. the influential Viennese psychiatrist Theodor Meynert (1833–1892), who chose 'illnesses of the forebrain' ('*Erkrankungen des Vorderhirns*') as the subtitle of his psychiatric textbook from 1884. This very strong position was later criticized as 'brain psychiatry', 'brain mythology' or 'psychiatry without the mental', e.g. by Karl Jaspers. Given our present day debate about the epistemological status of neuroscientific evidence for psychiatry, this, again, is convincing proof of the relevance of the historical perspective.

1.5   DEGENERATION THEORY

In the late 19th and early 20th century, degeneration theory was a highly influential psychiatric concept; this was an even more general way of thinking in the context of the zeitgeist. Degeneration theory had its roots in French psychopathology, especially in the writings of B.A. Morel (1809–1873) and V. Magnan (1835–1916). The central idea of this concept was that in 'degenerative' illness there is a steady decline in mental functioning and social adaptation from one generation to the next. For example, there might be an inter-generational development from a nervous character to major depressive disorder, then to overt psychotic illness and, finally, to severe and chronic cognitive impairment, i.e. dementia. It should be noted, however, that this theory has always been a vague and highly speculative concept, which was put forward decades before the rediscovery of Mendelian genetics and their application to medicine in general and psychiatry in particular [9, 10, 11, 12, 13].

Most of the influential psychiatric authors of that time used arguments derived from degeneration theory broadly. This, for example, is the case in Emil Kraepelin's (1856–1927) writings. He made special reference to degeneration theory with regard to manic-depressive illness, paranoia and personality disorders. His attitude towards degeneration theory was not unambiguously positive, however, but in some ways ambivalent. On the one hand, Kraepelin can be seen as an early forerunner of evolutionary biology, which was strongly reactivated in Konrad Lorenz's writings in the 20th century. The concept of disease – especially chronic mental disease – fitted very well into this framework, insofar as these phenomena were regarded as signs of an evolution in the wrong direction, as 'degeneration': a 'degenerative' process in this sense leaves the usual path of nature. So far, Kraepelin was clearly advocating degeneration theory.

Kraepelin continued to be sceptical about oversimplistic versions of this concept, how-ever; although he commented approvingly on the basic ideas of Cesare Lombroso's 'criminal anthropology', he did not accept the idea of overt '*stigmata degenerationis*', by which individual persons could be identified as being 'degenerated' simply by their physical appearance [14, 15].

There is an important reason that degeneration theory is a very sensitive issue in psychiatric history and should be dealt with as thoroughly and scientifically as possible. From its beginnings until the end of World War II, National Socialism used the central ideas of degeneration theory, social Darwinism and eugenics to pseudo-justify their barbaric world view and – as an ultimate consequence – the killing of people whose lives were defined as 'unworthy'. It is of utmost importance that historians of psychiatry follow the line that runs from the early concepts of degeneration theory to the unprecedented cruelties of National Socialism. But it must not be forgotten that the concept of degeneration was always vague and heterogeneous. Morel, for example, argued from a position of moral philosophy, whereas Magnan tried to link the idea of degeneration with empirical science. In the following decades, authors also addressed quite different issues when using the term 'degeneration'. So, there is definitely a line that runs from degeneration theory to National Socialism, but – as is so often the case in the history of ideas – it is by no means a simple and direct one. From a political point of view, there have been right wing and left wing supporters of the ideas of degeneration, social Darwinism and eugenics in many countries; but the National Socialists in Germany were the only group with the political power not only to *think* those ideas but also to *put them into action* on a large scale, up to the final, cruel consequences. This topic will be addressed again later.

1.6   EARLY TWENTIETH CENTURY

1.6.1   Seminal Clinicians

Around the turn of the 20th century, a number of seminal clinicians shaped major psychiatric concepts in a way that is still relevant nowadays. Some of them are covered here.

Kahlbaum and Kraepelin

Karl Ludwig Kahlbaum (1828–1899) and, a generation later, Emil Kraepelin (1856–1926) emphasized the importance of describing and evaluating the course of illness in a clinical and pragmatic way. Both were sceptical about orientating psychiatric nosology mainly at the actual clinical picture with its constant fluctuations. With 'progressive paralysis of the insane' as an example, Kahlbaum explained the way from the 'syndrome-course unit' ('*Syndrom-Verlaufs-Einheit*') to the – postulated – etiologically-based 'disease entity' ('*Krankheitseinheit*').

Kraepelin followed Kahlbaum in taking this central idea of psychiatric 'disease entities', and expanded his position further. He postulated that the essential features of all psychotic disorders will eventually be classified in a 'natural' (i.e. primarily biological) system, no matter what scientific method is applied; anatomy, etiology and symptomatology, if developed sufficiently, will necessarily converge in the same 'natural disease entities'. The most influential result of this basic idea was Kraepelin's nosological dichotomy, dividing the area of major psychotic illnesses into the two areas of 'dementia praecox' (markedly bad prognosis) versus 'manic-depressive insanity' (markedly better prognosis).

Kraepelin's nosology showed a remarkable stability over time. From the second to ninth editions of his textbook (i.e. from 1887 to 1927), Kraepelin did not change the central postulate. This strong hypothesis is limited to a certain extent, however, in three of his theoretical papers, written between 1918 and 1920: 'Ends and means of psychiatric research'(*Ziele und Wege der psychiatrischen Forschung*) [16]; 'Research on the manifestations of mental illness' (*Die Erforschung psychischer Krankheitsformen*) [17]; and 'Clinical manifestations of mental illness' (*Die Erscheinungsformen des Irreseins*) [18]. Here, Kraepelin took into account contemporary arguments by Karl Birnbaum (the differentiation between pathogenetic and pathoplastic factors in mental illness) and Robert Gaupp (the possibility of psychogenic delusions). He now acknowledged the value of defining certain *syndromes* as a medium level between nosologically unspecific symptoms and specific diseases. But – and this is the essential point – at no time did he abandon his postulate of underlying distinct and natural disease entities [19, 20].

Kretschmer

Ernst Kretschmer (1888–1964) developed the concept of a multidimensional approach to psychiatry, taking psychopathological, biographical and somatic findings into consideration, especially concerning the relationship between body habitus and personality traits or even distinct types of mental illness.

Wernicke

Carl Wernicke (1848–1905) suggested a psychiatric nosology that in some respects resembled the classification of neurological disorders. He, and the later authors of his school, such as Karl Kleist (1879–1960) and Karl Leonhard (1904–1988), regarded Kraepelin's dichotomy of the major psychoses as too narrow. Taking forward the line of thought of association psychology from earlier in the 19th century, they subdivided mental life into different functions that may be disturbed separately or in various combinations. This led, for example, to the sophisticated, albeit psychopathologically stimulating, nosological model proposed by Karl Leonhard, which has just the opposite basic intention (i.e. a multitude of clearly distinct psychotic illnesses) to Griesinger's unitary psychosis.

Bonhoeffer

Karl Bonhoeffer (1868–1948) postulated the *nosological unspecifity* of psychopathological syndromes. He saw the reason for this in the limited number of reaction types the brain can display when confronted with any given irritation. Thus, it is not possible to draw direct conclusions from the clinical picture to its etiology.

Bleuler

The Swiss psychiatrist *Eugen Bleuler* (1857–1939) published his influential work *Dementia praecox oder Gruppe der Schizophrenien* in 1911 [21]. He agreed with Kraepelin in some important respects; e.g. the dichotomy between dementia praecox and manic-depressive illness, and the generally naturalistic attitude towards mental illness. But, in marked contrast to Kraepelin, Bleuler integrated the psychological (also in the sense of hermeneutical) perspective into clinical psychiatry. He was the only prominent academic psychiatrist at that time who not only read Sigmund Freud's (1856–1939) works, but accepted and implemented his ideas, although he later came up with remarkably critical arguments against certain parts of the psychoanalytic school. Bleuler was especially interested in the psychiatric applicability of Freud's concept of unconscious mental events that can be made recognizable by means of interpretation.

Bleuler regarded the course of schizophrenic illness to be highly heterogeneous, departing definitely from Kraepelin's highly pessimistic point of view. His main argument to switch from dementia praecox to schizophrenia was that the disease does not always become a *dementia*, and it does not always appear *praecociter*. Recently, Christian Scharfetter [22] has given Eugen Bleuler's scientific and personal thinking a thorough overview and interpretation.

1.6.2 Behaviourism

The school of *behaviourism*, founded by J. Watson in the early 20th century and later continued by E. L. Thorndike und B. F. Skinner, was in many respects the counterpart of the

Freudian approach. It was not the subjective interpretation of any mental phenomenon, but rather the objective description of behaviour, that was placed at the centre of psychological and psychopathological activities, in diagnosis and therapy as well as in research. Since many psychiatric entities (e.g. phobic disorders) were regarded as conditioned by disturbed learning processes, therapy was the task of reversing, 'deconditioning', them. It took a considerable amount of time for both the psychoanalytical and the behavioural school to gain some influence in practical clinical psychiatry, Eugen Bleuler in Zurich being an exemption.

1.6.3   Jaspers

Karl Jaspers' (1883–1969) book, *General Psychopathology (Allgemeine Psychopathologie)* [23] must still be called a cornerstone of psychiatric conceptualization. He regarded psycho-pathology as a central, practical and research tool for the psychiatrist, and tried to establish it as both an empirical and theoretical scientific field. For Jaspers, it is not possible to completely describe or even explain human mental life by objective and quantitative procedures alone. One of his central arguments is that our access to the mental events of other people is never direct but indirect, and necessarily involves intersubjectivity insofar as we depend on the person's expressions through their language, non-verbal communication, behaviour patterns, even their literary or other pieces of art. As for the concept of mental illness in general, Jaspers regarded the Kraepelinian idea of natural psychiatric disease entities as practically relevant, but – according to the theoretical arguments above – not in the realistic sense of entities existing completely independently from the patient and the psychiatrist.

1.6.4   Schneider

Like Jaspers', part of the Heidelberg psychopathological tradition, Kurt Schneider (1887–1967) explicitly acknowledged that neurobiological factors play a major role in the etiology and pathogenesis of mental disorders, but added that this does not rule out other factors, e.g. psychological and social ones. He insisted that psychiatric diagnoses are by no means objective, 'naturalistic' statements, but conceptual constructs based on empirical data [24]. In his attempt to differentiate and sharpen the diagnostic process, for example by his subtle description of 'first and second rank symptoms of schizophrenia', Kurt Schneider may well be regarded as a precursor of modern operationalized diagnostic manuals like ICD-10 or DSM-IV-TR.

1.6.5   The Impact of National Socialism

Before we turn to developments from the end of World War II to the present time, the unprecedented and barbaric *abuse of psychiatric power* by National Socialist Germany has to be mentioned briefly. This has not to do with any differentiated concept of mental illness, being the topic of this chapter, but – on the contrary – has to do with very rude and unscientific, albeit powerful, simplifications that dramatically illustrate the potential vul-nerability and weakness of a clinical and scientific field.

Long before 1933, social Darwinist and eugenic concepts became influential, not just in psychiatry but in medicine and even social politics in general. Against the background of 'degeneration theory' (see above), a number of overtly racist positions arose. One such was Alfred Ploetz's concept of 'racial hygiene', which regarded it as a prominent duty of the state to ensure that 'healthy' people have offspring – and to prevent 'ill' people from doing so, in order to continuously improve the social and biological status of society. In this context, a strong, increasingly cruel anti-Semitism forced many Jewish psychiatrists and psychoanalysts to emigrate. These included F. J. Kallmann (1897–1965), a genetician and psychiatrist, who in 1936 emigrated to New York, where he founded a genetic research unit at the Institute of Psychiatry.

From 1934, the sterilization of mentally ill people intensified in Germany. In later years, for some of the psychiatrists who actively supported National Socialism, there seem to have been no ethical or humanitarian barriers whatsoever. Besides sterilization, uncontrolled and cruel 'scientific trials' were carried out with psychiatric patients, patients with epilepsy or severe neurological disorders, physically or mentally disabled people, homosexuals and a number of other groups. It is estimated that about 360 000 individuals were sterilized between 1934 and 1945. Finally, 'euthanasia' was the cynical term for the killing of mentally ill or handicapped individuals; this cost between 80 000 and 130 000 people their lives, mainly in the years 1940 and 1941 [25].

1.7   DEVELOPMENTS TO THE PRESENT DAY

1.7.1   Anthropological Psychiatry

Following the horrifying crimes of the Nazi period, with their crude, pseudoscientific background, it is not surprising that biological, especially genetic, research in psychiatry practically came to a standstill in Germany for quite a long time. Until the early 1960s, academic psychiatry adhered to a completely different perspective. This was the era of anthropological psychiatry, which was decisively oriented towards existential philosophy and focused strongly on the idiographic and biographical aspects in the pethogenesis and etiology of mental disorders.

In particular, the existential school of Daseinsanalyse, founded by Ludwig Binswanger (1881–1966), declined any elementaristic approach (as opposed to association psychology) and tried to get access to the complete mental act and its inner structure ('*Ganzheit*'). In this perspective, psychosis, for example, is not only the appearance of isolated symptoms like delusions and hallucinations, but a specifically human disorder of shaping one's life. On the one hand, this disorder may severely diminish degrees of freedom and personal autonomy, and lead to 'loss of natural awareness of the world' ('*Verlust der natuerlichen Selbstverstaendlichkeit*') and to 'an inability to change perspectives deliberately' ('*Unfaehigkeit zum Perspektivenwechsel*') [26, 27]. On the other hand, to view psychotic (and other psychiatric) states not only as mere deficits, but also – albeit pathological and creating significant suffering – as carrying meanings with regard to the person's life and self-understanding, may open up psychotherapeutic options.

1.7.2 Gestalt

Basic Gestalt psychology ideas reached psychiatry through the work of Klaus Conrad (1905–1961). His approach was oriented to a subtle psychopathological perspective and the course of illness, especially in schizophrenic psychoses. He tried to establish this concept as a 'third way' between classical description (which he believed to be too static and not sufficiently differentiated) and strictly hermeneutical methods (which he believed were not reliable enough and often too speculative) [28].

The Heidelberg psychopathologist Werner Janzarik followed these lines and differentiated them further, and markedly, in his concept of 'structural dynamics' ('*Strukturdynamik*'). The *dynamic* component of any mental event (normal or pathological) includes affectivity and drive, whereas the *structural* component addresses longstanding and characteristic psychological features of the individual person, e.g. value systems, interactional styles or, in general, personality traits [29]. This basic idea was then fruitfully applied to different nosological areas like psychotic and personality disorders. Although this model is a genuinely psychopathological one, and therefore does not directly contribute to diagnostic, nosological or therapeutical issues, it proved (and will continue) to be a rich source of arguments and critical questions that have to be debated *within* psychopathology if this field claims to be an indispensable scientific tool for psychiatry [30].

1.7.3 Anti-Psychiatry

Fundamental questions of psychiatry (e.g. the notion of mental illness itself or the mind-body relationship) are by no means 'only theoretical'. They bear profound practical and ethical implications. This was proven by anti-psychiatry, a heterogeneous group of authors who, from about 1960, formulated a fundamental critique of classical psychiatric concepts. The core issue here was (and, in a more differentiated way, still is) the assertion that psychiatry claims to be a scientific medical field, objectively dealing with (neurobiological) illnesses; but in reality is a powerful instrument of society (or of politics) to deal with people who may exhibit strange behaviour without, however, being ill or in need of any treatment [31]. Such a critique (and many other less dramatic problematic issues within psychiatric practice and research) will only be answered in a convincing manner if psychiatry does not exclude or underestimate 'philosophical' or 'theoretical' topics.

1.7.4 Neurobiological Findings

In recent years, the enormous progress in neurobiological findings on the structure and function of the brain has also gained significance for psychiatric diagnosis in two respects. First, the efficacy of a certain drug with its neuropharmacological properties was regarded as diagnostically relevant information ('*diagnosis ex juvantibus*'), e.g. positive response of neuroleptics suggests a psychotic disorder. Second, new imaging, neurophysiological or biochemical techniques (fMRI, endophenotypes, pharmacogenomics) tend to leave the area of research and enter the clinical, especially the diagnostic field. Whether this process will already affect the upcoming versions of our diagnostic manuals (ICD-11 and DSM-V) remains to be seen.

1.7.5 Operationalized Psychiatric Diagnosis

Finally, the concept of operationalized psychiatric diagnosis itself should be mentioned. Situated in the epistemological tradition of logical empiricism and analytical philosophy, ICD-10 and DSM-IV-TR lay the emphasis on descriptive psychopathological elements that are delineated by explicit criteria and (wherever possible) stay clear from etiological presuppositions. This critical, even puristic attitude towards psychiatric (and especially diagnostic) terms has its merits, given the many incompatible and often idiosyncratic diagnostic and nosological systems our field has seen in the last two centuries. But one has to acknowledge the limitations of this approach, too; if quantification and reliability on the level of operationally defined single symptoms become the only points of reference for the diagnostic process, complex (albeit therapeutically relevant) psychopathological and intersubjective phenomena might be overlooked, underestimated or even regarded as unscientific (e.g. patient-doctor relationship; complex delusional experiences; specific affective qualities in severe depression). This, again, would create an unjustified restriction and simplification of psychopathology.

1.8 CONCLUSION

In concluding this brief historical and conceptual overview of the highly heterogeneous concepts of mental disorders, it can be stated that, for a number of reasons, psychiatry's self-understanding is (and will probably stay) more fragile than that of other medical specialities. In order to prevent future psychiatry from dissolving in a number of methodically defined subunits, and to further strengthen person-centred diagnostic approaches [32], we strongly need the historical perspective. Each psychiatric concept – be it of naturalistic, descriptive, hermeneutical, anthropological or sociological orientation – is necessarily (albeit often implicitly) linked with theoretical presuppositions.

But this is also true of the notion of the *person* or *personhood* itself. Of course, this issue leads us into the centre of philosophical debate. Not a few psychiatrists, both historically and today, were and are decisively sceptical about the benefits of such philosophical arguments for their field. However, if we do not want to reduce the notion of the person just to a single (usually the prevailing) scientific perspective, we will have to enter the debate on what is or what we call a person, and whether personhood can be affected by mental illness. One of the radical positions on this issue was developed by transcendental philosophers like Immanuel Kant and Johann Gottlieb Fichte, for whom the concept of an irreducibly autonomous and responsible subject was not (only) a matter of empirical science, but the prerequisite of any scientific approach to the *conditio humana*. These complex philosophical theories – and many others from the 18th and 19th centuries – have been criticized in recent decades, especially following the linguistic turn in philosophy in the 20th century and its (usually underestimated) consequences for psychiatry. Nonetheless, the issue of personhood and its relationship to the diagnosis and treatment of mental illness is far from being settled. So, if person-centredness is to become *the* essential framework for psychiatry, the philosophical debate needs to be specifically reflected upon and integrated into psychiatry. This, no doubt, is a demanding task for the future.

Already today, it is obvious that the questions of how mental health and mental disorder should be conceptualized and how one can be differentiated reliably from the other, cannot not be answered sufficiently without taking the history of psychiatric concepts into account. And this is what makes history of psychiatry a practically relevant scientific field.

NOTE

1. Paracelsus' real name was Philippus Aureolus Theophrastus Bombastus von Hohenheim.

REFERENCES

[1] Hoff P. [Leib & Seele, Gehirn & Geist, Gesundheit & Krankheit: Die Psychiatrie als Schnittstelle medizinischer, philosophischer und gesellschaftlicher Kontroversen]. In: Hermanni F, Buchheim T. (eds.) [Das Leib-Seele-Problem. Antwortversuche aus medizinisch-naturwissenschaftlicher, philosophischer und theologischer Sicht]. Munich: Wilhelm Fink; 2006a. pp. 39–67.
[2] Benzenhöfer U. [Psychiatrie und Anthropologie in der ersten Haelfte des 19. Jahrhunderts]. Stuttgart: Pressler; 1993.
[3] Marx OM. German romantic psychiatry, Part I. History of Psychiatry 1990;1: pp. 351–381.
[4] Marx OM. German romantic psychiatry, Part II. History of Psychiatry 1991;2: pp. 1–25.
[5] Schmidt-Degenhard M. [Zum Melancholiebegriff JCA Heinroths]. In: Nissen G, Keil G. (eds.) [Psychiatrie auf dem Wege zur Wissenschaft]. Stuttgart: Thieme; 1985. pp.12–18.
[6] Griesinger W. [Die Pathologie und Therapie der psychischen Krankheiten]. 2nd ed. Stuttgart: Krabbe;1861.
[7] Hoff P, Hippius H. [Wilhelm Griesinger (1817-1868) – sein Psychiatrieverstaendnis aus historischer und aktueller Perspektive]. Nervenarzt 2001;72: pp. 885–892.
[8] Roessler W. [Wilhelm Griesinger und die gemeindenahe Versorgung]. Nervenarzt 1992;63: pp.257–261.
[9] Dowbiggin I. Degeneration and hereditarianism in French mental medicine 1840-1890 – psychiatric theory as ideological adaptation. In: Bynum WF, Porter R, Shepherd M (eds.) Anatomy of Madness, Volume I: People and Ideas. London: Tavistock; 1985. pp.188–232.
[10] Chamberlin E, Gilman S. (eds.) Degeneration. The dark side of progress. New York: Columbia University Press; 1985.
[11] Hermle L. [Die Degenerationslehre in der Psychiatrie]. Fortschr Neurol Psychiatr 1986;54: pp. 69–79.
[12] Liegeois A. Hidden philosophy and theology in Morel's theory of degeneration and nosology. History of Psychiatry 1991;2: pp. 419–427.
[13] Pick D. Faces of degeneration: a European disorder 1848–1918. Cambridge: Cambridge University Press; 1989.
[14] Hoff P. Kraepelin and degeneration theory. Eur Arch Psychiatry Clin Neurosci 2008; 258 (Suppl. 2): pp.12–17.
[15] Zubin J, Oppenheimer G, Neugebauer G. Degeneration theory and the stigma of schizophrenia (editorial). Biological Psychiatry 1985; 20: pp. 1145–1148.
[16] Kraepelin E. Ends and means of psychiatric research [Ziele und Wege der psychiatrischen Forschung] . Zeitschrift für die gesamte Neurologie und Psychiatrie 1918; 42: pp. 169–205.
[17] Kraepelin E. Research on the manifestations of mental illness [Die Erforschung psychischer Krankheitsformen]. Zeitschrift für die gesamte Neurologie und Psychiatrie 1919;51: pp. 224–246.
[18] Kraepelin E. Clinical manifestations of mental illness [Die Erscheinungsformen des Irreseins]. Zeitschrift für die gesamte Neurologie und Psychiatrie 1920;62: pp. 1–29.

[19] Hoff P. [*Emil Kraepelin und die Psychiatrie als klinische Wissenschaft. Ein Beitrag zum Selbstverstaendnis psychiatrischer Forschung*]. Berlin: Springer; 1994.

[20] Hoff P. *Kraepelin – Clinical Section*. In: Berrios GE, Porter R. (eds.) *A History of Clinical Psychiatry. The Origin and History of Psychiatric Disorders*.London: Athlone; 1995. pp. 261–279.

[21] Bleuler E. [Dementia praecox oder Gruppe der Schizophrenien]. In: Aschaffenburg G. (ed.) [*Handbuch der Psychiatrie*]. Spezieller Teil. 4. Abteilung. 1. Hälfte. Leipzig Wien: Deuticke; 1911.

[22] Scharfetter C. [*Eugen Bleuler 1857–1939. Polyphrenie und Schizophrenie*]. Zurich: vdf Hochschulverlag; 2006.

[23] Jaspers K. *General Psychopathology [Allgemeine Psychopathologie]*. Berlin: Springer; 1913.

[24] Schneider K. [*Klinische Psychopathologie*] 14th ed. Stuttgart: Thieme; 1992.

[25] Holdorff B, Hoff P. [Neurologie und Psychiatrie in der Zeit des Nationalsozialismus]. In: Schliack H, Hippius H. (eds.) [*Nervenärzte*]. Stuttgart: Thieme; 1997. pp. 173–184.

[26] Binswanger L. [*Wahn*]. Pfullingen: Neske; 1965.

[27] Blankenburg W. [*Der Verlust der natuerlichen Selbstverstaendlichkeit*]. Stuttgart: Enke; 1971.

[28] Conrad K. [*Die beginnende Schizophrenie: Versuch einer Gestaltsanalyse des Wahns*]. Stuttgart: Thieme; 1958.

[29] Janzarik W. [*Strukturdynamische Grundlagen der Psychiatrie*]. Stuttgart: Enke; 1988.

[30] Hoff P. [Warum noch Psychopathologie?]. In: Schneider F. (ed.) [*Entwicklungen der Psychiatrie*]. Heidelberg: Springer; 2006b. pp. 151–157.

[31] Szasz TS. *The Myth of Mental Illness*. New York: Hoeber Harper; 1961.

[32] Mezzich JE. Institutional consolidation and global impact: towards a psychiatry for the person. *World Psychiatry* 2006;5: pp. 65–66.

CHAPTER 2

Philosophical Perspectives on Health, Illness and Clinical Judgement in Psychiatry and Medicine

Tim Thornton
Professor of Philosophy and Mental Health and Director of Philosophy,
University of Central Lancashire, UK
KWM (Bill) Fulford
Professor of Philosophy and Mental Health, University of Warwick, UK; Fellow of
St Cross College and Member of the Philosophy Faculty, University of Oxford;
Honorary Consultant Psychiatrist, University of Oxford, UK;
Co-Director, Institute for Philosophy, Diversity and Mental Health,
University of Central Lancashire, UK;
National Fellow for Values-Based Practice, Department of Health, London, UK;
George Christodoulou
Professor of Psychiatry, Athens University, Greece;
Standing Committee on Ethics, World Psychiatric Association;
European Division, Royal College of Psychiatry;
Honorary President, Hellenic Psychiatric Association;
President, Hellenic Center for Mental Health & Research, Athens, Greece

2.1   INTRODUCTION

Mental health care raises as many conceptual questions as empirical ones. For that reason, and given the recent rapid developments in psychiatry driven by both medical research and public policy initiatives, there has been a resurgence in philosophical work on issues of illness, health and mental health care, which has application throughout medicine. Such work has been carried out by a partnership of psychiatrists and philosophers deploying both the traditions of, and innovations in, both disciplines.

Psychiatric Diagnosis: Challenges and Prospects   Edited by I.M. Salloum and J.E. Mezzich
© 2009 John Wiley & Sons, Ltd

The conceptual issues of health and illness are of paramount theoretical and clinical importance, as they are closely related to the mission and obligations of the physician and the psychiatrist. We do not intend to cover the immense area of this subject, but will try to delineate the problems that are associated with this issue and draw some conclusions that might be useful to the practicing physician.

One example of the resurgence of philosophy of psychiatry has been the development of values-based practice. As has been described elsewhere [1], Fulford *et al.* 2008 [2], values-based practice is based on the tradition of Oxford analytic philosophy [3, 4] and represents a primarily skills-based response to complex and conflicting values, particularly as these are evident in mental health care [5], although with growing applications to the rest of medicine (see, for example, [6] and [7]).

The thorough articulation of the nature of value judgements and the development of consequent practical training materials is a good example of the contribution that philosophy can make to psychiatric practice, especially when carried out in a partnership. It is, perhaps, the most worked out example from the 'new philosophy of psychiatry' based largely on Anglo-American or analytic philosophy [8]. But it is still only one example of the rich resources of the field (e.g. Fulford, Stanghellini and Broome 2004 [9]) and, of course, it is something of a latecomer compared with phenomenology and the other great traditions of Continental philosophy (e.g. [10]). Furthermore, even within the analytic tradition of philosophy, clinical judgement is just one aspect of mental health care that can be investigated and the role of values is just one aspect of that.

In the rest of this short chapter, we will focus on the light that philosophy can help shed on clinical judgement in particular; thus, we will not touch on the growing literature on taxonomy, validity and evidence-based medicine as applied to psychiatry, for example. We will outline some of the aspects of clinical decision-making, outside judgements of values, that are important in mental health care and that can be usefully examined in the context of traditional and recent philosophical developments.

First, we will outline the way the complexities of the concepts of health and illness going back to ancient Greece place weighty demands on the role of clinical judgement in medicine and psychiatry.

2.2 CONCEPTS OF HEALTH AND ILLNESS
IN ANCIENT GREECE

Ancient Greek philosophers and physicians (notably Socrates and Plato) considered illness in its holistic sense. Plato's dialogue, *Charmides* (in [11]), in which Socrates urges the physicians of his time to consider their patients in a non-fragmented way and underlines the need to treat the whole person and not merely part of the body (the eyes, in Socrates' paradigm) is characteristic.

These concepts are important, because modern vistas on holism and psychosomatic medicine are based on them. They have infiltrated psychiatric and also medical thinking, and they constitute an integral part of personified medicine and psychiatry.

However, these ideas have not been accepted uncritically and universally. The philosopher Popper, in his *Poverty of Historicism*, criticizes holism and holists as 'carelessly pseudo-scientific, uncritical and incapable of real scientific scrutiny'. Yet, medical practice faces the dilemma of either being an applied, non-person oriented science or using only partly generalized scientific findings but being in essence person-oriented [12].

Aristotle has dealt extensively with concepts of illness and personified medicine. His teaching is not only relevant but also visible in contemporary concepts of holistic medicine, personified medicine and ethics [13].

Aristotle advocates a focus on the health of a specific person rather than on health as a concept ('*την υγείαν ανθρώπου τούδε*') and believes in individualized medicine on the basis of each person's needs ('*καθ' έκαστον γαρ ιατρεύει*'). Practical reason (phronesis, or *φρόνησις*) occupies a cardinal position in his teaching and plays a major role in clinical judgement. On the basis of *φρόνησις*, decisions on the appropriate management of a specific patient are based on the specific circumstances that exist at a specific time ('*δει δ' αυτούς αεί τους πράττοντας τα προς τον καιρόν σκοπείν*'). The balance (*το μέσον*) is another concept in medical treatment that Aristotle advocates. Not hyperbole (*υπερβολή*) but also not too little (*έλλειψις*).

It is interesting (but not controversial) that Aristotle considers practical reason (*φρόνησις*) subordinate to wisdom (*σοφία*) and ethical virtue (*αρετή*) in the same way that he considers health to occupy a higher hierarchical position than medical practice, because medical practice only sees to it that the necessary actions to permit health to realize itself are carried out ('*η Ιατρική ου γαρ χρήται αυτή τη υγιεία αλλ' ορά όπως γένηται*') [13]. This hierarchical placement, however, by no means invalidates the primacy of practical reason and personified medicine over scientific, research-oriented medicine (Novak, 1986 [12]).

2.3 HEALTH AND ILLNESS

According to most modern definitions (including the old but very relevant WHO definition), health is not identical to absence of illness. Something more is needed, and this is the '*ευ εχειν*' (well-being) identified as a basic component of health, originally by the Ancient Greeks [14, 15]. If this is true about medicine in general, it is certainly particularly true about psychiatry (the medicine of the psyche).

If we accept that the well-being of the patient is an integral component of health, what inevitably follows is that the task of the physician is not only to treat the patient with the purpose of relieving him (her) from the illness but, additionally, to guarantee the quality of the patient's life.

Is that possible? Is this really the purpose of medicine and psychiatry? Would this not be unrealistic, especially in our times when technocracy prevails and humanistic values are hardly considered? It is true that Hippocrates thought of the physician as '*ισοθεος*' ('equal to God') but is this not a very heavy burden, in addition to being unrealistic?

Answering these questions is not easy and there are certainly many disagreements about them among physicians. There are those who feel that the role of the physician should be restricted to the treatment of illness, aiming at the restoration of physical health; and that well-being, psychological problems and psychopathological conditions, even when they arise as a result of somatic pathology, should be dealt with by mental health professionals (the 'I do not want to know' approach). There are others who feel that somatic and psychological pathology are the two sides of the same coin, that there is cross-talk between them, that the well-being of the patient is determined by the acquisition of a somato-psychic equilibrium and that, consequently, it is within the sphere of the doctor's responsibility to guarantee the well-being of the patient (the psychosomatic approach). The 'Psychiatry for the Person' movement represents a third approach aiming at focusing attention on the need for personified psychiatry and medicine [16]. It does not deal especially with quality of life, but its orientation and aims implicitly focus towards this end.

We feel that the well-being of each person is a personal issue and does not obey general rules. It depends on the psychic synthesis of each one of us, on our hereditary endowment, the influences that have been dynamically integrated in each person's psyche, our conditioned predisposition, our defence strategies, the perpetual interaction with the environment, the multitude of choices and the choice of 'battlefields' that each of us has identified and selected in our lives, our own personal concepts of achievement and a multitude of other factors that cannot be generalized and possibly cannot be fully identified. Therefore, 'well-being' is a very personal matter.

If we accept the above, then well-being cannot be considered as a task or an obligation of the physician or the psychiatrist. Yet, the physician does have an obligation and this is the obligation to guarantee the well-being of the patient *to the degree that this well-being is linked with the patient's health*. This is, indeed, a physician's task and responsibility.

Prevention is yet another area that has not been given the priority it deserves. Psychiatric prevention is historically a psychosocial concept, yet its importance has been highlighted only when it became evident that biological methods of prevention, exemplified by lithium prophylaxis, were effective [17]. With reference to biological preventive methods, an issue of importance (clinical and ethical) is the divergent concepts of health among society, clinician, relatives and carers and, eventually, the recipient of services, the patient. A patient with bipolar illness stabilized on lithium often finds his or her pharmacologically-included health of very low quality, not so much because of the undesirable effects of the treatment but mainly because he or she misses the 'highs' of the manic or hypomanic episodes. This is in contrast with the people in the patient's entourage, who are relieved and grateful for the prophylactic result achieved by mood stabilizers.

The importance of a focus on the particular circumstances of individuals to address their illnesses and to promote health and well-being in a way sensitive to their specific wishes suggests that clinical judgement is a key skill for physicians and, especially, psychiatrists. We will now examine some philophical perspectives on this issue.

2.4   THE HISTORY OF PHILOSOPHY AS A RESOURCE FOR CLINICAL JUDGEMENT

Philosophy has long studied the kind or kinds of judgement found in good clinical practice. Aristotle (384–322 BC), for example, distinguished *phronesis* from general scientific knowledge or episteme and technical knowledge or know-how: *techne*. Phronesis is practical wisdom; practical in the sense of concerning how to change aspects of the world. That is its intended aim or output, and suggests that it serves as a good model for medical practice. But its inputs are particular states of affairs. It is 'concerned with particulars as well as universals, and particulars become known from experience . . . [thus] some length of time is needed to produce it'. [18, p.160] This stress on responses to individual circumstances is a promising start to thinking about clinical judgement.

In fact, phronesis is particularly relevant to values-based practice because it was explicitly described by Aristotle in relation to value judgements (although the strict separation of values from facts is a modern phenomenon). Insofar as values-based practice is a response to the uncodifiable complexities of particular situations, it can be thought of as a modern exemplification of Aristotelian phronesis.

The concentration on making judgements about particular cases with a practical aim, however, serves as a model for clinical judgement more broadly. To put the matter rather abstractly, clinical judgement involves skilled coping with individual cases: both people and their situations. But the nature and demands of such judgement is, in fact, better first approached not through Aristotle's account of phronesis but through a distinction from a much later philosopher, Immanuel Kant (1724–1804).

In his third major work, the *Critique of Judgement*, Kant draws an important distinction between what he calls 'determinate' and 'reflective' judgement. He describes these in this way:

> 'If the universal (the rule, principle, law) is given, then judgment, which subsumes the particular under it, is determinate . . . But if only the particular is given and judgment has to find the universal for it, then this power is merely reflective.'

[19, p.18]

The model at work here is of judgement as having two elements: a general concept and a particular subject matter. Judgement subsumes a particular under a general concept. The contrast between determinate and reflective judgement is then between an essentially general judgement, when the concept is already given, and a particular or singular judgement, which starts only with a particular. The former, determinate judgement, appears to be relatively mechanical and thus unproblematic. The idea that if a general principle is already given then judgements that deploy it are relatively unproblematic can be illustrated through the related case of logical deduction where a general principle is already given. If, for example, one believes that:

1. All men are mortal; and
2. Socrates is a man; then it is rational to infer that:
3. Socrates is mortal.

One reason this can seem unproblematic is the following thought. If one has accepted premises 1 and 2, then one has, *ipso facto*, already accepted premiss 3. To accept that all men are mortal is to accept that Tom, Dick, Harry *and Socrates* are mortal. So, given 1 and 2, then 3 is no step at all (though see [20] and [21, pp. 98–105]). Furthermore, some central forms of deductive judgement, at least, can be codified using Frege's logical notation. Given the codification, one can inspect the *form* of a deductive inference to determine whether true premises could ever lead to a false conclusion. (In fact, neither of these reasons for taking deduction, and thus determinate judgement, to be conceptually simple is quite so straightforward. For the moment, however, the *perceived* relative straightforward nature of determinate judgement is what matters.)

By contrast, for reflective judgement, there is a principled problem in how to get from the level of individuals to the level of generalities, or how to get from brute things to the general concepts that apply to them. This is not a matter of deduction because the choice of universal or general concept is precisely what is in question. To move from the particular to the general that applies to it is somehow to gain information, not to deploy it. Reflective judgement thus calls for philosophical clarification.

Because clinical judgement has to respond to individuals or particular cases, it inherits this apparently deep principled difficulty. By examining specific models of judgements aimed at particular or individual cases, light can be shed on clinical judgement in general. We will mention three kinds of particular judgement towards which philosophical attention has already been directed but which are worthy of further investigation. We will then return to question Kant's distinction and thus suggest that there is not such a great contrast between particular and general forms of judgement. This in turn suggests that the contrast between particular clinical judgement and generally codified evidence-based medicine is not, in principle, as great as it might seem.

The three forms of particular judgement are:

1. Idiographic judgement
2. Empathy
3. Tacit knowledge.

2.4.1   Idiographic Judgement

Idiographic judgement, like reflective judgement, is defined in opposition to a (conception of a) general form of judgement. In this case, the general conception is called 'nomothetic', because it concerns laws of nature. The inventor of the terms 'idiographic' and 'nomothetic', the neo-Kantian philosopher Wilhelm Windelband (1848–1915), defines it in this passage:

> 'In their quest for knowledge of reality, the empirical sciences either seek the general in the form of the law of nature or the particular in the form of the historically defined structure. On the one hand, they are concerned with the form which invariably remains constant. On the other hand, they are concerned with the unique, immanently defined content of the real event. The former disciplines are nomological sciences. The latter disciplines are sciences of process or sciences of the event. The nomological sciences are concerned with what is invariably the case. The sciences of process are concerned with what was once the case. If I may be permitted to introduce some new technical terms, scientific thought is nomothetic in the former case and idiographic in the latter case.'
>
> [22, pp. 175–6]

Idiographic judgement looks to be tailored to addressing the nature of individuals. Whilst nomothetic judgements subsume individuals under general kinds, idiographic judgements are supposed to be directed at 'the uniqueness and incomparability of their object' [22, p. 182]. For that reason, it has been an important concept in recent discussion of psychiatry, notably the WPA's Institutional Program on Psychiatry for the Person [23]. If psychiatry is aimed at understanding individuals, it might seem that a form of one-off or singular judgement is the perfect vehicle to do that.

There are, however, reasons to be suspicious of idiographic judgement. The very idea of judgement tailored only to individuals and making no implicit comparison between cases threatens to undermine the key virtue of psychiatric assessment and diagnosis: validity. The idea of a form of judgement that is so essentially one-off that it eschews generalized conceptual elements in its efforts to track the nature of individual subjects smacks of what the philosopher Wilfrid Sellars (1912–89) describes as the 'Myth of the Given' (Sellars 1997 [24]). Sellars argues, however, that the idea of a form of judgement that does not itself depend on a more general conception is incoherent.

In a nutshell, his argument is that if a subject is to take a perceptual experience to be an indication of the nature of something objective, some feature of the world, then the experience must have a kind of authority for the subject. But, for a perceptual experience to have authority, it must not only actually be a reliable indicator of the state of the world but, according to Sellars, its subject must *know* that it is reliable. Such knowledge makes any judgement based on a perceptual experience also depend more generally on the subject's worldview, in particular how his or her experiences are brought about by worldly features. Thus the idea of a genuinely singular or one-off judgement is incoherent because it would be a form of judgement unconnected with the background beliefs. But Sellars argues that these are necessary in the very idea of a perceptually based judgement.

This suggests that strictly idiographic judgement is impossible. But, in fact, in recent discussion, 'idiographic' is often used interchangeably with 'narrative' [25]. Narrative judgement can escape Sellars' argument because it need not be genuinely one-off in the way so far described. That is, it can approach individuals using general concepts and thus by making implicit comparisons. But, nevertheless, its underlying logic is distinct from the nomological or nomothetic approach of inductive and statistical sciences. It can provide distinct insight into individual case histories. On one view, at least, narrative understanding compares cases to meaningful ideals rather than subsuming them under universal generalisations. This has consequences for how exceptions are accommodated. An exception to a universal law undermines the law. An exception to an ideal of rationality merely demonstrates less than ideal reasoning by a fallible human subject.

Some important questions about narratives remain, however, such as whether there is any essential connection between being a person and being describable in a narrative [26]. But there need be no threat to the validity of a clinical judgement couched in narrative terms from Sellars' argument. There is thus need for further investigation of the apparent role of idiographic judgement in psychiatric assessment and whether it might instead be played by something strictly distinct from it, such as a narrative judgement (see e.g. [27]).

2.4.2 Empathy

Empathy is another form of particular judgement tied to understanding the nature of individual human subjects. According to Karl Jaspers, empathy lies at the heart of psychological psychiatric understanding:

'Whereas the rational understanding is only an *aid* to psychology, empathic understanding *is* psychology itself.'

[28, p. 83]

Jaspers' view of empathy puts significant weight on the role of fellow feeling. Rather than deploying a theoretical and context free form of judgement, Jasperian empathy is mediated by psychological aspects of the empathic judge him or herself. Thus, judgement of the particulars of a case is made possible by the fact that a clinician shares common mental attributes with the person whom she or he aims to understand:

'Subjective symptoms cannot be perceived by the sense-organs, but have to be grasped by transferring oneself, so to say, into the other individual's psyche; that is, by empathy. They can only become an inner reality for the observer by his participating in the other person's experiences, not by any intellectual effort.'

[29, p. 1313]

Unlike Windelband's definition of idiographic judgement, Jaspers' characterisation of empathy is not so much concerned with its nature or logic as with its method of delivery. This, however, raises the question: would that method deliver a distinct *kind* of judgement. Is empathy genuinely distinct in its form or its content from other approaches to judgements of individuals and thus a distinct addition to psychiatric diagnostic knowledge? Or is it, rather, that empathic understanding is a shortcut to knowledge that would, in principle, be available by other means.

A clue to this issue comes from the debate in contemporary philosophy of mind between two rival accounts of knowledge of other people's minds [30]. Some philosophers, especially those influenced by and influencing cognitive psychology, have argued that knowledge of other minds is theoretical and akin to knowledge of unobservable entities in the physical sciences. Behavioural evidence is used as the basis for a theoretical inference about its underlying mental causes. Such 'theory theorists' are opposed by 'simulation theorists' who argue that it is not necessary to *know* a theory of mind to have knowledge of others' minds. One needs merely to *have* a mind oneself and imaginatively put oneself in the other's position, so to speak. Simulation theory thus promises to shed light on empathy.

The mere distinction between simulation theory and theory theory does not in itself explain how empathy might be a source of genuinely distinct knowledge of individuals, however. In fact, the two sides of the modern debate are in some danger of collapsing together. The theory that, according to theory theorists, explains knowledge of other minds seems, largely, to be a tacit or implicit theory. If so, tacit knowledge of a theory might not be so very different from the ability to simulate. Further, the ability to simulate could perhaps be set out or described in a series of principles in much the way that the rules of chess codify legal play whether or not they are actually appealed to by skilled players. If so, again, the two sides might collapse together and thus fail to provide an account of a distinct role for empathy. But two ideas help keep the sides apart and thus indicate a potentially genuinely distinct role for empathy in psychiatry.

Firstly, if understanding depends centrally on making rational sense of one another and if, plausibly, the demands of rationality cannot – outside well regulated areas such as logic – be codified, then theory theory must fail. Mutual understanding would instead depend on shared but open ended patterns of reasoning rather than the application of a theory. Such an argument would place shared rationality at the heart of empathy and thus would contradict what Jaspers himself says when he says:

> 'When the contents of thoughts emerge one from another in accordance with the rules of logic, we understand the connections *rationally*. But if we understand the content of the thoughts as they have arisen out of the moods, wishes, and fears of the person who thought them, we understand the connections psychologically or empathetically.'
>
> [28, p. 83]

It is possible, however, that Jaspers' took 'rationality' to refer only to codifiable aspects of rationality and thus overly restricted his view of its importance.

Secondly, it is difficult to capture in any theory the way in which individuals' experiences of the world carry a particular perspective. Theories are set out as though from no perspective, a view from nowhere. Empathy might thus be construed not so much as the route to what thoughts people are thinking, but as the way they think those thoughts from a particular perspective [31]. Both of these are promising lines of inquiry that agree with

Jaspers' assessment of the key importance of empathy for psychiatry. But both substantially develop what Jaspers himself has to say.

2.4.3 Tacit Knowledge

In addition to knowledge of explicitly codified theory, there has been recent work on the importance of tacit knowledge or 'know-how' in science. The first substantial recent work was by the chemist turned philosopher of science Michael Polanyi [32, 33] but his work has been complemented by that of the historian Thomas Kuhn [34] and the sociologist of science Harry Collins [35]. What is particularly relevant for psychiatry is that this work highlights the role of a tacit dimension for both theoretical and applied science. It thus promises to unite clinical judgement and more evidence-based research [36].

Tacit knowledge looks to be another instance of a contrast with determinate judgement. Whilst tacit knowledge need not be one-off (riding a bicycle or determining the gender of a chicken are general abilities: they apply to lots of bikes and chickens), its application is not a matter of explicit derivation from principles. Thus it is not, like determinate judgement, a matter of derivation from a universal concept (though see below). This conception of knowledge raises a number of questions. We will flag two.

Firstly, since, by its very definition, tacit knowledge is not explicitly governed by principles, can it be conceptually informed? In effect, this is to ask whether, although it is not a matter of derivation from general principles, it might still be a case of tacit subsumption under concepts. It seems intuitive to think that the skilled coping that characterizes much tacit knowledge is 'mindless' and thus cannot be regarded as the exercise of a conceptually structured and informed capacity [37]. If so, that might seem to rule out a role for tacit knowledge in informed clinical judgement. But that assumption appears to be questionable. It is also possible to see in the skilled but almost instantaneous movement as the application of a concept in action akin to its application in speech or thought:

> 'When a rational agent catches a frisbee, she is realizing a concept of a thing to do. In the case of a skilled agent, she does not do that by realizing other concepts of things to do. She does not realize concepts of contributory things to do, in play for her as concepts of what she is to do by virtue of her means-end rationality in a context in which her overarching project is to catch the frisbee. But she does realize a concept of, say, catching this. (Think of a case in which, as one walks across a park, a frisbee flies towards one, and one catches it on the spur of the moment.) When a dog catches a frisbee, he is not realizing any practical concept; in the relevant sense, he has none. The point of saying that the rational agent, unlike the dog, is realizing a concept in doing what she does is that her doing, under a specification that captures the content of the practical concept that she is realizing, comes within the scope of her practical rationality.'
>
> [38, p. 368]

Secondly, if tacit knowledge is not governed by explicit principles, in what sense can it be correct or incorrect, assessed or evaluated? Collins assumes that such assessment is at least problematic. He says:

> 'Experimental ability has the character of a skill that can be acquired and developed with practice. Like a skill it cannot be fully explicated or absolutely established.'
>
> [35, p. 73].

Collins appears to assume that what is not explicitly codified cannot be explicated or established either. But this depends on assuming significance for the contrast between what can be codified and what cannot, which, as we will mention below, can be questioned.

Like the idea that there is a role for idiographic judgement and for empathy in psychiatric clinical judgement, so the idea that it has a tacit dimension raises questions the answers to which will contribute to a fuller understanding of clinical judgement. But having introduced these forms of judgement – which may be important for clinical practice – as akin to Kant's concept of reflective judgement, it is worth returning to Kant's distinction to reflect, in particular, on the relation of clinical judgement and generalized forms of judgement such as those found in evidence-based medicine.

2.4.4 Kant's Distinction again, and Evidence-Based Medicine to fit normal practice

Kant introduces the idea of reflective judgement in the context of the following problem. To take a simple non-medical example, imagine that someone has judged correctly, by looking, that there is a cow in front of them. If so, various things will follow from that judgement in combination with their other knowledge. Cows are relatively slow moving, are poor climbers, do not respond to verbal commands and so forth. Thus it follows that the subject can judge that there is something slow moving, that is a poor climber and that will not respond to verbal command. But whilst deriving these judgements from the judgement that it is a cow to the fore is apparently unproblematic, there is a preliminary issue. How, in the face of visual appearances, can one make the preliminary judgement that there is a cow present?

The problem is that the most natural solution creates a vicious regress. One can imagine that a subject knows a rule that connects a particular kind of appearance with a word – 'cow', in this case – in virtue of the word's meaning. But the rule would have to refer to the *range* of appearances that justify the application of the word. This begs the question of how such a 'visual concept' is justifiably applied to any particular cow. Is there a further rule linking a range of appearances to the 'visual concept'?

Kant touches on this problem in the 'schematism' chapter of the first *Critique*. He suggests that an intermediary is needed between concepts and objects but which is not an image:

'[I]t is schemata, not images of objects, which underlie our pure sensible concepts . . . The concept of 'dog' signifies a rule according to which my imagination can delineate the figure of a four footed animal in a general manner, without limitation to any single determinate figure such as experience, or any possible image that I can represent in concreto, actually presents.'

[39, pp. 182–183]

This does not answer the problem, however. Firstly, it is not clear what the figure of a 'four footed animal in general' might be like. Secondly, for any general schematic figure, the question of what determines that *it* applies to any particular dog would return. Kant recognizes that this account does not really address the problem, commenting:

'[T]his schematism of our understanding, in its application to appearances and their mere form, is an art concealed in the depths of the human soul, whose real modes of activity nature is hardly likely ever to allow us to discover.'

[39, p. 183]

If an account couched in general terms – such as general rules for applying concepts – merely replicates the problem, what solution is there? One clue to disarming the problem is the way in which the problem presupposes a distinction between understanding a concept or general rule and knowing when to apply it [40]. Whilst that distinction seems plausible if one assumes that concepts are something like representations in the mind, as cognitivist psychiatry might have it, it is a potentially misleading picture [41]. A second and related clue comes from a closer examination of what it is, instead, to understand a concept or to follow a general rule. Taken together, these two clues suggest that the initial contrast between reflective and determinate judgement is not in the end as great as it seemed.

Whilst there is insufficient space to describe the argument in detail, the central message of Wittgenstein's discussion in the *Philosophical Investigations* [42] of following a rule – an instance of determinate judgement – is that even deductively applying a general principle requires that a judging subject makes a contribution to the derivation, sees what a relevant similar way of going on would be. Even further explication of the rule governing adding two, which says: the units always go '0, 2, 4, 6, 8, 10 and so on', requires that one can connect that very short symbol to an infinite number of cases written in all sorts of specific ways. Thus, an account of how one knows how to follow a rule that attempts to explicate it in purely mechanical terms looks to initiate an infinite regress. However the rule for adding two is 'unpacked' or interpreted, there will always be a question of how to apply the last such interpretation to any actual number. There will always be a potential gap between the interpretation and its application.

Wittgenstein's conclusion is that it is a mistake to think of understanding a rule (such as how to apply it) as having an interpretation in mind. Instead, understanding is always a piece of know-how:

> 'What this shews is that there is a way of grasping a rule which is not an interpretation, but which is exhibited in what we call 'obeying the rule' and 'going against it' in actual cases.'
>
> [42, section 202]

This argument suggests that even explicitly codified or theoretical knowledge – 'knowledge that' – rests on a bedrock of practical ability or know-how. In turn, it suggests that the contrast (mentioned above) on which Collins relies to suggest that tacit knowledge is capricious is undermined because conceptual judgement itself relies on a tacit ability. This suggests that general forms of judgement that are normally contrasted with clinical expertise share, at a deeper level, the same grounding in a practical ability.

The Kantian contrast between determinate and reflective judgement is a useful way of focusing critical attention on the difficulties of clinical judgements about individuals. But in fact, closer attention to it suggests that judgement as a whole relies on an ability to make skilled, one-off judgements. This applies not only to clinical judgements about individual people and their situations, but also to derivations from general principles. This suggests that the same kind of ability is in play in following the general guidelines that partly constitute evidence-based medicine. Further philosophical reflection on the assumptions that lie behind the Kantian distinction will shed light on clinical judgement across the whole of mental health care.

2.5   CONCLUSIONS

The rise of the new philosophy of psychiatry shows the value of a partnership between psychiatry and philosophy for developing, first a better theoretical understanding of the concepts of health and illness, and then practical tools to aid our application of them in developing good mental health care. Influenced and informed by cutting edge psychiatric practice and by philosophical analysis and theories, the partnership has already been evident in the development of the theory and practice of values-based practice, now exported to other areas of medicine. But other aspects of mental health care and, in particular, of clinical judgement are ripe for further reflection to underpin developments in mental health care in the 21st century.

REFERENCES

[1] Fulford KWM. Values-Based Practice: A New Partner to Evidence-Based Practice and a First for Psychiatry? Editorial. In: Singh AR, Singh SA (eds.) Medicine, Mental Health, Science, Religion, and Well-being. *Mens Sana Monographs* 2008;6(1): pp. 10–21.

[2] Fulford KWM, Woodbridge K. Practicing Ethically: Values-Based Practice and Ethics-Working Together to Support Person-Centred and Multidisciplinary Mental Health Care. In: Stickley T, Basset T (eds.) *Learning About Mental Health Practice*. London: John Wiley & Sons, Ltd.; 2008. Chapter 5, pp. 79–103.

[3] Fulford KWM. *Moral Theory and Medical Practice*. Cambridge: Cambridge University Press; 1989, reprinted 1995 and 1999.

[4] Fulford KWM. Ten Principles of Values-Based Medicine. In: Radden J. (ed) *The Philosophy of Psychiatry: A Companion*. New York: Oxford University Press; 2004. pp 205–234.

[5] Woodbridge K, Fulford KWM. *Whose Values? A workbook for values-based practice in mental health care*. London: Sainsbury Centre for Mental Health; 2004.

[6] Fulford KWM, Campbell AV, Cox J. (2006) Introduction: At the Heart of Healing. In: Cox J, Campbell AV, Fulford KWM. (eds.) *Medicine of the Person: Faith, Science and Values in Health Care Provision*. London: Jessica Kingsley Publishers; 2006. pp. 17–29.

[7] Petrova M, Dale J, Fulford KWM. Values-Based Practice in primary care: easing the tensions between individual values, ethical principles and best evidence. *British Journal of General Practice* September 2006: pp. 703–709.

[8] Banner NF, Thornton T. (2007) The philosophy of psychiatry: the past, the present and the future: A review of the Oxford University Press series, 'International Perspectives in Philosophy and Psychiatry'. *Philosophy Ethics and Humanities of Medicine* 2007;2(9).

[9] Fulford KWM, Stanghellini G, Broome M. 'What can philosophy do for psychiatry?' *World Psychiatry* 2004;3(3) pp. 130–135.

[10] Stanghellini G. *Deanimated bodies and disembodied spirits. Essays on the psychopathology of common sense*. Oxford: Oxford University Press; 2004.

[11] Christodoulou GN. Preface in Christodoulou GN (ed) *Psychosomatic Medicine*. New York: Plenum Press; 1986.

[12] Novak P. Holistic concepts of Illness in Ancient Greece and in Contemporary Medicine. In: Christodoulou GN. (ed.) *Psychosomatic Medicine*. New York: Plenum; 1987. pp. 1–8.

[13] Aristoteles. *Ethica Nicomachea*. London: Oxford University Press; 1959.

[14] Christodoulou GN, Kontaxakis VP. *Topics in Preventive Psychiatry*. Basel: Karger; 1994.

[15] Christodoulou GN, Lecic-Tosevski D, Kontaxakis VP. *Issues in Preventive Psychiatry*. Basel: Karger; 1999.

[16] Mezzich JE. Psychiatry for the person: articulating medicine's science and humanism. *World Psychiatry* 2007;6(2).

[17] Christodoulou GN. (ed.) *Aspects of Preventive Psychiatry*. Basel: Karger; 1981.

[18] Aristotle *Nicomachean Ethics*. Trans Irwin T. Indianapolis: Hackett; 1985.

[19] Kant I. *Critique of judgment*. Indianapolis: Hackett; 1987.
[20] Carroll L. 'What The Tortoise Said To Achilles' *Mind* 1895;(4): pp. 278–280.
[21] Fulford KWM, Thornton T, Graham G. *The Oxford Textbook of Philosophy and Psychiatry*. Oxford: Oxford University Press; 2006.
[22] Windelband W. History and natural science. *History and Theory & Psychology* 1980;19: pp. 169–185.
[23] IDGA Workgroup, WPA. IGDA 8: Idiographic (personalised) diagnostic formulation. *British Journal of Psychiatry* 2003;18(suppl 45): pp. 55–57.
[24] Sellars W. Empiricism and the Philosophy of Mind, Cambridge, Mass: Harvard University Press; 1997.
[25] Phillips J. Idiographic Formulations, Symbols, Narratives, Context and Meaning. *Psychopathology* 2005;38: pp.180–184.
[26] Thornton T. Psychopathology and two varieties of narrative account of the self. *Philosophy Psychiatry and Psychology* 2003;10(4): pp. 361–367.
[27] Thornton T. Should comprehensive diagnosis include idiographic understanding? *Medicine, Healthcare and Philosophy* 2008;11: pp. 293–302.
[28] Jaspers K. Causal and 'Meaningful' Connections between Life History and Psychosis [1913]. Trans Hoenig J. In: Hirsch SR, Shepherd M. (eds.) *Themes and Variations in European Psychiatry*. Bristol: Wright; 1974. pp. 80–93.
[29] Jaspers K. The phenomenological approach in psychopathology [1912]. *British Journal of Psychiatry* 1968;114: pp. 1313–1323.
[30] Carruthers P, Smith PK. (eds.) *Theories of Theories of Mind*. Cambridge: Cambridge University Press; 1996.
[31] Ayob G. *Empathy*. Unpublished manuscript.
[32] Polanyi M. *Personal Knowledge. Towards a Post Critical Philosophy*. London: Routledge; 1958.
[33] Polanyi M. *The Tacit Dimension*. London: Routledge & Kegan Paul; 1967.
[34] Kuhn T. *The Structure of Scientific Revolutions*. Chicago: University of Chicago Press; 1962.
[35] Collins H. *Changing Order: Replication and Induction in Scientific Practice*. London: Sage; 1985.
[36] Thornton T. Tacit knowledge as the unifying factor in EBM and clinical judgement. *Philosophy Ethics and Humanities of Medicine* 2006;1(2).
[37] Dreyfus HL. Overcoming the Myth of the Mental: How Philosophers Can Profit from the Phenomenology of Everyday Expertise (APA Pacific Division Presidential Address 2005) *Proceedings and Addresses of the American Philosophical Association* 2005;79(2).
[38] McDowell J. Response to Dreyfus. *Inquiry* 2007;50: pp. 366–370.
[39] Kant I. *Critique of pure reason*. London: Macmillan; 1929.
[40] Thornton T. An aesthetic grounding for the role of concepts in experience in Kant, Wittgenstein and McDowell? *Forum Philosophicum* 2007;12(2): pp. 227–245.
[41] Thornton T. Thought insertion, cognitivism and inner space. *Cognitive neuropsychiatry* 2002;7(3): pp. 237–249.
[42] Wittgenstein L. *Philosophical Investigations*. Oxford: Blackwell; 1953.

CHAPTER 3

Culture and Mental Illness: Social Context and Explanatory Models

Laurence J. Kirmayer

Professor & Director, Division of Social & Transcultural Psychiatry, McGill University, Culture & Mental Health Research Unit, Sir Mortimer B Davis–Jewish General Hospital, Montreal, Quebec, Canada

Dinesh Bhugra

Professor of Social & Cultural Psychiatry, Institute of Psychiatry, London, UK; President, Royal College of Psychiatrists, UK

3.1   INTRODUCTION

There is wide recognition that cultural models influence how individuals interpret the signs and symptoms of illness, including psychiatric disorders. The processes of interpreting and ascribing meaning to one's bodily sensations, thoughts, feelings and behaviour are mediated by cognitive models and social interactions with others, which in turn reflect cultural knowledge and practices. Social scientists have distinguished between the biomedical concept of *disease*, the patient's subjective experience of *illness*, and the social meanings of *sickness*, each of which may be based on different explanatory models [1, 2]. However, pathophysiology, individual psychology and social responses interact. The cultural mediation of illness meaning, therefore, not only shapes the social manifestations of distress through symptom reports and help-seeking, but also influences the underlying psychophysiological processes that contribute to psycho-pathology and illness experience. In this chapter, we provide some examples of how social context and explanatory models influence common psychiatric conditions, including somatization, dissociation, mood, and anxiety disorders, as well as psychotic experience. Our aim is to demonstrate the important role played by explanations in the mechanisms of psychopathology as well as in clinical illness behaviour. Explanatory models are therefore an important target of research, clinical assessment, and intervention.

Psychiatric Diagnosis: Challenges and Prospects   Edited by I.M. Salloum and J.E. Mezzich
© 2009 John Wiley & Sons, Ltd

3.2   UNDERSTANDING AND ELICITING EXPLANATORY MODELS

The notion of explanatory models was introduced by Kleinman and colleagues [3], building on work on schemas in cognitive psychology and medical anthropological studies of illness experience. Kleinman's view of explanatory models emphasized the parallels with clinicians' biomedical models of disease, which typically include specific names or labels located within a diagnostic system notions of causation, theories of underlying mechanisms, expectations for outcome or prognosis, and recommended or appropriate treatment. Kleinman and colleagues [3] devised a simple set of questions to elicit patients' explanatory models (Table 3.1). In an effort to draw clinical attention to what was at stake for patients, they included the question: 'What do you fear most about the illness?'. The explanatory model approach has stimulated a substantial body of research in medical anthropology and, along with a parallel body of work in health psychology on symptom and illness schemas and attributions, has influenced clinical training and practice.

Various other interviews and self-report questionnaires have been devised to elicit explanatory models and symptom or illness schemas. Eisenbruch [4] developed the Mental Distress Explanatory Model Questionnaire (MDEMQ), which asks respondents to rate the potential causes of mental illness on a list of 45 causes drawn from the earlier classification of theories of illness causation by Murdock and colleagues [5]. Subsequent work has also confirmed Murdock's broad distinction between natural and supernatural causes as two clusters that are differentially associated with mental disorder, with both common and severe mental disorders often attributed to spiritual or supernatural agents or influences [6]. A simple checklist can elicit some aspects of patients' explanatory models for common mental disorders, including causal attributions to social or spiritual causes that correlate with treatment preferences [7].

Following closely on Kleinman's work, Weiss developed the Explanatory Model Interview Catalogue (EMIC), a research method for systematically eliciting EMs and quantitatively scoring for specific content [8, 9]. Sections of the EMIC are adapted for specific research contexts and questions to address: (i) patterns of distress; (ii) perceived causes; (iii) help-seeking behaviour and treatment; (iv) general illness beliefs; and (v) disease-specific queries. The EMIC has proved useful for research (e.g. [10–12]) but is too long and cumbersome for use in large-scale surveys or clinical practice [13]. The Short Explanatory Model Interview (SEMI) [14]), developed for use in epidemiological studies, includes five sections, with open-ended questions assessing: (i) the patient's personal sociocultural background; (ii) the nature of the presenting problem (reason for consultation,

Table 3.1   Explanatory model interview (Kleinman *et al.* 1978).

(1) What do you call your problem?
(2) What causes your problem?
(3) Why do you think it started when it did?
(4) How does it work?
(5) What is going on in your body?
(6) What kind of treatment do you think would be best for this problem?
(7) How has this problem affected your life?
(8) What frightens or concerns you most about this problem or treatment?

Adapted from [3].

causes, consequences, severity); (iii) help-seeking behaviour; (iv) interaction with the clinician; and (v) attitudes toward mental health and illness, elicited by brief vignettes. The SEMI has been used to study explanatory models among patients and community health workers in a variety of settings [15].

There has been much interest, in the field of health psychology, on the role of explanatory models in illness experience, symptom regulation, and coping with chronic illness [16]. The Illness Perception Questionnaire (IPQ) [17], based on Leventhal's self-regulation model of illness cognition [18], assesses five dimensions of illness models: identity (symptoms, nature of condition), causal component (cause/causes), time-line component (perception of the duration of problem), consequences component (severity and impact on functioning), and cure component (extent to which problem is amenable to cure). The IPQ has been applied mainly to the study of physical illness but recent studies have applied it to psychiatric disorders [19], including depression [20] and schizophrenia [21, 22]. A revised version, the IPQ-R, improves the psychometric properties of the subscales and demonstrated that the cognitive and emotional aspects of illness representations can be distinguished [23]. There is also a brief, nine-item version that taps the basic attitudinal dimensions and elicits causal attributions but does not explore specific content or meaning [24]. To date, there has been little cross-cultural application of these measures.

3.3   CULTURE, CONTEXT AND EXPLANATION

Despite its utility, the notion of explanatory models is based on a problematic theory of knowledge and action. Young characterized the emphasis on explanatory models as the 'rational man' approach to subjectivity, with its assumption that patients have explicit 'logical' models to account for their illness [25]. Drawing from his ethnographic research on illness explanations, Young argued that many people do not have coherent models of the type sought for with the EM questions, but rather have a complex array of fragmentary explanations borrowing from multiple sources, including salient individual or cultural prototypes, and sequences of events or actions that are habitual or sedimented in institutional practices and procedures. These different knowledge structures are used to construct illness narratives using both logical arguments and the cognitive devices of metaphor and metonym (Table 3.2) [26].

Table 3.2   Types of knowledge structure underlying illness narratives.

	Chain complexes	Prototypes	Explanatory models
Structure	metonymical	analogical	schematic
Production system	contiguity	images and metaphors	propositional logic
Representation	events	prototypes	causal sequences, mechanisms
Mode of elicitation	'What happened around the time you developed your symptoms?'	'Have you ever had anything like this before?' 'Do you know anyone/Have you heard of anyone who had something similar?'	'What caused your symptoms?'

Adapted from [67].

In fact, many patients do not have well worked out explanations for their illness, particularly when it is acute. Over time, individuals develop coherent illness narratives, but these are not all based on explanatory models. Some knowledge of illness is procedural, involving learned dispositions to respond, automatically expressed skills, and habits that the individual may not be able to articulate or describe. These underlying models can be discerned by observing the individual's behaviour and social interactions, and by analyzing the structure of their illness narratives. In addition, much illness behaviour is governed by interactional processes with implicit rules that are distributed among participants so that the individual's behaviour can be understood not in terms of their own cognitive models but as an outcome of interactions with others.

The McGill Illness Narrative Interview (MINI), based on Young's earlier work, is an open-ended, semi-structured interview designed to elicit chain complexes, prototypes and explanatory models [27]. The models elicited are not simply individual representations but are embedded in an illness narrative that is *situated*, responding to the nature of the interlocutor and unfolding over the course of the interview.

Research with the MINI and with other ethnographic methods confirms that many individuals have multiple models that they use to answer different questions [28, 29, 30]. Different models may be accessed or elicited in different social contexts or particular moments in a clinical interview, depending on the patient's perception of the physician's expectations. This diversity of models extends to the patients' family and entourage, whose members may have different models; in some instances, the model of a relative or significant other may be more important than that of the patient for determining illness behaviour and outcome, especially in cultural settings where identity is sociocentric or kinship based [31].

Illness models may be tentative at first, and become stabilized and consolidated over time. Models can be contested by others and re-entrenched in response to challenges. Patients, also, may hold several inconsistent or contradictory models, without being troubled by the contradiction. The availability of multiple explanations creates additional possibilities for meaning and contributes to what Good has called a 'subjunctive' stance [32], in which the meaning and implications of symptoms and illness are deliberately kept open to allow for positive outcomes. The need for consistency varies across cultures [33] and is particularly important in some overarching systems, like biomedicine or religious doctrines, which insist that individuals work to reconcile contradictions and reject incompatible explanations. Faced with the ambiguity of many clinical conditions, demands for diagnostic certainty, closure and consistency — on the part of either clinician or patient — may increase the possibility of conflict in the clinical encounter [34].

In sum, explanatory models are not fixed, static products of cognitive schemas or representations, but fluid, dynamic and changeable strategies for making sense of affliction. At any given moment, the explanatory models offered by (or elicited from) patients will reflect their efforts to understand their predicament, deal with their own fears and concerns, communicate their needs to the clinician, and position themselves in the clinical relationship and in larger institutional and social contexts in which every explanation has specific consequences. The observation that illness narratives, and the explanatory models they contain, depend on social context means that the information provided by brief questionnaires or structured interviews must be understood in terms of this more dynamic, interactional view of illness meaning and experience.

3.4   HOW REASONS BECOME CAUSES: EXPLANATIONS AND LOOPING EFFECTS

The ways that people interpret and respond to sensations, symptoms and behaviours can feed back into the physiological and psychological processes that give rise to sensations, symptoms and behaviours in the first place [35]. This sets the stage for cycles of symptom amplification that may intensify and maintain symptoms so that they reach thresholds of severity and chronicity. These amplifying loops can extend into the social world so that symptoms and behaviours lead to specific social responses, which in turn influence the symptoms and behaviours (Figure 3.1). A particular set of 'looping effects' acts to stabilize our categories of experience so that psychiatric diagnostic categories, which are tentative constructs, become socially reified and enacted by patients [36, 37]. In this way, psychiatric theory becomes self-confirming. In this section, we present some brief examples of how culturally mediated explanations and social contextual factors shape the causes, course and outcome of psychiatric disorders.

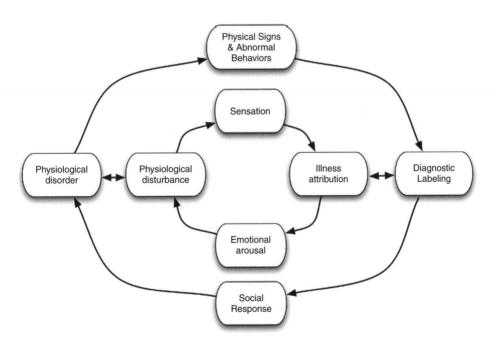

The inner loop represents the cognitive-emotional amplification of distress. The outer loop represents the social amplification of deviant behaviour. Other loops may cross these levels with circuits linking cognitive-emotional processes to social interaction. Culture influences every step in these cycles, but has particularly well studied effects at the levels of illness attributions (based on cultural models) and diagnostic labeling (based on systems of healing).

Figure 3.1   How reasons become causes: a typology of looping effects.

3.4.1 Somatoform Disorders

Research on illness behaviour has demonstrated how cognitive schemas, emotional states and social responses to bodily experience shape the experience and expression of distress. Ordinary physical sensations may be viewed as symptoms of illness and prompt worry and help-seeking. Symptoms of an illness may be misinterpreted as ordinary sensations, and minimized or ignored, leading to delayed help-seeking or rejection of treatment. Even when sensations are recognized as unusual they may be interpreted in markedly different ways.

Many patients in primary care present with medically unexplained symptoms [29]. While most patients acknowledge psychosocial factors as contributors to their distress, some adamantly deny any causal connection [10]. In current nosology, these patterns of illness behaviour are classified as somatoform disorders, implying a specific form of psychopathology. Many common somatic symptoms reflect cultural idioms of distress used to express a wide range of personal concerns [38]. People in many parts of the world employ *sociosomatic* theories that link adverse life circumstances to physical and emotional illness. The pattern of symptom attribution or mode of explanation influences clinical presentations [39, 40]. However, patients' disclosure of the emotional and social dimensions of their predicament depends on their views of what is appropriate to express to others within the family, in the community or in health care settings. Social and emotional dimensions of distress may be suppressed or hidden because of the potential for social stigmatization, while somatic symptoms and illness may be more acceptable to express [28, 41]. The category of somatoform disorders — which implies psychological causation that is evident to the clinician but denied by the patient — thus, reflects both the persistent mind-body dualism of biomedicine, patients' patterns of symptom attribution, and the clinician's difficulty in accessing the social meanings of the patient's suffering [34, 42, 43]. A contextual view would argue for dissolving the somatoform disorders as a discrete category in favour of attention to the ways in which social context, cognitive and emotional processes shape the individual's response to bodily distress. In place of discrete disorders, we might have a typology of psychological, interpersonal and social looping effects that contribute to amplifying somatic distress [35].

3.4.2 Dissociative Disorders

Dissociative disorders have also been viewed as a distinct form of psychopathology reflecting a lack of normal integration of experience. However, around the world, dissociative experiences are extremely common and usually do not indicate pathology [44]. Trance and possession commonly occur as part of religious and healing cults and practices, where such behaviour is prescribed and follows cultural scripts [45]. In such contexts, dissociation may communicate a message about one's distress, lack of control and lack of culpability by showing that the person is somehow controlled by or speaking for an 'other' [46]. In many cultures, this other is a god, spirit, or ancestor; in Western societies, the 'other' tends to be understood as a fragment of one's own personal history or imagination. Dissociation may be evidence of psychopathology when it falls outside the range of locally accepted behaviour, but this judgment requires careful consideration of multiple social contexts, including the setting where the behaviour first emerged, the demand characteristics of the clinical situation, and the larger cultural meanings given to dissociative behaviours.

Dissociation involves interpreting or attributing behaviours that are normally self-directed to agencies external to the self. The monological self assumed by Western folk psychology does not provide a place for the multiplicity of identity and multiple centres of agency that characterize human behaviour [47]. As a result, dissociation tends to be viewed as a maladaptive psychological coping mechanism or defence, rather than as socially scripted behaviour for managing fractures of identity, contradictions and social entrapment. A contextual view would put as much emphasis on the contexts in which dissociation occurs as on any psychological mechanism [48]. The observation that rates of dissociation are changing in response to increased industrialization and urbanization reflects this sensitivity to social context and needs to be explored further in cross-cultural studies.

3.4.3   Depressive and Anxiety Disorders

While major depression and anxiety disorders can be identified around the world, their symptoms, clinical presentation, and expected treatment vary substantially [39, 49, 50]. The development of individuals' self-representations and self-esteem are shaped by cultural norms and values and this may contribute to their vulnerability or resistance to depression [51]. Notions of guilt and shame also vary across religions and cultures, altering the cognitive schemas and specific symptoms associated with depressed mood [49, 52]. In many cultures, the psychological symptoms of depression are not recognized as a health problem but explained in sociomoral or spiritual terms [53].

Differences in the interpretation and causal explanation of events can also contribute to the processes that exacerbate depression and anxiety. The cognitive theories of depression and anxiety emphasize the role of specific attributions of behaviour and experience in creating vicious circles. A general self-enhancing attributional bias may help individuals maintain self-esteem [54]. However, the meaning of these attributions depends on cultural concepts of the person. For example, in individualistic cultures, attributing failures to one's self and success to others can precipitate or exacerbate depression, while in more sociocentric cultures such self-blame may be evidence of one's social responsibility [51].

Our understanding of the nature of depression and anxiety, and their effective treatment, is strongly influenced by the economic context of psychiatric practice [55]. Recent work has shown how the DSM criteria for depression have served to pathologize responses that can be understood as ordinary grief, sadness or demoralization [56, 57].

In some instances, a specific cultural model may be central to the development of a disorder. A growing body of work shows how the vicious circles of excessive self-awareness and expectations of catastrophe that drive panic disorder and other anxiety disorders (including the forms of health anxiety labelled 'hypochondriasis') may be mediated by culture-specific understandings of physical sensations that occur either as normal events or as a consequence of physiological dysregulation [58]. Clinical interventions targeting these specific attributions in ways that are culturally consonant can be effective [59].

3.4.4   Psychotic Disorders

Both the causes and the course of psychotic illness are influenced by social and cultural context. Psychotic experiences are deeply perplexing and prompt a search for meaning that often results in invoking spiritual or other extra-ordinary explanations [60, 61]. The explanations that patients consider may be tentative and shift over time [62]. Explanations also vary across cultural groups [63]. Explanations that centre on brain dysfunction, while consonant with biomedical theory, may result in loss of self-esteem and social stigmatization that contribute to chronicity [64]. Religious and other cultural systems of meaning may allow the person to imbue psychotic experience with positive meaning, maintain social integration and, hence, contribute to better outcome. Although impaired insight is often viewed as intrinsic to psychotic disorders, it can also be understood in interpersonal or interactional terms as the failure of the patient to agree with the clinician's account [65]. The success or failure of the negotiation of meaning depends on the quality of the clinician-patient relationship — which may, of course, be influenced by a host of social and psychological factors, including the nature of the patient's psychopathology, but also the larger social contexts from which illness receives meaning.

3.5 CONCLUSION: CULTURE, CONTEXT AND MEANING IN PSYCHIATRIC NOSOLOGY

The recognition that both patients and clinicians have explanatory models is an important preliminary to successful clinical assessment, treatment negotiation and intervention. However, there remains a tendency to view patients' models as simply misguided or ill informed, so that the clinician's task is to replace these inaccurate models with the medically correct label and explanation. From this point of view, patients' explanatory models are important mainly as potential barriers to clinical communication and adherence to treatment. This view ignores the crucial function of explanations as ways of interpreting the social and moral meaning of affliction. It also ignores the cognitive and social effects of explanations, which not only govern illness behaviour but which can contribute directly to psychopathology, constituting social or psychological problems in their own right, and also provide strategies for coping, adaptation and recovery. Explanatory models, then, are not merely *post hoc* attempts to explain or rationalize illness experience but are themselves constitutive of psychiatric disorders and of the psychological and social response to psychopathology. Research on explanatory models suggests that cultural meanings may participate directly in psychological or social loops or vicious circles that lead to specific forms of psychopathology. Psychiatric nosology can incorporate this insight by developing a typology of looping effects relevant to specific types of disorder [35]. These looping effects may contribute to many types of disorders and so might be placed on a separate diagnostic axis reflecting the clinical assessment of illness cognition and behaviour.

The cultural formulation in DSM-V provides an outline of some of the basic information needed to understand diagnosis in social and cultural context [66]. The cultural formulation canvases four broad domains: (i) identity; (ii) illness meanings; (iii) social functioning, stresses and supports; and (iv) the relationship with the clinician. Of course, the domains of cultural influence and experience tapped by the cultural formulation are not independent. Anthropological studies make it clear that explanatory models interact with identity, family and social functioning, and the clinician-patient relationship. Illness explanations may reflect the individual's cognitive representations but they may also be distributed among family members and others in their lifeworld or larger social contexts. In addition to explicit explanatory models, illness meanings may be based on situated experiences and personal or cultural prototypes, Specific modes of clinical inquiry and observation are needed to access these knowledge structures [27, 68].

Explanations, then, are not simply cognitive schemas or representations that can be accessed with a few direct questions, but acts of positioning, strategies for meaning-making, and ways of creating possibilities for recovery. Clinical assessment and treatment, therefore, must track the evolving meanings of distress throughout the clinical encounter, from diagnostic assessment to treatment negotiation and follow-up over the course of the illness. In this way, cultural models and explanations can become guides to diagnosis, a basis for empathic understanding, and resources for effective intervention.

REFERENCES

[1] Eisenberg L. Disease and illness: Distinctions between professional and popular ideas of sickness. *Culture, Medicine and Psychiatry* 1977;1: pp. 9–23.

[2] Young A. The anthropologies of illness and sickness. *Annual Review of Anthropology* 1992;11: pp. 257–285.

[3] Kleinman A, Eisenberg L, Good B. Culture, illness, and care: clinical lessons from anthropologic and cross-cultural research. *Annals of Internal Medicine* 1978;88: pp.251–258.

[4] Eisenbruch M. Classification of natural and supernatural causes of mental distress. Development of a Mental Distress Explanatory Model Questionnaire. *Journal of Nervous and Mental Disease* 1990;178: pp. 712–719.

[5] Murdock GP, Wilson SF, Frederick V. World distribution of theories of illness. *Ethnology* 1978;17: pp. 449–470.

[6] Minas H, Klimidis S, Tuncer C. Illness causal beliefs in Turkish immigrants. *BMC Psychiatry* 2007;7: p. 34.

[7] Bhui K, Rudell K, Priebe S. Assessing explanatory models for common mental disorders. *Journal of Clinical Psychiatry* 2006;67: pp. 964–971.

[8] Weiss M. Explanatory Model Interview Catalogue (EMIC): Framework for comparative study of illness. *Transcultural Psychiatry* 1997;34: pp. 235–263.

[9] Weiss MG, Doongaji DR, Siddartha S, Wypij D, Pathare S, Bhatawdekar M, Bhave A, Sheth A, Fernandes R. The Explanatory Model Interview Catalogue (EMIC): Contribution to cross-cultural research methods from a study of leprosy and mental health. *British Journal of Psychiatry* 1992;160: pp. 819–830.

[10] Henningsen P, Jakobsen T, Schiltenwolf M, Weiss MG. Somatization revisited: diagnosis and perceived causes of common mental disorders. *Journal of Nervous and Mental Disease* 2005;193: pp.85–92.

[11] Weiss MG. Cultural epidemiology: An introduction and overview. *Anthropology and Medicine* 2001;8: pp. 5–30.

[12] Lee R, Rodin G, Devins G, Weiss MG. Illness experience, meaning and help-seeking among Chinese immigrants in Canada with chronic fatigue and weakness. *Anthropology and Medicine* 2001;8: pp. 89–107.

[13] Bhui K, Bhugra D. Explanatory models for mental distress: implications for clinical practice and research. *British Journal of Psychiatry* 2002;181: pp. 6–7.

[14] Lloyd KR, Jacob KS, Patel V, St Louis L, Bhugra D, Mann AH. The development of the Short Explanatory Model Interview (SEMI) and its use among primary-care attenders with common mental disorders. *Psychological Medicine* 1998;28: pp. 1231–1237.

[15] Joel D, Sathyaseelan M, Jayakaran R, Vijayakumar C, Muthurathnam S, Jacob KS. Explanatory models of psychosis among community health workers in South India. *Acta Psychiatrica Scandinavica* 2003;108: pp. 66–69.

[16] Lyons AC, Chamberlain K. *Health psychology: a critical introduction*. Cambridge:Cambridge University Press; 2006.

[17] Weinman J, Petrie KJ, Moss-Morris R, Horne R. The illness perception questionnaire: a new method for assessing the cognitive representation of illness. *Psychology and Health* 1996;11: pp. 431–445.

[18] Leventhal H, Nerenz DR, Steele DJ. Illness representations and coping with health threats. In: Baum A, Singer J. (eds.) *A Handbook of Psychology and Health*. New Jersey: Erlbaum; 1984.

[19] Lobban F, Barrowclough C, Jones S. A review of the role of illness models in severe mental illness. *Clinical Psychology Review* 2003;23: pp. 171–196.

[20] Fortune G, Barrowclough C, Lobban F. Illness representations in depression. *British Journal of Clinical Psychology* 2004; 43: pp. 347–364.

[21] Lobban F, Barrowclough C, Jones S. Assessing cognitive representations of mental health problems. I. The illness perception questionnaire for schizophrenia. *British Journal of Clinical Psychology* 2005;44: pp.147–162.

[22] Lobban F, Barrowclough C, Jones S. Assessing cognitive representations of mental health problems. II. The illness perception questionnaire for schizophrenia: Relatives' version. *British Journal of Clinical Psychology* 2005;44: pp. 163–179.

[23] Moss-Morris R, Weinman J, Petrie KJ, Horne R, Cameron LS, Buick D. The Revised Illness Perception Questionnaire (IPQ-R). *Psychology and Health* 2002;17: pp. 1–16.

[24] Broadbent E, Petrie KJ, Main J, Weinman J. The brief illness perception questionnaire. *Journal of Psychosomatic Research* 2006;60: pp. 631–637.

[25] Young A. Rational men and the explanatory model approach. *Culture, Medicine and Psychiatry* 1982;6: pp. 57–71.

[26] Kirmayer LJ. Improvisation and authority in illness meaning. *Culture, Medicine and Psychiatry*, 1994;18: pp. 183–214.

[27] Groleau D, Young A, Kirmayer LJ. (2006) The McGill Illness Narrative Interview (MINI): an interview schedule to elicit meanings and modes of reasoning related to illness experience. *Transcultural Psychiatry*, 43, 671–91.

[28] Groleau D, Kirmayer LJ. Sociosomatic theory in Vietnamese immigrants' narratives of distress. *Anthropology and Medicine* 2004;11: pp. 117–133.

[29] Kirmayer LJ, Groleau D, Looper KJ, Dao MD. Explaining medically unexplained symptoms. *Canadian Journal of Psychiatry* 2004;49: pp. 663–672.

[30] Williams B, Healy D. Perceptions of illness causation among new referrals to a community mental health team: "explanatory model: or "exploratory map"? *Social Science and Medicine* 2001;53: pp. 465–476.

[31] Bhugra D. Migration, distress and cultural identity. *British Medical Bulletin* 2004;69; pp. 129–141.

[32] Good BJ. *Medicine, Rationality, and Experience: An Anthropological Perspective*. Cambridge: Cambridge University Press; 1994.

[33] Heine SJ. Self as cultural product: An examination of East Asian and North American selves. *Journal of Personality* 2001;69: pp. 881–906.

[34] Kirmayer LJ. Broken narratives: Clinical encounters and the poetics of illness experience. In: Mattingly C, Garro L. (eds.) *Narrative and the Cultural Construction of Illness and Healing*. Berkeley: University of California Press; 2000.

[35] Kirmayer LJ, Sartorius N. Cultural models and somatic syndromes. *Psychosomatic Medicine* 2007;69: pp. 832–840.

[36] Hacking I. The looping effect of human kinds. In: Sperber D, Premack D, Premack AJ. (eds.) *Causal Cognition: A Multidisciplinary Debate*. Oxford: Oxford University Press; 1995.

[37] Hacking I. *Mad Travelers: Reflections on the Reality of Transient Mental Illnesses*. Charlottesville: University Press of Virginia; 1998.

[38] Kirmayer LJ, Young A. Culture and somatization: clinical, epidemiological, and ethnographic perspectives. *Psychosomatic Medicine* 1998;60: pp. 420–430.

[39] Kirmayer LJ. Cultural variations in the clinical presentation of depression and anxiety: implications for diagnosis and treatment. *Journal of Clinical Psychiatry* 2001;62 (Suppl 13): pp. 22–28; discussion pp. 29–30.

[40] Bhui K, Bhugra D, Goldberg D. Causal explanations of distress and general practitioners' assessments of common mental disorder among Punjabi and English attendees. *Social Psychiatry and Psychiatric Epidemiology* 2002;37: pp. 38–45.

[41] Raguram R, Weiss MG, Channabasavanna SM, Devins GM. Stigma, depression, and somatization in South India. *American Journal of Psychiatry* 1996;153: pp. 1043–1049.

[42] Kirmayer LJ. Mind and body as metaphors: Hidden values in biomedicine. In: Lock M, Gordon D. (eds.) *Biomedicine Examined*. Dordrecht: Kluwer; 1988.

[43] Miresco MJ, Kirmayer LJ. The persistence of mind-brain dualism in psychiatric reasoning about clinical scenarios. *American Journal of Psychiatry* 2006;163: pp. 913–918.

[44] Kirmayer LJ. *Pacing the void: Social and cultural dimensions of dissociation*. In: Spiegel D. (ed.) *Dissociation: Culture, Mind and Body*. Washington: American Psychiatric Press; 1994.

[45] Leavitt J. Are trance and possession disorders? *Transcultural Psychiatric Research Review* 1993;30: pp. 51–57.

[46] Kirmayer LJ, Santhanam R. The anthropology of hysteria. In: Halligan PW, Bass C, Marshall JC. (Eds.) *Contemporary Approaches to the Study of Hysteria: Clinical and Theoretical Perspectives*. Oxford: Oxford University Press; 2001.

[47] Littlewood R. *Reason and necessity in the specification of the multiple self*. Royal Anthropological Institute of Great Britain and Ireland; 1996.

[48] Seligman R, Kirmayer LJ. Dissociative experience and cultural neuroscience: narrative, metaphor and mechanism. *Culture, Medicine and Psychiatry* 2008;32: pp. 31–64.

[49] Bhugra D. Depression across cultures. *Primary Care Psychiatry* 1996;2: pp. 155–165.

[50] Kirmayer LJ, Jarvis GE. Depression across cultures. In: Stein D, Schatzberg A, Kupfer D. (eds.) *Textbook of Mood Disorders*. Washington: American Psychiatric Press; 2005.

[51] Heine SJ, Lehman DR, Markus HR, Kitayama S. Is there a universal need for positive self-regard? *Psychological Review* 1999;106: pp. 766–794.

[52] Bhugra D, Gupta KR, Wright B. Depression in North India. *International Journal of Psychiatry in Clinical Practice* 1997;1: pp. 83–87.

[53] Karasz A. Cultural differences in conceptual models of depression. *Social Science and Medicine* 2005;60: pp. 1625–1635.

[54] Mezulis AH, Abramson LY, Hyde JS, Hanking BL. Is there a universal positivity bias in attributions? A meta-analytic review of individual, developmental, and cultural differences in the self-serving attributional bias. *Psychological Bulletin* 2004;130: pp. 711–747.

[55] Healy D. *Let them eat Prozac: the unhealthy relationship between the pharmaceutical industry and depression*. New York: New York University Press; 2004.

[56] Horwitz AV. *The Social Control of Mental Illness*. Orlando, CA: Academic Press; 1982.

[57] Wakefield JC, Schmitz MF, First MB, Horwitz AV. Extending the bereavement exclusion for major depression to other losses: evidence from the National Comorbidity Survey. *Archives of General Psychiatry* 2007;64: pp. 433–40.

[58] Hinton DE, Hinton L, Tran M, Nguyen M, Nguyen L, Hsia C, Pollack MH. Orthostatic panic attacks among Vietnamese refugees. *Transcultural Psychiatry* 2007;44: pp. 515–44.

[59] Hinton DE, Chhean D, Pich V, Safren SA, Hofmann SG, Pollack MH. A randomized controlled trial of cognitive-behavior therapy for Cambodian refugees with treatment-resistant PTSD and panic attacks: a cross-over design. *Journal of Traumatic Stress* 2005;18: pp. 617–629.

[60] Corin E. The "Other" of culture in psychosis: The ex-centricity of the subject. In: Biehl J, Good BJ, Kleinman A. (eds.) *Subjectivity: Ethnographic Investigations*. Berkeley: University of California Press; 2007.

[61] Saravanan B, Jacob KS, Johnson S, Prince M, Bhugra D, David AS. Assessing insight in schizophrenia: East meets West. *British Journal of Psychiatry* 2007;190: pp. 243–247.

[62] McCabe R, Priebe S. Assessing the stability of schizophrenic patients' explanatory models of illness over time. *Journal of Mental Health* 2004;13: pp. 163–169.

[63] McCabe R, Priebe S. Explanatory models of illness in schizophrenia: comparison of four ethnic groups. *British Journal of Psychiatry* 2004;185: pp. 25–30.

[64] Angermeyer MC, Matschinger H. Causal beliefs and attitudes to people with schizophrenia: Trend analysis based on data from two population surveys in Germany. *British Journal of Psychiatry* 2005;186: pp. 331–334.

[65] Kirmayer LJ, Corin E, Jarvis GE. Inside knowledge: Cultural constructions of insight in psychosis. In: Amador XF, David AS. (eds.) *Insight in Psychosis*. 2nd ed. New York: Oxford University Press; 2004.

[66] American Psychiatric Association. *Diagnostic and statistical manual of mental disorders: DSM-IV-TR*. Washington DC: American Psychiatric Association; 2000.

[67] Kirmayer LJ, Young A, Robbins JM. Symptom attribution in cultural perspective. *Canadian Journal of Psychiatry* 1994;39: pp. 584–595.

[68] Kirmayer LJ, Rousseau C, Jarvis GE, Guzder J. The Cultural context of clinical assessment. In: Tasman A, Maj M, First MB, Kay J, Lieberman J. (eds.) *Psychiatry*. 3rd ed. New York: John Wiley & Sons; 2008: pp. 54–66.

CHAPTER 4

Quality of Life in Illness and Health[1]

Heinz Katschnig
Professor, Ludwig Boltzmann Institute for Social Psychiatry, Vienna, Austria
Raluca Sfetcu
Professor, Babes-Bolyai University, Cluj-Napoca, Romania
Norman Sartorius
Professor, University of Geneva, Switzerland

4.1 INTRODUCTION

The earliest systematic approaches to empirically assessing quality of life (Qol) go back to the 1960s and 1970s. At a time when the welfare state was growing in Western nations and inequalities in the distribution of resources and well-being were increasingly recognized, research on 'social indicators', 'wellbeing', 'standard of living' and 'quality of life' was stimulated [1, 2, 3]. This research was more concerned with populations, including whole nations, than with the individual person. Around the same time, another relevant development started, called today 'positive psychology' and 'happiness research', which, in contrast to the studies just mentioned, concentrated exclusively on the well-being of individuals [4].

In this body of research, three dimensions can be distinguished: first, well-being and satisfaction with life; second, functioning in social roles; and, third, environmental conditions, including both the social environment (social network) and the material standard of living.

4.2 THE RISE OF THE QUALITY OF LIFE CONCEPT IN MEDICINE

The above-mentioned developments took place outside medicine. However, since health and illness are clearly factors that influence quality of life and well-being (*'ill*ness' as

Psychiatric Diagnosis: Challenges and Prospects   Edited by I.M. Salloum and J.E. Mezzich
© 2009 John Wiley & Sons, Ltd

opposed to '*well*ness') it is not surprising that – albeit with a certain time lag – medicine followed suit with research on health-related quality of life (HRQL). This development was also fuelled by the ever-increasing criticism that modern medicine gives more attention to technical issues than Qol issues.

The first documented use of the term 'quality of life' in a medical journal dates back to 1966 [5], when it was employed by Russel Elkinton in an editorial on transplantation medicine in the *Annals of Internal Medicine*. In referring to Francis Bacon's statement that 'the office of medicine is but to tune this curious harp of man's body and reduce it to harmony', Elkinton criticizes modern medicine as doing the tuning with 'unprecedented skill' but having 'trouble with the harmony'. He goes on to ask: 'What is the harmony within a man, and between a man and his world – the *quality of life* – to which the patient, the physician, and society aspires?' It is noteworthy that Elkinton stresses both the harmony within a person, and that between the person and his/her environment. We shall come back to this later.

Critics of mainstream medicine, from the cynical George Bernard Shaw ('the doctor's dilemma') to the provocative Ivan Illich ('medical nemesis'); from Elkinton's 'lack of harmony' to Engel's 'bio-psycho-social model'; and from alternative and complementary medicine to the myriads of self-help groups for all kinds of diseases, all maintain that medical practice is neglecting subjective, holistic and, more generally speaking, non-medical aspects of illness. These aspects can be subsumed under the term 'quality of life'. While they have been taken care of in the medical *research* literature for some time, as will be shown below, the criticism concerns the fact that they are not yet taken into account in any systematic way in medical *practice*.

In medicine, oncology was among the first to notice that adding 'years to life' does not necessarily imply adding 'life to years'. This is now common knowledge: in the 1992 novel *Paradise News* by David Lodge, when the protagonist is asked why she refuses chemotherapy for cancer, she says: 'I'd rather die with my own hair on'. For nearly every disease, Qol instruments have been developed over the last two decades, most of them focusing on subjective well-being and satisfaction. A MEDLINE search shows there were slowly increasing numbers of Qol articles before the 1990s but a steep rise thereafter, to more than 2000 publications in 1995, more than 7000 in 2004, and nearly 12 000 in 2007. Most publications relate to one of three topics: description of Qol in chronically sick populations; clinical trials, where Qol measures are increasingly employed in addition to medical variables; and health economic studies. In the 1980s and 1990s, a number of generic instruments (i.e. instruments that can be used in all types of diseases) were published, among them the SF-36 [6] and the World Health Organization's WHOQOL [7]. In 1992, a scientific journal, *Quality of Life Research: An International Journal of Quality of Life Aspects of Treatment, Care and Rehabilitation* was founded and, since then, an International Society of Quality of Life Research has organized annual conferences.

In contrast to all these scientific efforts, the Qol issue still seems to be underrepresented in clinical practice of treatment and rehabilitation – this might be a justification for including a quality of life axis in a multiaxial psychiatric classification and incorporating it into the person-centred integrative diagnostic model (PID) (see chapters 28 and 30, this volume). Also, the use of the Qol concept for mental health promotion and mental disorder prevention needs to be considered more seriously [8].

Furthermore, although the term Qol is much used in today's medical literature and Qol is 'measured' in all types of diseases, no agreed upon definition exists yet. While this is regrettable, the term 'quality of life' itself obviously has an intuitive appeal to all stake-holders involved in health and illness, who tend to agree that improving Qol matters in health care: the patients and their relatives (not only the individuals but also their self-help organizations), the professionals, the pharmaceutical industry, health administrators, poli-ticians and regulatory agencies (who, for instance, increasingly ask for a drug to improve not only symptoms but also Qol, or at least not to diminish it).

4.3 THE CONCEPT OF QUALITY OF LIFE IN RELATION TO MENTAL HEALTH

When it was shown in the mid-1970s that neuroleptic medication could prevent relapses in schizophrenia but that the price was often a crippling Parkinson's syndrome, an article in *The American Journal of Psychiatry* raised the question of whether, in maintenance antipsychotic medication, 'the cure was worse than the disease' [9]. This observation on the disturbed Qol in these patients has contributed to the development of the second-generation antipsychotics. Also, perhaps because psychiatry paid more attention to psy-chosocial issues, it was in the forefront of developing disease-specific Qol (and related) assessment instruments (e.g. [10, 11, 12, 13]).

Of the three components identified at the beginning of this article as being part of the sociological and the psychological Qol concepts, there is a tendency in health-related quality of life (HRQL) research – criticized for medicine in general by Rapley [14] – to concentrate on one component only, namely directly disease-related subjective well-being and satisfaction (often measured by a single index), and to disregard social functioning and environmental assets, like standard of living and social support.

The use of such a uni-dimensional, subject-centred concept is even less appropriate for the mental health field. If we talk about the Qol of persons suffering from mental disorders, we have to ask many questions, such as: how they live their daily lives; how 'good' or 'bad' this life is at some times or at others; how they view their lives, their well-being, their functioning and their resources; how satisfied they are with these aspects of their lives, but also how good their functioning and resources are by external standards. Finally, there is the question of how they integrate the 'symptoms' and the 'disorder' into their lives and how they deal with stigma.

This is a large number of topics, which, obviously, cannot be represented by a single measure reflecting mostly momentary well-being. In order to ensure that well-being will also be possible in the future, role functioning and environmental assets also have to be addressed. Consider the extreme example of a manic patient who feels very well, but who is not functioning appropriately in social roles and thereby undermines the basis for his future.

It is not only paramount for mental disorders that a wide array of domains are assessed – subjective well-being and satisfaction, as well as the environmental aspects mentioned above – but that the environmental aspects are also evaluated 'externally', e.g. by family members and professionals. Income, lack of autonomy (e.g. because of lack of money), ability to get or hold a job, role function as a mother in a family, low social support – all these and many other 'objective' facts determine how good or bad a patient's life is. Such external evaluation is the more important, since in chronic conditions the persons affected tend to downgrade their expectations over time and lower their standards.

It is obvious, though, that both an objective assessment – of the individuals' positions in life, their symptoms and their capacities – and a subjective assessment by the individuals themselves are important and complementary [15]. The strategy that the World Health Organization (WHO) adopted in its effort to develop cross-culturally-acceptable and applicable methods for the measurement of Qol exemplifies this position [16, 17]. The definition proposed by WHO is that Qol is the individuals' perception of their position in life in relation to their goals and in the framework of their culture and of value systems they have accepted and incorporated in their decision-making. This definition places primary importance on individuals' willingness and capacity to communicate and participate in the assessment of their Qol. In the WHO Quality of Life Instrument (WHOQOL), a number of domains of individuals' activities have been selected by consulting a large group of scientists and practitioners from different cultures. For each of the domains, a number of 'facets' have been defined and for each of these, an *objective assessment* (e.g. of the individuals' capacity to walk) and two *subjective assessments* (i.e. how the individuals feel about their capacity to walk and whether this influences their overall quality of life) have been sought.

If the evaluation of Qol is reduced to assessing subjective well-being and satisfaction, then a number of 'fallacies' are possible. The 'affective fallacy' is especially relevant here [18]: simply stated, when a patient is depressed, his well-being and satisfaction with life are low by definition; when he/she is manic it might be the other way around. When examining the items on well-being scales, it is obvious that many of them could also be present in depression rating scales – and calling such a score a measure for the severity of depression may be more appropriate than calling it a Qol measure. This refers especially to clinical trials of antidepressant medication, where it is sometimes claimed that a new drug not only improves depression but also Qol, which means that two labels are used for the same fact [19].

The WHO approach acknowledges the fact that a patient's Qol may be satisfactory in one area of life (such as family life),but not in another (such as work), and this matters for choosing an intervention. How many areas should be chosen for assessment is debatable but, clearly, several such areas should be assessed separately. Finally, without going into too much detail here, it has also to be considered that some areas may be regarded by a patient as more relevant than others, and this would also have to be taken into consideration.

4.4   FROM ASSESSMENT TO ACTION

Medicine and psychiatry are applied sciences. Assessing a psychiatric patient's quality of life cannot, therefore, be just an ivory tower exercise, but it should be related to interventions in clinical practice [20]. What is required, therefore, in the field of mental health and in other fields of medicine, is a well-structured and multifaceted concept of Qol with appropriate measurement methods that allow the assessment of a wide array of aspects of Qol, by patients, relatives, and professionals, and which should be linked to interventions.

A few instruments that have been developed in order to assess the needs of persons with mental disorders, without having been called Qol instruments, approach these ideas (Camberwell Assessment of Need (CAN) [21] and the Needs for Care Assessment instrument of the Medical Research Council unit in London (NCA-MRC) [22]). A specific Management Orientated Needs Assessment instrument (MONA) for use in a day hospital has been developed by Amering *et al.* in Vienna [23]. Only one Qol instrument available for psychiatric disorders was constructed along these lines (the Wisconsin Quality of Life Index (W-QLI) [24]).

These instruments are complex and time consuming to employ and they can hardly be incorporated into a multiaxial psychiatric diagnostic system. However, if the intention is to use the Qol concept as a guideline for interventions, a single index of subjective well-being and satisfaction is not very helpful for the comprehensive interventions required for psychiatric patients, especially for the many who have complex needs.

Katschnig *et al.* [25] have attempted to provide a manageable framework for action, as a kind of compromise between, on the one hand, the seemingly unmanageable complexity of comprehensive Qol information and, on the other hand, the straightforward uni-dimensional Qol scales with little implication for practical interventions. Details of this framework are presented in Figure 4.1. It indicates four possible points of intervention, two

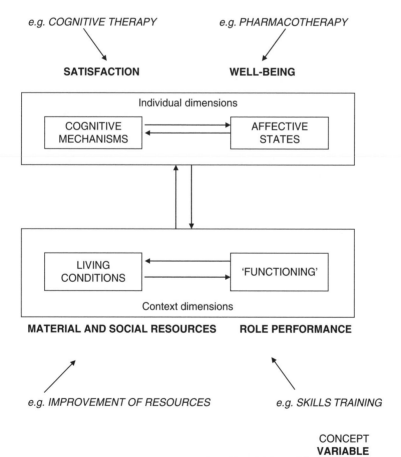

Figure 4.1 A comprehensive model of action oriented assessment of quality of life in depression (derived from Katschnig *et al.* [25]).

belonging to interventions on the individual level (cognitive mechanisms – satisfaction; affective states – well-being) and two relating to contextual aspects (role performance – functioning; material and social resources – living conditions). Each is illustrated by an example for intervention: cognitive therapy for satisfaction; pharmacotherapy for well-being; skills training for role performance; and, finally, increase of external resources for compensating for their absence.

This model, or similar ones, might be useful for systematizing information obtained by complex Qol instruments and channelling it towards appropriate interventions. As the graph indicates by the arrows between the four components, we can assume that a successful intervention for one component has positive influences on other components.

4.5 CONCLUSION

The term Qol is used with many different meanings. In relation to ill health, it is most often equated with reduced subjective well-being, and most Qol instruments for specific diseases focus on this aspect. It is argued here that, at least for mental health care, a complex concept of Qol, also including environmental aspects (such as functioning in social roles, social support, and standard of living) is more appropriate and that, in addition to having these aspects evaluated by patients themselves, external assessment is also required. Complex Qol models go hand in hand with the development of modern community psychiatry, and with the fact that, for patients living in the community, life in all its aspects becomes a possibility and that they need assistance in all areas of life in order to maximize their well-being. This situation requires multi-professional teams, implying that specialized team members are responsible for attending to the different aspects of patients' needs and quality of life. While waiting for this to be achieved, the incorporation of a simple assessment of the patient's subjective experience of Qol into the routine medical examinations and evaluations of effects of care interventions would be a great step forward likely to improve and humanize health care.

NOTE

1. Many issues dealt with in this article are more extensively discussed and referenced in Katschnig *et al.* [25].

REFERENCES

[1] Andrews FM, Withey SB. *Social Indicators of Well-Being*. America's Perception of Life Quality. New York: Plenum Press; 1976.
[2] Campbell A, Converse P, Rodgers W. *The Quality of American Life*. New York: Russell Sage; 1976.
[3] Albrecht GL, Fitzpatrick R. A sociological perspective on health-related quality of life research. In: Albrecht GL, Fitzpatrick R. (eds.) *Advances in Medical Sociology, Volume 5. Quality of Life in Health Care*. Greenwich, Connecticut: Jai Press Inc; 1994. pp. 1–21.
[4] Diener E, Suh EM, Lucas RE, Smith HL. Subjective well-being: Three decades of progress. *Psychological Bulletin* 1999;125: pp. 276–302.

[5] Elkinton J. Medicine and the quality of life. *Annals of Internal Medicine* 1966;64: pp. 711–714.

[6] Ware JE, Sherbourne CD. The MOS 36-Item Short-Form Health Survey (SF-36). *Medical Care* 1992;30: pp. 473–483.

[7] WHOQOL Group. The World Health Organization Quality of Life Assessment (WHOQOL): development and general psychometric properties. *Social Science & Medicine* 1998;46(12): pp. 1569–1585.

[8] Jané-Llopis E, Katschnig H. Improving Quality of Life Through Mental Health Promotion. In: Katschnig H, Freeman H, Sartorius N. (eds.) *Quality of Life in Mental Disorders*. 2nd ed. Chichester: John Wiley & Sons, Ltd; 2006. pp. 331–342.

[9] Gardos G, Cole JO. Maintenance antipsychotic therapy: Is the cure worse than the disease? *American Journal of Psychiatry* 1976;133: pp. 32–36.

[10] Malm U, May APR, Dencher SJ. Evaluation of the quality of life of the schizophrenic outpatient: a checklist. *Schizophrenia Bulletin* 1981;7: pp. 477–487.

[11] Baker F, Intagliata J. Quality of life in the evaluation of community support systems. *Evaluation and Program Planning* 1982;5: pp. 69–79.

[12] Bigelow DA, Brodsky G, Stewart L, Olson MM. The concept and measurement of quality of life as a dependent variable in evaluation of mental health services. In: Stahler GJ, Tash WR. (eds.) *Innovative Approaches to Mental Health Evaluation*. New York: Academic Press Inc; 1982. pp. 345–366.

[13] Lehman AF, Ward NC, Linn LS. Chronic mental patients: The quality of life issue. *American Journal of Psychiatry* 1982;139: pp. 1271–1276.

[14] Rapley M. *Quality of Life Research: A Critical Introduction*. London: Sage Publications; 2003.

[15] Sartorius N. Quality of Life in Mental Disorders – A Global Perspective. In: Katschnig H, Freeman H, Sartorius N. (eds.) *Quality of Life in Mental Disorders*. 2nd ed. Chichester: John Wiley & Sons, Ltd; 2006. pp. 321–327.

[16] Sartorius N. A WHO method for the assessment of health-related quality of life (WHOQOL). In: Walker SR, Rosser RM. (eds). *Quality of Life Assessment: Key Issues in the 1990s*. Dordrecht: Kluwer Academic Publishers; 1993. pp. 201–207.

[17] Skevington S, Sartorius N, Amir M, the WHOQOL Group. Developing methods for assessing quality of life in different cultural groups. The history of the WHOQOL instruments. *Social Psychiatry and Psychiatric Epidemiology* 2004;39: pp. 1–8.

[18] Katschnig H. How useful is the concept of Quality of Life in Psychiatry? In: Katschnig H, Freeman H, Sartorius N. (eds.) *Quality of Life in Mental Disorders*. 2nd ed. Chichester: John Wiley & Sons, Ltd; 2006. pp. 3–17.

[19] Katschnig H, Krautgartner M, Schrank B, Angermeyer MC. Quality of Life in Depression. In: Katschnig H, Freeman H, Sartorius N. (eds,): *Quality of Life in Mental Disorders*. 2nd ed. Chichester: John Wiley & Sons, Ltd.; 2006. pp.129–140.

[20] Katschnig H. Quality of life in mental disorders: challenges for research and clinical practice. *World Psychiatry* 2006;5: pp. 139–145.

[21] Phelan M, Slade M, Thornicroft G, Dunn G, Holloway F, Wykes T, Strathdee G, Loftus L, McCrone P, Hayward P. The Camberwell Assessment of Need: The validity and reliability of an instrument to assess the needs of people with severe mental illness. *British Journal of Psychiatry* 1995;167: pp. 589–595.

[22] Brewin CR, Wing JK, Mangen SP, Brugha TS, MacCarthy B. Principles and practice of measuring needs in the long-term mentally ill: The MRC Needs for Care Assessment. *Psychological Medicine* 1987;17: pp. 971–981.

[23] Amering M, Hofer E, Windhaber J, Wancata J, Katschnig H. *MONA – a new instrument for Management Oriented Needs Assessment*. Book of abstracts of the VI World Congress of the World Association for Psychosocial Rehabilitation. Hamburg; 1998. p. 28.

[24] Becker M, Diamond R, Sainfort F. A new client centered index for measuring quality of life in persons with severe and persistent mental illness. *Quality of Life Research*, 1993;2: pp. 239–251.

[25] Katschnig H, Freeman H, Sartorius N. (eds.) *Quality of Life in Mental Disorders*. Chichester: John Wiley & Sons Ltd; 2006.

CHAPTER 5

Recovery and Resilience

Michaela Amering [1]
Professor, Department of Psychiatry and Psychotherapy,
Division of Social Psychiatry, Medical University of Vienna, Vienna, Austria
Margit Schmolke [1]
German Academy for Psychoanalysis, Munich, Germany; Co-Chair, World
Psychiatric Association Section on Preventive Psychiatry

5.1 REMISSION AND RECOVERY

In 2005, a group of eminent schizophrenia experts in the US formulated remission criteria for schizophrenia [2], with an affirmative response from Europe [3]. This is a major challenge to ongoing statements about the inevitability of persistent and life-long symptoms of schizophrenia, statements that have been exposed as flying: '... in the face of evidence, collected over a century of research, that there is a high level of heterogeneity in the course and outcome of schizophrenia and that symptomatic remission is common'. [3]

Traditional predictions of generally poor outcome have been overstated, while, since Kraepelin's hypothesis of the incurability of dementia praecox, all the data have consistently shown that a sizeable proportion of people diagnosed with schizophrenia can and do recover. This, of course, has always been known to persons with a lived experience of such mental health problems. With more people telling their stories of recovery, and conceptualizing and contextualizing their experience, it can no longer be ignored. Clearly, however, recovery as defined by the people who are experiencing it themselves shows some major and noteworthy differences to the traditional clinical definitions of remission and recovery.

'Recovery does not refer to an end product or result. It does not mean that one is "cured" nor does it mean that one is simply stabilized or maintained in the community. Recovery often involves a transformation of the self wherein one both accepts ones limitation and discovers a new world of

Psychiatric Diagnosis: Challenges and Prospects   Edited by I.M. Salloum and J.E. Mezzich possibility. This is the paradox of recovery i.e., that in accepting what we cannot do or be, we begin to discover who we can be and what we can do. Thus, recovery is a process. It is a way of life.'

Pat Deegan [4, p. 67]

Pat Deegan [4] was one of the first people to describe eloquently how she and other people with the experience of psychosis and a diagnosis of schizophrenia have moved beyond a patient role to live in recovery, build meaningful lives and enjoy success and a great deal of health, rather than a life 'in the sometimes desolate wastelands of mental health programs and institutions'. Recovery is not a return to a 'premorbid' state, but rather a development of personal growth and the overcoming of the often negative personal and societal implications of receiving a diagnosis, especially the traditionally attached prognosis, which can hinder this process and the full use of coping strategies and resilience. Mental health services can be helpful if they succeed in fostering control, choice and hope, but harmful if they undermine self-determination and convey pessimism and hopelessness.

The movement of people in recovery makes clear that recovery refers to an individual process concerning subjective values and aspirations, rather than 'objective' criteria. Against this background, much of the scientific literature today talks about two different concepts:

1. the reduction of symptoms and disabilities;
2. the efforts and successes of leading a meaningful, self-determined life, with or in spite of certain symptoms, disabilities, vulnerabilities and idiosyncrasies.

These definitions have been referred to as service-based versus user-based [5]; clinical versus rehabilitative [6]; and symptom-focused versus person-centred [7].

Recovery concepts are not limited to schizophrenia, as described in detail in Amering and Schmolke's book on recovery [42]. Mary Ellen Copeland [8] was one of the first people to develop recovery concepts from her own experience with a diagnosis of bipolar illness. Her expertise not only stems from her own experience and her work in self-help, but also has important roots in the life story of her mother, who recovered after long years in hospital, where she and her family had been shocked by the hopeless prognosis. Andreas Knuf's call for a development 'from demoralizing pessimism towards rational optimism' clearly includes the discourse on borderline personality disorders [9]. Recovery is well established as a demand for integrating mental health and addiction services [10]. Also, for most common mental disorders, the course is variable. Remissions are possible, as are recurrences and long-term disabilities. Research struggles with the problems of definitions of types of courses, and the methodological problems of long-term studies. The clinical use of prognostic indicators and determinants of remission, recurrence and long-term courses for individual patients is limited. Many patients hesitate to understand their mental health problems within a model of medical care for chronic conditions [11]. As a result, a considerable proportion of their efforts towards coping and finding meaning in their struggle for recovery occur outside the patient-clinician relationship. A collaborative approach, allowing for individualized interventions and accommodating hopes, fears and subjective evidence in a personalized context, might be better suited to combine the resources of patients, their families and friends, and professional helpers with different professional backgrounds. The recovery model, with its emphasis on mental health promotion, subjective quality of life, self-determination of the patient, and choice, has a lot to offer in terms of the collaborative management of disorders with highly variable courses and little prognostic certainty.

England, Wales, Ireland, Scotland, Australia, New Zealand and the USA have been introducing recovery policy in mental health services, and most professional bodies concerned with mental health have endorsed recovery orientation as a key component in their work.

5.2   RECOVERY AND CLINICAL AND SCIENTIFIC RESPONSIBILITIES

'Each person's story of recovery is unique. Each person must find what works for him- or herself. This means that we must have the opportunity to try and fail and to try again. In order to support the recovery process mental health professionals must not rob us of the opportunity to fail. Professionals must embrace the concept of the dignity of risk and the right to failure if they are to be supportive of us.'

Pat Deegan [4, p. 67]

While much of recovery is lived outside clinical settings, clearly there are important responsibilities for clinicians in supporting and assisting persons with mental health problems in their efforts towards making full use of their health and resilience, and achieving their goals in life. For services and mental health workers, recovery orientation means not only fighting for a system that is able to offer all evidence-based interventions (currently only realized for a small proportion of people with severe mental illness [12]) but also accepting that what is essential for one person's recovery is not necessarily what has been proven to work in a majority of a large group of patients. Sometimes it is very specific individual approaches that are most effective.

In the long-term, patient self-determination, individual choice of flexible support and opportunities, interventions to promote empowerment, and hope, are also new indicators of quality of services, as is assistance in situations of calculated risk. Moving beyond a deficit model of mental illness to include a focus on health promotion, individual strengths and resilience, a shift from demoralizing prognostic scepticism towards a rational, optimistic attitude towards recovery, and broadening treatment goals beyond symptom reduction and stabilization, needs specific skills and new forms of co-operations between clinicians and patients, between mental health workers of different backgrounds, and between psychiatry and the public. New rules for services (e.g. user involvement and person-centred care) and new tools for clinical collaborations (e.g. shared decision making and psychiatric advance directives) are being complemented by new proposals regarding more ethically consistent anti-discrimination and involuntary treatment legislation, as well as participatory approaches to evidence-based medicine and policy [13].

Marianne Farkas and William Anthony from Boston University's Center for Psychiatric Rehabilitation are among those established professionals who have endorsed the recovery concept from its beginnings. In the era of evidence-based psychiatry, they have been pioneers in defining a recovery orientation for services in this context.

In several publications and as part of state and federal advisory committees, Anthony and Farkas have applied their scientific backgrounds to develop ideas and proposals that capture the recovery concept meaningfully and promote its application in research and services. Several of their publications have been co-authored with user/survivor activists, such as Judi Chamberlin from the National Empowerment Center in Lawrence, Massachussets [14].

The authors make clear that one important implication of recovery orientation for evaluation and research is that it is not sufficient to assess the impact of one component of a particular programme, such as medications or a day treatment programme, but that the basic attitude of the programme staff, their mission statement, self-definition and values, must be captured by any research endeavour. There are some indications that these values have a greater impact than any single component of the programme or questions such as how much of a particular element can have what kind of effect. Most likely, what we are calling the recovery orientation of a service is largely contained in these basic values. Farkas *et al.* [14] refer to earlier publications in their definition and description of four key values that they see as indispensable ingredients of a recovery orientation: person orientation; person involvement; self-determination and choice; and growth potential.

5.2.1   Person Orientation

A person-centred orientation implies that the services are primarily defined according to the needs of an individual, with all of his/her strengths, talents and interests, as well as their limitations. This is in stark contrast to the focus on an individual as a 'case', along with the signs and symptoms of an illness and a diagnosis, which determine the services to be delivered. Many recovery concepts and plans place a major emphasis on the way people are being approached. Davidson and Strauss [15], Pat Deegan [4] and many others have pointed out that people are always more than just patients and that it serves them well to be seen as whole human beings. They should not merely be viewed and understood in their patient role, but rather in their many roles, along with their possibilities and limitations. Deegan underlines explicitly that professional service providers who deny such a holistic view to the people they encounter as patients, are causing them harm.

5.2.2   Person Involvement

Services are concentrating on the right to a partnership in all relationships pertaining to recovery. This includes the right of the people who are supposed to be assisted in their recovery to have input in the planning, organization and evaluation of the services they use. Rehabilitation research teaches us that people are more likely to be successful when they have been meaningfully involved in the organization and evaluation of their services. User-involvement is increasingly seen as a benchmark for quality in organization, planning and evaluation [16].

5.2.3   Self-determination and Choice

Services should place an emphasis on the rights of all persons to make individual decisions and choices in all aspects of their recovery. This includes, among other things, treatment goals and the choice of the support that should assist them in reaching those goals, as well as when and whether to make use of services. The literature has repeatedly cautioned that compliance (i.e. simply going along with interventions suggested by professionals) should not be overestimated. It may very well be that such compliance might weaken a person who finds him/herself dependent on the decisions of others.

5.2.4 Growth Potential

Services should focus on the inherent potential for recovery for every person, irrespective of whether he/she is currently overwhelmed by the illness or disability, struggling with adversity or living with disadvantages. It cannot be stated too often: hope is an essential ingredient of any recovery orientation. Concentrating on the potential of every person to grow implies a dedication to sustain hope by the professional service providers as well as by the recipients. For the services, this means that they need to assess themselves according to the amount of hope and belief in possibilities that is being promulgated. It also means that the work has to be provided in such a manner that progress is being recognized.

Recovery orientation might require a fundamental change in the way services are offered and organized, and would need to be reflected in guidelines, procedures and quality assurance efforts, as well as in staffing, training, leadership and supervision.

Such a recovery-oriented form of practice might contribute to a more successful realization of already existing aims in evidence-based mental health services. On the other hand, additional goals that are more directly linked to recovery might emerge. These could include enhancing self-worth, empowerment and subjective well-being. A clear outline of the recovery orientation within a service agency would enable potential consumers and other interested parties to evaluate the service. It would also help administrators in determining their strengths and weaknesses in the area of recovery orientation. Researchers might be able to specifically investigate the implications of the recovery concept for evidence-based mental health services.

Mike Slade's [17] example of a necessary debate regarding an intervention that is known to reduce symptoms but that also fosters dependency and loss of hope, gives an indication of what kind of research is necessary if recovery outcomes are to be captured in a valid way.

He calls for the identification of the 'active ingredients' in recovery-focused mental health services, work that would include finding out not only 'what they do' but also 'how they do it'. Fidelity scales would then allow evaluation of just how successful services have been in promoting recovery. Regarding outcome measures that can capture recovery, Slade draws our attention to the fact that they would need to reflect personal preferences and that research design must make the best use of both quantitative and qualitative approaches as well as user-led approaches.

Self-determination, empowerment and hope are crucial elements of recovery processes, as is knowing about your own strengths and reserve capacities, and the opportunities of using and developing resilience:

> 'Being diagnosed with mental illness/distress does not preclude someone from the ability to build resilience. Identifying too fully with mental illness and its implicit limitations may prevent someone developing their personal meaning and responses to negative emotions and experiences.' [18]

5.3 RESILIENCE

The term 'resilience' originally stems from engineering, with the following meanings: impact-strength, resistance, stability or durability of a material vis-à-vis the forces of weight, physical assault, pressure, friction, centrifugal power and other potentially disturbing or destructive forces [19]. 'Resilience' also means elasticity, malleability, tension, bounce, flexibility and pliancy ('bending rather than breaking') – all terms used in technical areas.

In clinical psychology and psychotherapy, the term 'resilience' has been used increasingly in recent years. Here, it implies the power to resist; mental and emotional elasticity; and regaining one's former mental stability following a stressful period or event.

According to various researchers in this field, resilience is understood as:

- an interactive concept that refers to a relative resistance to environmental risk experiences, or the overcoming of stress or adversity; as such, it differs from both social competence or positive mental health [20];
- elastic capability for resistance [21];
- motivational power [22];
- the process by which children, adolescents and adults resist challenges and are able to bounce back or recover from those stressful conditions [23];
- a couple of phenomena characterized by positive results despite severe threat to mental adaptation or development [24];
- the capability to become stronger and equipped with even greater resources after most adverse life conditions than would have been the case without those difficult conditions [25].

It has been emphasized that resilience is not a matter of an individual directing rigid forces against noxious influences from outside, but rather a flexible and dynamic energy developed adequately in specific situations; in other words, a bio-psycho-social competency [26].

According to the German resilience researcher Lösel [27], psychic resilience can be understood as analogous to biological processes, such as processes of protection (e.g. the immune system), processes of repair (e.g. the healing of wounds), and processes of regeneration (e.g. sleep).

5.3.1 The Concept of Resilience and Its Research

Since the 1980s, the conceptual development and empirical understanding of resilience has occurred primarily within the fields of developmental psychology, psychopathology and pedagogy. Prominent researchers are Sir Michael Rutter [28] in England, Emmy Werner [29] and Norman Garmezy [30] in the USA, and Friedrich Lösel [31] and Günther Opp, Michael Fingerle and Andreas Freytag [32] in Germany, to name just a few.

There are many stories of people who have succeeded in functioning well socially in spite of being challenged by the symptoms of a physical or mental condition, or who have bounced back after a period of extreme stress. The study of resilience involves a scientific analysis of such biographical accounts. This implies an attempt to understand the biographies of such individuals and retrace how they were able to overcome their difficulties and live productive, fulfilled lives. Learning from these experiences and applying this knowledge to an improvement of prevention and treatment programs, is an essential goal of such efforts [23].

According to Edith Henderson Grotberg [33, p.3], resilience means:

'...the personal and community qualities that enable us to rebound from adversity, trauma, tragedy, threats, or other stresses – and to go on with life with a sense of mastery, competence, and hope. We now understand from research that resilience is fostered by a positive childhood and includes positive individual traits, such as optimism, good problem-solving skills and treatments. Closely-knit communities and neighbourhoods are also resilient, providing support for their members.'

The psychology and psychiatry of childhood [24, 32] have recognized specific factors that contribute to protection and resilience in situations where a developing individual is facing massive mental, physical and psychosocial stressors. These factors include:

- positive self-esteem (self-efficacy);
- positive social behaviour and active coping;
- an intact home;
- positive relationships to other competent and caring adults;
- good intellectual capabilities;
- attractiveness;
- conviction of the meaningfulness of life and belief/spirituality;
- good education;
- socio-economic advantages.

Rutter [20, p.10] suggests three broad research implications that derive from resilience findings:

1. Because resilience is not a general quality that represents a particular trait of the individual, research needs to focus on the processes underlying individual differences in responding to environmental hazards, rather than resilience as an abstract entity.
2. Because resilience in relation to adverse childhood experiences may stem from positive adult experiences, it is necessary to adopt a lifespan trajectory approach that can investigate later turning-point effects.
3. Because of the importance of gene-environment interaction, it will be necessary to combine psychosocial and biological research approaches and to use a diverse range of research strategies. These should include functional imaging of cognitive processing, neuroendocrine studies, investigation of mental sets and models, and the use of animal studies of various kinds.

5.3.2 Implications for Practice

For resilience researchers, resilience is not a trait that people either have or do not have. Some people are able to use and benefit actively from their existing capacities; others may need support to increase their resilience.

In the field of *pedagogics*, the early strengthening of the child's self-esteem and ability to cope is of utmost relevance for resilience development. For example, the American Psychological Association (APA) aims for specially trained experts to educate children to cope with the unavoidable adversities of life. They train children in resilience behaviour by supporting them to cope constructively with daily stress situations and not to capitulate to severe problems such as neglect, the divorce of parents or violence [34].

Research results on resilience show important implications for *early prevention*. The foundations of resilience can be laid very early in human development if there is a secure attachment relationship between the infant and the primary attachment figure. The early promotion of a secure attachment implies a successful affect regulation and expansion of coping abilities, which guarantees the mental health of the infant [35].

Clear implications can be found for *psychotherapeutic and psychiatric treatment*. Resilience is not a static, given entity, but the result of active adaptation and coping processes that are often painful and difficult and may change the life of an individual more or less significantly. Empathic support and company from the clinician during these subtle and complex processes are indicated.

As the resilience researcher Ann Masten [24] has clearly pointed out, resilience is not the result of magic powers and extraordinary capabilities that are restricted only to a few people; it is rooted in the minds, brains and bodies of individuals, their families and the communities in which they live. This means that clinical interventions can be directed to these areas. Resilience can be developed, restored and learned, if the individual in adverse situations is supported to activate the necessary protective factors. These protective factors may be found:

- within the person (e.g. hope);
- in the social or treatment context (e.g. peers, sensible professionals trained in knowledge on resilience and recovery);
- in the macro-social context (e.g. outpatient and inpatient facilities whose staff members are oriented not exclusively to psychopathology but also to the promotion of mental health).

Finally, resilience provides an antidote against stigmatization. Many stigmatized persons with a mental illness gain strength from the experience, and learn valuable lessons for their lives, thus developing resilience when confronted with the negative consequences of a mental illness [36, 37, 38, 39].

5.3.3   Implications for Diagnostic Assessment

It would be seductive to assess resilience from a single observable trait, by using a questionnaire or interview method. This would be a misleading approach, however, since resilience is not a single quality, as has been pointed out by Rutter [20]. Information about the context is crucial; people may be resilient in some environmental risk situations but not in others, and at one period in their life but not at others.

The challenge of assessing resilient persons, therefore, is much more complex. It seems to be useful to assess the interaction of various risk factors, the differences in individual levels of vulnerability to adverse influences, and the coping capacity of a person for certain experiences. Of high significance is the assessment of experiences in the person's biography (e.g. positive turning points in adult life, despite traumatic or other stressful factors in early childhood) and of specific patterns of social interaction within and outside the person's family. The diagnostician should pay attention to the existence of resilience in some areas and its non-existence in others. A risk is implied in being too fascinated of and overestimate a person's resilience visible in one special area and this way in overlooking the person's specific needs for help and support.

5.4   CONCLUSIONS

Recovery concepts have travelled rapidly from marginal movements to mainstream psychiatry in recent years. Recovery advocacy has been joined by recovery research, resulting in new information on the long-term perspectives of people experiencing severe mental health problems. Emerging data on recovery outcomes, as well as processes, are bringing about a paradigm shift from prognostic scepticism and a focus on maintenance therapies, towards an optimistic outlook and recovery-oriented interventions and services. The dynamic complexities of recovery and resilience have the ability to take biological, psychological, social and political developments in the direction of modern integrated and subject-oriented psychiatry. The WPA Institutional Program on Psychiatry for the Person (IPPP) has set out to affirm the whole person of the patient in context, as the centre and goal of clinical care and health promotion, and at both individual and community levels [40].

In the United States, a vision of resilience and recovery orientation in mental health has been ambitiously formulated in the Executive Summary of the President's New Freedom Commission on Mental Health [41, p.1], which reads as follows:

'We envision a future when everyone with a mental illness will recover, a future when mental illnesses can be prevented or cured, a future when mental illnesses are detected early, and a future when everyone with a mental illness at any stage of life has access to effective treatment and supports – essentials for living, working, learning, and participating fully in the community.'

REFERENCES

[1] Amering M, Schmolke M. *Recovery. Das Ende der Unheilbarkeit*. Bonn: Psychiatrie-Verlag; 2007.
[2] Andreasen NC, Carpenter WT, Kane JM, Lasser RA, Marder SR, Weinberger DR. Remission in schizophrenia: proposed criteria and rationale for consensus. *American Journal of Psychiatry* 2005;162: pp. 441–449.
[3] van Os J, Burns T, Cavallaro R, Leucht S, Peuskens J, Helldin L, Bernardo M, Arango C, Fleischhacker W, Lachaux B, Kane JM. (2006) Standardized remission criteria in schizophrenia. *Acta Psychiatrica Scandinavica* 2006;113: pp. 91–95.
[4] Deegan P. Recovery as a journey of the heart. In: Davidson L, Harding C, L Spaniol. (eds.) *Recovery from severe mental illnesses: research evidence and implications for practice* Vol 1. Boston: Center for Psychiatric Rehabilitation, Trustees of Boston University; 2005. pp. 57–68.
[5] Schrank B, Slade M. Recovery in Psychiatry. *Psychiatric Bulletin* 2007;31: pp. 321–325.
[6] Davidson L, Lawless MS, Leary F. Concepts of recovery: competing or complementary? *Current Opinion in Psychiatry* 2005;18: pp. 664–667.
[7] Schrank B, Amering M. Recovery in der Psychiatrie. (Recovery in Psychiatry) *Neuropsychiatrie* 2007;21: pp. 45–50.
[8] Copeland ME. www.mentalhealthrecovery.com [Accessed 10 january 2008].

 [9] Knuf A. Vom demoralisierenden Pessimismus zum vernünftigen Optimismus. Eine Annäherung an das Recovery-Konzept. *Soziale Psychiatrie* 2004;1: pp. 38–41.
[10] Davidson L, White W. The concept of recovery as an organizing principle for integrating mental health and addiction services. *Journal of Behavioral Health Services & Research* 2007; 34: pp. 109–120.
[11] Lester H, Gask L. Delivering medical care for patients with serious mental illness or promoting a collaborative model of recovery? *British Journal of Psychiatry* 2006;188: pp. 401–402.
[12] Anthony W, Rogers ES, Farkas M. Research on evidence-based practices: future directions in an era of recovery. *Community Mental Health Journal* 2003;39: pp. 101–114.
[13] Rose D, Thornicroft G, Slade M. Who decides what evidence is? Developing a multiple perspectives paradigm in mental health. *Acta Psychiatrica Scandinavica* 2006;113(Suppl 429): pp. 109–114.
[14] Farkas M, Gagne C, Anthony W, Chamberlin J. Implementing recovery oriented evidence based programs: identifying the critical dimensions. *Community Mental Health Journal* 2005;41: pp. 141–158.
[15] Davidson L, Strauss JS. Sense of self in recovery from severe mental illness. *British Journal of Medical Psychology* 1992;65: pp. 131–145.
[16] Wallcraft J, Schrank B, Amering M. (in press) Handbook of Service User Involvement in Mental Health Research.Wiley-Blackwell, London.
[17] Slade M. Recovery, psychosis and psychiatry: research is better than rhetoric. *Acta Psychiatrica Scandinavica* 2007;116: pp. 81–83.
[18] Glover H. (2003) www.mentalhealth.org.uk [Accessed 24 August 2006].
[19] Fengler J. Resilienz und Salutogenese – Wie wir den Helferberuf ertragen, gestalten und genießen können. In: Gunkel S, Kruse G. (eds.) *Salutogenese und Resilienz – Gesundheitsförderung, nicht nur, aber auch durch Psychotherapie?* Hanover: Hannoversche ärzte-Verlags-Union; 2004. pp. 349–368.
[20] Rutter M. Implications of resilience concepts for scientific understanding. *Annals of the New York Academy of Sciences* 2006;1094: pp. 1–12.
[21] Bender D, Lösel F. Protektive Faktoren der psychisch gesunden Entwicklung junger Menschen: Ein Beitrag zur Kontroverse um saluto- und pathogenetische Ansätze. In: Margraf J, Siegrist J, Neumer S. (eds.) *Gesundheits – oder Krankheitstheorie? Saluto- versus pathogenetische Ansätze im Gesundheitswesen*. Berlin: Springer; 1998. pp. 145–177.
[22] Richardson G. Mental health promotion through resilience and resiliency education. *International Journal of Emergency Mental Health* 2002;4 (1): pp. 65–76.
[23] Coatsworth JD, Duncan L. *Fostering Resilience. A Strenghts-Based Approach to Mental Health. A CASSP discussion paper*. Harrisburgh, PA: Pennsylvania CASSP Training and Technical Assistance Institute; 2003.
[24] Masten AS. (2001) Ordinary magic: Resilience processes in development. *American Psychologist* 2001;56: pp. 227–238.
[25] Walsh F. *Strengthening Family Resilience*. New York: Guilford Press; 1998.
[26] Gunkel S, Kruse G. Salutogenese und Resilienz – Gesundheitsförderung, nicht nur, aber auch durch Psychotherapie? In: Gunkel S, Kruse G. (eds.) *Salutogenese, Resilienz und Psychotherapie. Was hält gesund? Was bewirkt Heilung?* Hanover: Hannoversche ärzte-Verlags-Union; 2004. pp. 5–68.
[27] Lösel F. Resilienz in Kindes- und Jugendalter. *Paper at Internationaler Kongress zum Thema 'Resilienz – Gedeihen trotz widriger Umstände', Ausbildungsinstitut für systemische Therapie und Beratung*. Zürich, 9–12 February 2005.
[28] Rutter M. Resilience in the face of adversity. Protective factors and resistance to psychiatric disorder. *British Journal of Psychiatry* 1985;147: pp. 598–611.
[29] Werner EE. Risk, resilience and recovery: Perspectives from the Kauai longitudinal study. *Development and Psychopathology*, 1993;5: pp. 503–515.
[30] Garmezy N. Resiliency and vulnerability to adverse developmental outcomes associated with poverty. *American Behavioral Scientist*, 1991;34: pp. 416–430.
[31] Lösel F. Resilience in childhood and adolescence. *Children Worldwide* 1994;21: pp. 8–11.
[32] Opp G, Fingerle M, Freytag A. (eds.) *Was Kinder stärkt. Erziehung zwischen Risiko und Resilienz*. Munich: Ernst Reinhardt; 1999.

[33] Grotberg Henderson E. *Implications of the Shift from Diagnosis and Treatment to Recovery and Resilience for Research and Practice.* Washington DC: Georgetown University; 2006.

[34] Murray B. Rebounding from losses. *APA Monitor on Psychology* 2003;34(11): pp. 1–4. [Online]. Available from: www.apa.org/monitor/dec03/ [Accessed 21 November 2008].

[35] Schore A. Effects of a secure attachment relationship on right brain development, affect regulation, and infant mental health. *Infant Mental Health Journal* 2001;22(1-2): pp. 7–66.

[36] Shih M. Positive stigma: Examining resilience and empowerment in overcoming stigma. *Annals AAPSS* 2004;591: pp. 175–185.

[37] Linley PA, Joseph S. Positive change following trauma and adversity: A review. *Journal of Traumatic Stress* 2004;17(1): pp. 11–21.

[38] Joseph S, Linley PA. Growth following adversity: Theoretical perspectives and implications for clinical practice. *Clinical Psychology Review* 2006;26(8): pp. 1041–1053.

[39] Calhoun LG, Tedeschi RG. *Facilitating Post-traumatic Growth: A Clinician's Guide.* London: Erlbaum; 1999.

[40] Mezzich JE. Psychiatry for the Person: articulating medicine's science and humanism. *World Psychiatry* 2007;6 (2): pp. 1–3.

[41] U.S. Presidential Commission on Mental Health. Achieving the Promise: Transforming Mental Health Care in America. Final Report. DHHS Pub N: SMA-03-3832. Rockville, Maryland: Department of Health and Human Services; 2003. Available from: www. MentalHealthCommission.gov [Accessed 21 November 2008].

[42] Amering M, Schmolke M (in press) Recovery in Mental Health. Reshaping Scientific and Clinical Responsiblities. Wiley-Blackwell, London.

CHAPTER 6

Positive Health and Health Promotion: The WPA Institutional Programme of Psychiatry for the Person in a European Public Health Perspective

Wolfgang Rutz

Professor, University Hospital, Uppsala, Sweden; University for Applied Sciences, Coburg, Germany

Motto: 'I am I and my circumstances' (Ortega y Gasset)

6.1   INTRODUCTION

Today, there are still aspects of and problems relating to public mental health that are hardly recognized in health care policies, both in Europe and elsewhere in the world. There are a number of causes of this: the fragmentation of health care services; a lack of human rights from the perspective of mental health and populations who are vulnerable in terms of mental health; and ignorance about the essential importance of mental health to the public health of societies. This ignorance is triggered and maintained by stigmatisation, taboos and defense mechanisms, in the political layers of society as well as the whole population. A further reason for the lack of recognition and awareness of public mental health issues is that there is a focus on individual treatment and disorder, which, in situations where there is economic scarcity, is often a substitute for efforts that should be urgently directed at health care systems and health care factors on the basis of the population [1].

Consequently, in most countries, a big gap can be seen between the efforts that should and could be done (due to the real mental health problems in the country, and evidence-based

Psychiatric Diagnosis: Challenges and Prospects   Edited by I.M. Salloum and J.E. Mezzich
© 2009 John Wiley & Sons, Ltd

professional knowledge) and what is *actually* done. This gap is reflected by the fact that the care costs related to mental ill health often exceed 50% of the total health care expenditure in a society, whereas the budget for care related to mental health often is less than 10% [2].

Consequently, since the turn of the century, the United Nations and the World Health Organization have increasingly focused on the need for awareness of and investment in mental health issues. Thus, in the aftermath of the United Nations Year of Mental Health 2001 and the World Health Report 2001, the World Health Organization collected worldwide evidence on determinants of health and mental health. This evidence, presented in the World Health Report 2001 [1], the European WHO Report on Mental Health 2001 [3] and the WHO/EURO Publications 'The Solid Facts' [5] and 'Health for All 2000' [4], can be allocated to four areas:

1. A **sense of cohesion** is needed by human beings to keep healthy and to avoid dysfunction and disorder, both physically and mentally. This is described as access to a feeling of destiny and spirituality – a sense of being involved in an over-individual context of meaningfulness.
2. An experience of being **in control**, to be in charge in one's own life, the feeling of mastery and not feeling helpless.
3. A sense of **social significance** – to care and to be cared for.
4. A feeling of **caseness**, **ipseity** or **person-ness** – to be an individual, 'a person' in one's own right. This includes feelings of identity, status and dignity, and plays a major role in the onset of mental ill health in men. Results show that males are especially sensitive to violations of integrity, identity and social hierarchical status, whereas women are often more sensitive to the loss of social significance, to be needed, and the ability and opportunity to care for others [5, 6, 7].

In clients' histories of morbidity and disorder, these factors have to be viewed and assessed against the background of an individual, 'personal', biological and genetic vulnerability. Knowledge about them has been disseminated in different publications, meetings and worldwide conferences held by the WHO and other international organizations, focusing on public mental health, primary prevention, health promotion, salutogenesis and resilience.

A further message was that the United Nations and the World Health Organization not only considered access to health and treatment to be a human right, but considered access to the above described determinants of health and mental health to be a human right as well – a really political message [8].

6.2   CONSEQUENCES OF STRESS AND SOCIETAL TRANSITION

In the years during which there was heavy and traumatic societal transition, especially in those eastern European countries where there was dramatic political turmoil, stress factors linked to individual as well as population stress led to loss of identity and status, loss of existential meaning, loss of family cohesion and other societal cohesion, helplessness, loss of human rights, social exclusion, social detachment and increasing gaps. All of these losses resulted in dramatic socio-economic inequalities. They dramatically afflicted the mental health and public health of whole populations and, in some countries, led to mortality crises due to stress-related deaths that, politically, were declared to be national emergencies.

During the 1990s, life expectancy in some of these countries decreased by 10 to 15 years, violent youth criminality increased by 300% and there was a three- to fivefold increase in cardiovascular deaths, deaths by external causes including suicide, traffic accidents and family violence, hypertonia-related cerebral mortality and even deaths related to alcohol intoxication. These increases were even more pronounced for only the males in the population.

Most dramatically, homicides of adults and even infants increased eightfold during the 1990s, from a level that at the beginning of the decade was close to the European Union average and that stayed quite unchanged in the EU during this period.

Thus, we can identify a societal stress-related 'community syndrome' that consists of suicide, aggression, violence, addiction, dangerous behaviour and dangerous lifestyles, as well as stress-related vascular morbidity and mortality. This can be found in populations at risk and in transition, such as Inuits in Greenland, Indians in Canada, farmers in Ireland and youngsters in Scandinavia; but also in whole societies in eastern Europe. It leads to mortality crises, depopulation and stress-related societal 'moral insanity', increases dramatically in times of societal stress and turnover, and most heavily afflicts the males in the population.

The good news is that this stress-related mortality and morbidity is reversible. If hope, identity, predictability, dignity and social cohesion return to the society (as was the case in the Baltic states at the end of the 1990s, when the process of moving towards the European Union stabilized and continued), mortality figures decrease again and the societal levels of violence, addiction and destructivity are diminished. Even in Russia, the stress-related community syndrome became less dramatic again in the first years of this century [9].

The described societal syndrome of stress-related morbidity and mortality increases dramatically and seismically when stress levels in a society are increasing; and decreases again when positive societal and salutogenic factors return to the population. The syndrome consists of depression, suicide, aggression and violence, risk-taking and self-destructive lifestyles including alcohol and other abuse, as well as morbidity and mortality related to cardiovascular and cerebrovascular disorder. It also includes homicide and manslaughter, and seems related to something that could be described as a syndrome of 'moral insanity' in stress-afflicted societies.

Often, the factors behind this community stress are unpredictability and insecurity; the dilution of social cohesion; the loss of existential spiritual meaning in life; economic problems related to increasing gaps between the highest and lowest incomes; and careless lifestyles and behaviour (e.g. in the workplace and when driving).

6.3 INTERNATIONAL REACTIONS

International concerns about increasing weaknesses in mental health in the affected countries generated a strong international commitment, facilitated by the World Health Organization, European Union and the United Nations Organization. The World

Health Report 2001 [1] focused on mental health and the necessity of synergistic multi-factorial, intersectorial and multiprofessional action in the field of public mental health. Several WHO ministerial conferences, ending with a conference on mental health in Helsinki 2005, focused on the facts that there was 'no health without mental health', that mental health in any society and all societal sectors should be 'everybody's business', that mental health could not be separated from public health and that physical and mental health were mutually interlinked and interactive.

In 2005, under a WHO European declaration on mental health combined with a European action plan [10], governments in Europe undertook to invest in health and mental health, and to stimulate 'mental health impact awareness' and 'mental health impact assessment' strategies in governments, amongst political and other decision makers, with the focus on the importance of mental health determinants being of equal strength to the focus on other economical influences in the societal structure.

Following the WHO initiatives on mental health between 2001 and 2005, and the European Union's green book on mental health, the World Psychiatric Association launched its Institutional Program on Psychiatry for the Person (IPPP) in 2007. This offers a basis for further scientific development and societal efforts for public mental health. It emphasizes the value, dignity and individual 'personas' of human beings, the urgency for public action in the fields of mental health and the need for partnerships and intersectorial integration in these activities. Hereby, positive and negative mental health have to be seen in a biological, social, cultural and spiritual framework; and public health and individual mental health, as well as mental and physical health, have to be seen as an indivisible, not separable and causally interlinked holistic unity [10, 11, 12].

As the above described health determinants are evidently the same for physical and mental health as they are for recovery and primary prevention and health promotion, strong action towards the promotion of population and community mental health, as well as individual mental health, presupposes an increase in the ability of individuals and societies to acquire a sense of mastery, social connectedness, meaning and spiritual cohesion in life, and to gain access to integrity, dignity, individuality and cultural identity. Here, the main focus is mental health. Directed activities have to be moved from treatment to promotion, from disorder to health and function, from pathogenesis to salutogenesis and from risk factors to protection. Furthermore, individual health responsibility and individual 'healthy choices' have to be concommitted by the political and societal responsibility of politicians, governments and decision makers, to facilitate a psychosocial environment that allows people to be able to make these individual choices, but even to make the right political choices themselves, that gain the health and mental health of populations exposed to their decisions and policies.

Here, individuals at risk must be seen as 'persons' in their 'circumstances', as well as risk populations in different societies have to be health promoted according to their individual panorama of risks but also their protective assets and strengths [13].

6.4   MENTAL HEALTH PROMOTION – EFFECTIVE AND PERSONAL

There is evidence today that mental health promotional programmes are effective, as they save lives, reduce costs and reduce the suffering of patient's relatives and friends, as well as society as a whole. Promotional programmes, however, have to be designed individually, and adapted to the population they address. Gender, age and life course factors have to be taken into consideration, and new arenas and strategies, selected 'for the person' have to be established in a cultural, age and gender specific way. Thus, there are 'windows of opportunity' to be used in perinatal family care, in schools and workplaces, and establishing programmes aimed at finding, screening and assisting aggressive, depressive and suicidal males who do not seek help (e.g. in military services, the criminal system or police forces).

Examples of such activity are to be found in somatic health promotional programmes such as the Finnish Karelia Project on cardiovascular disorders that has been evaluated and showed positive affects; or American projects aimed at depressive and suicidal men in the military forces [14, 15].

6.5 SUICIDE PREVENTION 'FOR THE PERSON' – AN EXAMPLE OF PUBLIC ACTION ON HEALTH PROMOTION

Suicide prevention is health promotion; factors that improve the health and mental health of populations and individuals create resilience and are suicide preventive at the same time. Therefore, because there are increasing suicide problems in many societies, it seems easier, more timely and more feasible today to create long-lasting awareness about and real interest in public health promotion and mental health issues in political decision makers and governments. In some societies in Europe, the situation is quite dramatic. Thus, we find some of the highest suicide figures in the world in some European countries, resulting in the insight that efforts on suicide prevention, even politically, are urgent and necessary – from the UN, the European Union and national governments. This political awareness and interest, together with the fact that everything that promotes mental health is also suicide preventive, has already facilitated the establishment of mental health promoting programmes of suicide prevention in several countries.

In some cases, these programmes have gained important national visibility, and are adapted to the needs of different risk populations (e.g. farmers in Portugal, Ireland and Lithuania, youngsters in Switzerland and France, indigenous people in Denmark, and immigrant populations and female adolescents in Scandinavia). Other programmes focus on job insecurities and role transition in rural areas or on divorced men and elderly women who have lost their social significance and cohesion.

Hereby, an empathic analysis of the personal biological, psychosocial and existential individual 'circumstances' has to be done, to assess positive and protective, as well as negative, risk factors amongst risk individuals and risk populations. The access to 'personal' public health support is hereby crucial and an individualistic, intersubjectivistic approach, in which help-seekers and helpers encounter each other as subject to subject and person to person, must be applied on both an individual and a population level. Focus could be given to identity, empowerment and dignity, unpredictability, social cohesion and the lack of existential meaning among risk groups of women, males, youngsters and the elderly, analyzing the possibilities and responsibilities of politicians and professionals to (re-)create and reassure the necessary preconditions for (re)gaining access to the determinants of mental health promotion, for individuals and populations at risk [16].

Some challenging and feasible examples are:

- the need to diagnose atypically depressive, suicidal men in time, and to help them in spite of their incapacity to ask for help and show compliance;
- assistance to young girls who are in a situation of a value migration, from the familiar, culturally traditional value systems of their home countries, to being exposed to new, often completely different and contrary value demands in their new society;
- early health promoting, protective and preventive intervention in families in a difficult psychosocial situation in the prenatal and postnatal phase around the delivery of a newborn child.

6.6   OBSTACLES

Obstacles to these strategies can be found in the stigma around mental health issues that is still found in many populations, leading to a disturbing gap between professional knowledge and real political implementation. Other impediments consist of adverse and ignorant public opinions about mental issues, often triggered by irresponsible mass media activities. Furthermore, an evidence conceptualization focusing mainly on quantitative evidence, based on statistical and preferably randomized controlled trials as the golden standard, is often used by politicians and other decision makers as an excuse for a lack of action and the insufficient allocation of resources, and thus becomes a hindrance to implementing well-known and well-researched qualitative evidence.

Bearing in mind that suicide prevention, health and mental health promotion, the knowledge of users and families as well as their participation in care, prevention and promotion strongly demand the acceptance and implementation of qualitative evidence approaches, and that many of the greatest progresses in medicine and health care are based on qualitative research, our conceptualization of evidence should be widened and redefined to give stronger importance to the inclusion of qualitative methodology on an equal basis. Only then can individual, subjectivistic and person-centred public health strategies based on 'health promotion for the person' be facilitated in order to meet today's societal demands in areas of positive and negative health in a modern and timely way.

6.7   A STRATEGIC OUTLOOK

Strategies to realize person-centred public mental health promotion include the assessment of risks and assets on a population and society level, with the engagement of the whole society. Even sectors outside the structures of the health care sector should be included, in an approach that engages all stakeholders in the public mental health mental field in a country. That means that families, networks, non-political and non-governmental idealistic organizations, professionals, civil servants and the private and public sectors, as well as political and other decision makers, have to be involved. Efforts are needed that can be compared with the physical environmental ecological movement that has gained strength during the last decade. In this case, however, they should be directed at the human – and mental – ecological aspects of health, well-being and the survival of the human species.

Actions are to be taken that involve public and political policies, legislation, public services and the employment sector, as well as decision makers responsible for internal and health security. An apparent risk exists today, that measures are taken in the name of public safety and health protection that reinforce non democratic societal structures and dynamics, profoundly counteracting human basic needs of autonomy, integrity, social cohesion and existential self-directedness.

Moreover, awareness raising activities include the establishment of professional curricula in the fields of community mental health and public mental health promotion, as well as the sensitization and education of decision makers and administrators in public services, the private sector and on all political levels. Public mental health activities should be integrated in all types of environment and health programmes. Public investment has to be made in the mental health of the population, as one of society's most valuable types of capital. Awareness of the impact of political decisions and policy changes on the mental health of citizens has to be disseminated, and mental health has to be recognized and respected as both a human right and a democratic essential in society.

6.7 CONCLUSION

To invest in public mental health and to stimulate countrywide societal activities on public mental health promotion, adapted to the needs of both individual risk persons and aggregated risk populations, in a integrated, synoptic and holistic view, is today inevitable and essential in order to re-humanize both psychiatry and society. Furthermore, this will increase the development and maintenance of democracy by counteracting the societal regression that leads to the scapegoating, marginalization and exclusion of the deviant, societal splits, black and white thinking and regressive demands for simple solutions, strong leaders and totalitarian fundamentalism. A bio-psycho-societal and spiritual approach will hereby be the basis of a new, holistic, human, ecological movement, applying existing evidence about basic human conditions and directed at human ecological public health strategies 'for the person'.

Two quotations illustrate the timelessness, timeliness and urgency of an human ecological and person-directed public mental health approach: 'Medical science is a social science and politics are nothing else than medical science applied in the greater context' (Rudolf Virchow, 1848) [17] and 'The societies we have created generate mental ill health . . . and . . . mental ill health is Europe's unseen killer' (Kyprianou, European Commissioner for Health, 2005) [18].

Knowing what we know today about the human condition, and considering new (neuro)psychiatric as well as sociologic and anthropological evidence about the basic and essential position of mental and public health for survival and health, professions and politicians in the mental health sector cannot abdicate any longer from their societal responsibility to actively and politically engage as both advisors and actors in the establishment of effective structures of mental health and public mental health promotion. Climatic changes are not the only environmental threat to which, globally, humans and mankind are exposed today.

REFERENCES

[1] World Health Organization. *The World Health Report 2001. Mental Health: New Understanding, New Hope*. Geneva: WHO; 2001.
[2] World Health Organization. *Mental Health Atlas*. Geneva: WHO; 2005.

[3] WHO Regional Office for Europe: European Report on Mental Health. Copenhagen; 2001.

[4] World Health Organisation: WHO Office for Europe. "Health for All in the Year 2000". Copenhagen; 1998.

[5] Wilkinson R, Marmot M. (eds.) *Social Determinants of Health – the Solid Facts*. Copenhagen: WHO Regional Office for Europe; 1998.

[6] Cloninger CR. *Feeling Good. The Science of Well Being*. New York: Oxford University Press; 2004.

[7] Rutz W. A need to rethink social psychiatry in Europe. *The Lancet* 2004;363.

[8] World Health Organization. *Resource Book on Mental Health, Human Rights and Legislation*. Geneva: WHO; 2006.

[9] Rutz W. Mental Health in Europe: Problems, advances, challenges. *Acta Psychiatrica Scandinavica* 2001;419(Suppl): pp. 15–20.

[10] World Health Organization. *Conference Declaration and Action Plan. Helsinki Ministerial Conference on Mental Health*. Copenhagen: WHO Regional Office for Europe; 2005.

[11] European Commission. *EU – Green Book on European Mental Health*. Luxembourg: EU; 2006.

[12] Mezzich J, Salloum I. Clinical Complexity and person-centered integrative diagnosis. *World Psychiatry* 2008;7 (1): pp. 1–2.

[13] Amering M, Mezzich JE, Rutz W. Psychiatry for the Person and Public Health. Submitted, 2008.

[14] Puska P, Tuomilehto J, Nissinen A *et al. The North Karelia Project*. In: World Health Organization. *Successful prevention of non-communicable diseases*. Copenhagen: WHO Office for Europe; 1988.

[15] Knox KL, Litts DA, Talcott GW *et al.* Risk of suicide and related adverse outcomes after exposure to a suicide prevention programme in the United States Air Force: a cohort study. *British Medical Journal* 2003;327 pp. 1376–1380.

[16] Rutz W. Psychiatry for the Person - a person centered approach of suicide prevention. Summary, European Psychiatry, AEP, Nice 2008.

[17] Rudolf Virchow. "Die öffentliche Gesundheitspflege". In: *Die Medizinische Reform*, Berlin 1848.

[18] EU Health Directorate. Kyprianou, K: Introductory speech. Introducing the "European Unions Green Paper on Mental Health". Luxemborg, 2005.

PSYCHOPATHOLOGY

CHAPTER 7

Dementia

Olusegun Baiyewu

Professor of Psychiatry, College of Medicine, University of Ibadan, Nigeria

7.1 INTRODUCTION

Dementia is a chronic brain disease characterized by cognitive decline, functional impairment and behaviour symptoms. Berrios [1] observed that various terminologies related to dementia had been used in European languages for many centuries. Such descriptions include 'without mind', 'madness' and 'extravagance'. However, modern definitions are those used in the Diagnostic and Statistical Manual 4th Edition (DSM-IV) [2] and the International Classification of Diseases 10th Revision (ICD-10) [3] classificatory systems.

Dementia is a disease of old age, which has important public health impact. An important concern is the cost of care for the family of the patient with dementia, as well as for each nation [4].

7.2 EPIDEMIOLOGY

Studies from communities, hospital settings and nursing homes have given various prevalence and incidence rates of dementia. Alzheimer's disease is the most common type of dementia. Depending on the methodology, various estimates in Europe and North America put the prevalence rate of dementia at between 5% and 10% [5].

The prevalence rate increases with age, and rates double every 5.1 years [6]. The incidence of dementia also increases exponentially with age, doubling every five years [7].

Dementia and Alzheimer's disease have been reported to have lower prevalence and incident rates in some developing societies [8, 9].

In a comparative study of African Americans in Indianapolis and Nigerians in Ibadan, Nigerians had lower rates; environmental factors were thought to be responsible for the differences [8]. The importance of the environment was demonstrate in a Swedish twin study which estimates the environmental influence, potentially modifiable, to be 20–35% [10] in Alzheimer's disease.

Psychiatric Diagnosis: Challenges and Prospects   Edited by I.M. Salloum and J.E. Mezzich
© 2009 John Wiley & Sons, Ltd

Apolipoprotein E (APOE) polymorphism, a genetic factor, accounts for 40% of population attributable risk factors [11].

Alzheimer's disease (AD) constitutes about 60% of all dementias, followed by vascular dementia (VaD) (20%), dementia with Lewy bodies (DLB) (16%), with fronto-temporal dementia (FTD) and other dementias accounting for the rest.

Various studies indicate that dementia is more common in females than males, probably because women live longer. In these studies, AD has received a proportionally higher degree of attention and it is only recently that criteria for diagnosis of other subtypes have become operationalized.

One area of controversy is in the estimates of dementia in different populations using screening instruments developed originally for middle class Euro-American families. Some have suggested that these instruments are not valid for all cultures, largely because of education bias. The most frequently used screening test is the Mini Mental State Examination (MMSE) [12]. Many studies have observed that this instrument has a floor and ceiling effect due to education, and this has led to the use of modified MMSE in different cultures, as seen in the Hindi version [13]. As a result of this phenomenon, studies have been carried out to generate normative data that specifically takes care of age, ethnicity and education, not only for MMSE but for other neuropsychological tests as well [14, 15]. A more comprehensive screening interview is the Community Screening Interview for Dementia (CSI-D) [16]. The CSI-D was designed for screening for dementia in desperate populations. It incorporates items from many questionnaires already in use in dementia research, but has little education effect and has been used in many surveys on dementia in many countries and cultures [17].

7.3 DIAGNOSIS OF DEMENTIA

A great deal of controversy has been generated over the adequacy of the DSM and ICD diagnostic criteria. This was highlighted in a recent review by Reisberg and Sartorious [18] looking at DSM-IV-TR [19] and ICD-10. The following observations were made:

1. ICD-10 uses the term 'organic', indicating that there is also 'non-organic'. This terminology has been jettisoned in DSM-IV.
2. The DSM-IV definition of dementia does not specify that it is an acquired condition, thus not distinguishing it from mental sub-normalities that start early in life.
3. Memory impairment is not always present early in some forms of dementias, such as vascular dementia and fronto-temporal dementia.
4. Dichotomies of early onset/late onset AD in both ICD-10 and DSM-IV are not supported by current scientific evidence.
5. Symptoms like aphasia, agnosia and apraxia are often more associated with stroke and head injury. In AD, for example, they do not show till late in the course of the illness.

Of equal importance is the work of Erkinjuntti *et al.* [20] who reclassified subjects who had consensus diagnosis in the database of the Canadian Study on Health and Aging [21], using DSM-III-R [22]), DSM-IV, ICD-10 and the Cambridge Examination for Mental Disorders in the Elderly (CAMIDEX) [23] and found a lot of discrepancies. This raises the issue of reliability of diagnosis across research projects, and criticisms have followed this important finding relating to the validity of the two most important diagnostic systems for dementia.

A number of consensus statements have been developed for diagnosis in subtypes of dementia: for AD, the National Institute for Neurological and Communicative Disorders and Stroke – Alzheimer's Disease and Related Disorders Association (NINCDS-ADRDA) [24]; for dementia with Lewy bodies [25]; and for fronto-temporal dementia [26].

There are five diagnostic criteria in use for vascular dementia (VaD):

1. National Institute of Neurological Disorders and Stroke and Association Internationale pour la Recherche et l'Enseignement en Neurosciences (NINDS-AIREN criteria [27];
2. ICD-10;
3. The California AD Diagnosis and Treatment Center Criteria (ADDTC) (California Criteria) [28];
4. Modified Hachinsk Ischemic Score (HIS) [29];
5. DSM-IV criteria.

These criteria for VaD have low sensitivities and moderately high specificities. Part of the explanation is that there are mixed pathologies in the clinical diagnosed VaD, as many of them have neuritic plaques and neurofibrillary tangles characteristic of AD, and diagnosis of mixed dementia may be entertained. There could be large or small infarcts in various regions of white or grey matter, leading to the phenomenon of multi-infarct dementia. At the other end of the spectrum, there may be leukoaraiosis characterized by white matter hypertensities on MRI. These do not represent frank infarcts but associated cerebrovascular pathology [30]. Distinguishing between AD and DLB may also present some difficulties because of mixed pathology. These criteria, according to the opinion of their authors, need constant review.

7.4 PATHOLOGY

The gold standard for diagnosis in dementia is neuropathological findings at autopsy. Reports indicating agreement in the region of 80% for AD are in literature, but such reports are from a biased selection of patients who had undergone repeated evaluation during their lifetime and had reached a severe stage of the illness; this might have little to do with normal clinical situations, especially the diagnostic difficulties experienced in the early stages of AD [31].

In a typical clinical situation, the story might be different. Of the 382 consecutive persons with dementia who had an autopsy at the State of Florida Brain Bank between 1992 and 2000, 145 (38%) had more than one central nervous system post-mortem diagnosis: among 294 with AD pathological diagnosis, 159 (54%) had pure AD; others had mixed pathology [32]. Camberwell Dementia Case Register also had 55% pure AD and 34% mixed pathologies [33].

For AD, neuritic plaques and neurofibrillary tangles are the hallmarks of diagnosis; however, these have also been found in the brains of persons without dementia. A correlation was established between the severity of plaque deposition and cognitive performance on ADL [34]. Recently, Terry [35] observed that, while plaques could be found in the neocortex and hippocampal enthorhinal region of the normal elderly, neurofibrillary tangles are extremely rare in people without dementia.

The typical distribution of plaques and tangles is in the mediotemporal limbic areas, posterior inferior temporal areas, adjoining the parieto-occipital lobes and posterior cingulated gyrus [36].

Braak and Braak [37] established clinico-pathological classification of AD based on neuritic plaques and neurofibrillary tangles. The severity of AD is divided into six stages, which have been grouped into low, intermediate and severe [38].

7.5 BIOLOGIC MAKERS

In dominantly inherited familial AD, amyloid precursor protein (APP) plays a critical role in amyloid deposition. The APP molecule is cut at a different site than usual, at position 42 instead of 40. By this method, the production of β-amyloid peptides (Aβ) increases, leading to deposition. Neuronal cell death occurs in old age but this is increased in AD by increased amyloid deposit and phosphorylated tau proteins. These lead to cell death and neuronal loss [39]. Low $A\beta_{1-42}$ has been demonstrated in CSF of sporadic AD patients and individuals with MCI [40].

CSF $A\beta_{1-42}$ differentiates AD from normal elderly controls and patients with other forms of dementia, giving specificity of 81% and 59% respectively [41]. Thus, while it could distinguish between AD and normal controls, it is not efficient in distinguishing between AD and other dementias. CSF total tau also distinguishes AD from normal controls, but its ability to distinguish AD from non-AD dementia is poor [41].

Another maker is phosphorylated tau (p-tau), which has been documented to increase in AD CSF relative to normal controls, but has been reported to discriminate between AD, FT and LBD [42, 43]. When $A\beta_{1-42}$ and p-tau are combined, sensitivity of detecting AD and specificities for excluding other dementing disorders rise to between 80% and 90% [40].

Many other biomakers have been reported in the literature, using measurements in urine, serum and platelet, but none has shown the promise seen in tau and beta amyloid.

Schipper [44] has suggested that:

1. Biologic makers should not at this stage be included in the battery of tests used by primary physicians to evaluate memory loss.
2. Even though useful for the specialist, biologic makers in isolation are not sufficient to diagnose or exclude AD but could be useful in distinguishing between AD and FTD.

7.6 NEUROIMAGING

The general uses of neuroimaging are:

1. to eliminate cases of pseudodementia, like tumours and space-occupying lesions;
2. to distinguish different subtypes of dementia (AD, FTD, vascular and DLB).

This is supported by a number of consensus statements that indicate the need for neuroimaging in the diagnosis of dementia. Two forms of neuroimaging are generally available:

1. structural imaging, consisting of computerized tomographic scan (CT Scan) and magnetic resonance imaging (MRI);
2. functional imaging, consisting of single photon emission computed tomography (SPECT) and positron emission tomography (PET) Scan.

MRI is useful in distinguishing mild AD from mild cognitive impairment (MCI). If patients with MCI are followed up longitudinally, those that will convert to AD show atrophy in the entorhinal cortex and the hippocampus [45].

On PET scans, patients with DLB show evidence of deficit in temporal, parietal, occipital and cerebella regions of the brain. Those with FTD show frontal deficit, while those with Parkinson's dementia show parietal, frontal, lateral temporal and visual cortex deficit [46]. PET has been used to correlate clinical diagnosis with post-mortem neuropathological changes in AD patients giving sensitivity of 94% and specificity of 73–78% [47].

In a review of published articles, SPECT discriminated between AD, VaD and FTD, and non-dementia control (PC). Pooled sensitivity was lowest for AD vs PC (65.7%) and highest for AD vs FTD (71.5%). Specificity was lowest for AD vs VaD (75.9%) and highest for AD vs PC (79.1%) [48].

A new approach to DBL diagnosis now uses SPECT imaging with a dopamine transporter scan. In a European multi-centre study, this method discriminated between possible DBL and AD at rates between 84% and 87% [49].

7.7 BEHAVIOUR SYMPTOMS IN DEMENTIA

There are three important aspects of clinical dementia: cognition, functioning and behaviour. While a lot of attention has been paid to cognition, both in clinical practice and in research, correspondingly less attention has been paid to behaviour. The term 'behavioural and psychological symptoms in dementia' has been used to describe behaviour in dementia [50]. Various other terminologies exist, however. These include behavioural disturbance and non-cognitive changes, among others. With the aid of factor analysis, the symptoms were broadly classified into psychosis, depression, anxiety and sleep difficulties, by researchers [51, 52]. Behavioural symptoms are found in all stages of dementia but are probably highest in the middle stage when symptoms are moderate to severe. At the terminal stages of dementia they are much reduced, probably because the patient shows more apathy and communicates less.

Assessment of behaviour in patients with dementia can be carried out through a number of rating scales, but two have widespread use in research: BEHAVE- AD [53] and the Neuropsychiatric Inventory (NPI) [54].

Most studies have concentrated on behaviour disorders in AD, but behaviour symptoms are part of other subtypes of dementia, like VaD, DLB, FTD and Parkinson's Disease Dementia.

DSM-IV has no specific criteria for the diagnosis of behaviour disorders; these are subsumed under additional coding, like 'with delusion', 'with depression', etc. The symptoms may be fleeting, however, not reaching the severity seen in schizophrenia, with disorganized speech and behaviour or equivalent symptom severity, as seen in major depressive disorder.

Sixty-one percent of AD patients assessed [55] had at least one behaviour symptom, but O'Brien *et al.* [56] reported 46% psychosis in hospitalized patients with vascular dementia. About 40–45% of patients with DLB may experience well-formed visual hallucinations [57] compared with 25% in pure AD [58]. Aberrant behaviour change is a diagnostic feature of FTD, which may include symptoms like hyperorality and hypersexuality [59].

Depression as a syndrome is also common in dementia. In AD, syndromal depression is about 15–25% and an additional 20–30% might be sub-syndromal [60].

Agitation has been reported in 20–60% of patients with AD, depending on the criteria used in various studies [61], and sleep disturbance has been found in 19–44% of patients with AD [62].

There had been attempts to devise criteria that incorporate behaviour syndromes into diagnosis in dementia. Diagnostic criteria for psychosis of AD was put forward by Jeste and Finkel [63] and that has been accepted for use by the United States Federal Drug Administration. Other criteria for depression of AD [64] and AD-associated affective disorder [52] have been published.

A number of neuroimaging, genetic and post-mortem studies have given indications that there are differences between AD patients with psychosis, depression and agitation when compared with those without these symptoms [65].

7.8 FUNCTIONING

Assessment of functioning in dementia patient is of great importance. In both ICD-10 and DSM-IV, diagnosis of dementia can only be made if there is evidence of impairment of activities of daily life (personal or instrumental) that is of such severity that it affects the daily functioning of the individual. Instrumental Activities of Daily Living (IADL) items include leisure activities, food preparation, handling medicine, transportation, finances and using the telephone. Activities of Daily Life (Personal Care) (ADL) items include dressing, eating and toileting. It has been observed that the most sensitive indicators for early dementia are for IADL items of handling medication, finances, telephone and transportation [66]. Driving by people with dementia has been of public health concern in industrialized societies [67].

When the subtypes of dementia are examined, functional impairment differs across categories. Subjects with VaD seem to have slower functional decline when compared to those with AD [68], but mixed AD/VaD patients appear to decline at the same rate as AD patients .

Various instruments are available for the assessment of functional impairment in patients with dementia, such as the Blessed Dementia Rating Scale [34] and the Disability Assessment in Dementia Scale [69].

7.9 MILD COGNITIVE IMPAIRMENT

In recent times, mild cognitive impairment (MCI) has received the attention of researchers and clinicians. It was previously conceived to be a transitional stage between normal aging and AD, but recently the concept has been broadened to include other forms of dementia

[70]. While some authors have argued that MCI is a prodromal stage of AD, in that everyone with MCI would eventually develop AD if they lived long enough [71], other workers, especially those using community based samples, have found that not all subjects with MCI convert to dementia; some revert to normal while others remain MCI [72, 73]. This possibility of reversal may affect the need for treatment, or even operationalization as a disease process. The current classification of MCI includes amnestic MCI, in which the majority of subjects would probably become AD; and non-amnestic MCI, which is believed to lead to other dementia subtypes such as FTD, DLB and VaD. In amnestic MCI, memory complaints predominate, while in nonamnestic MCI, cognitive complaints other than memory predominate. In all forms of MCI, functioning must be preserved or only mildly affected. MCI subjects should ordinarily not score more than 0.5 on Clinical Dementia Rating Scale (CDR) [74]. Indeed, the criteria for vascular cognitive impairment has been operationalized [56] while that of MCI preceding dementia with Lewy bodies has been laid out [75].

Amnestic MCI progresses to AD at a rate of 10–15% per annum [76] and it is associated with increased risk of death [77]. APOE4 carrier status and atrophic changes in hippocampal volume on magnetic resonance imaging predict rapid progression to AD [78, 79].

At present, diagnosis of MCI is by clinical criteria; neuropsychological tests will help, but, as with AD, there are no cut-off scores to determine MCI [70]. Neuropathological studies also show amnestic MCI to be midway between normal aging and AD [80].

7.10 CARE OF THE PERSON WITH DEMENTIA

Two issues are involved here: the first is the treatment of the patient with dementia, which itself consists of pharmacological and non-pharmacological treatment; the second concerns the well-being of the carer. Caregivers of people with dementia experience a heavy psychological burden, and it is important to address this along with the treatment plan for the individual with dementia. The burden of care, which is often due to the behavioural problems of dementia, influences early institutionalization and leaves the carer at the risk of developing depression and other emotional and physical disorders.

Common drugs used in the treatment of dementia consist mainly of cholinesterase inhibitors and memantine. Other treatments, like vitamins E and C, and Ginkgo biloba, which are available in many countries, have limited value [81].

Management can be divided in two:

1. the management of MCI and mild to moderate dementia;
2. the management of severe dementia.

There is controversy about the value of treating MCI, as some drug trials produced no overall benefit in patients being treated over a period of three years, even though there initially appeared to be some benefit [82]. For mild to moderate dementia, cholinesterase inhibitors are the drugs of choice. Various drug trials have consistently reported their significant benefits over a placebo in cognition and functioning, and they are useful in mild, moderate and severe AD [82, 83, 84]. Three of these – donepezil, galantamine and rivastigmine – are licensed in most countries. Both donepezil and galantamine have been found to be effective in VaD [85, 86]. Memantine, which is an uncompetitive antagonist to glutamate N-methyl-D-aspertate (NMDA) receptor, has been observed to be useful in moderate to severe AD, as well as in VaD [87]. Because they have different modes of action, a combination of cholinesterase inhibitors and memantine has been tried with beneficial effects.

Both the cholinesterase inhibitors and memantine have some positive effect on BPSD in patients with dementia; however, it is necessary at times to treat psychotic symptoms in dementia with antipsychotics. Meta-analysis of some drug trial studies showed that, while the newer atypical antipsychotics had better effects in treating behaviour symptoms, they are associated with higher risk of mortality in patients with severe dementia [88]. Based on a review of unpublished data, it has been suggested that antipsychotic drugs like resperidone, olanzepine, and qutiapine are associated with increased cardiovascular adverse events (CVAEs) [89]. This has made a number of health regulatory agencies warn of an increased risk of CVAEs and mortality in drug treated patients. However, other studies have shown that atypical antipsychotics do not show an increased risk of CVAEs and death [90, 91].

Anticonvulsants have been reported to be useful in BPSD but a recent review by Herrmann *et al.* [84] indicates a need for caution. For depressive symptoms, antidepressants, especially the serotonin-specific reuptake inhibitors (SSRIs) have been found to be effective in AD [92]. More importantly, citalopram has been reported in one study to perform better for agitation, aggression, and psychosis than a placebo [93].

Non-pharmacological modes of treatment are also available for patients with severe dementia. These include music therapy, aromatherapy, reminiscence, sensory stimulation, Snoezelen and the psychoeducation of caregivers on how to handle difficult behaviour. While some studies have reported positive benefits from some of these procedures, there have not been enough randomized clinical trials to determine their worth [84]. However, in mild to moderate AD, exercise, environmental manipulation, cognitive training, provision of vision and hearing aids, and treating comorbid illnesses are essential steps to be taken early in the management [81].

Caregivers' issues are of great importance in the treatment of dementia. Studies have shown that the physical and mental health of the caregiver could be worse than those of non-caregivers, and caregiving is associated with increased mortality [94, 95]. The burden of caregiving is related to placement in an institution [96]. Wimo *et al.* [4] have estimated the cost of care of patients with dementia for different countries, and cost increases with severity of illness. Intervention studies that include training have consistently shown a better outcome in experimental groups compared to control groups [97], and caregivers of patients treated with donepezil reported less difficulty with caregiving when compared with controls [98]. People with dementia whose spouses received psychoeducation, training and support had a better long-term outcome when compared with controls on routine treatment [99].

7.11   STUDIES FROM NON-WESTERN SOCIETIES

Most research on dementia comes from the Western nations but, in the last decade or so, a number of quality research reports have come from Africa, Latin America and Asia. Prince *et al* [17] validated the diagnosis of dementia in a multi-centre study from many sites in developing countries. Incidence rates for dementia and AD were lower in Yoruba than in African Americans [8]; similarly lower incidence rates for AD (when compared with reports from Western countries) were found in Indians [9]. More important is the fact that the most widely accepted risk factor for AD, the APOE4 allele, has been reported not to have an association with AD in Nigerians [100], or the conversion of cognitively impaired subjects to AD. The rate of conversion is also lower than seen in Western societies [101]. With BPSD, however, it would appear that presentation and clinical course are similar the world over. These studies, however, need replication in other centres of the developing world.

REFERENCES

[1] Berrios G. Dementia historical overview. In: Burns A, O'Brien J, Ames D (eds.) *Dementia*. 3rd ed. London: Hodder Arnold; 2005.

[2] American Psychiatric Association. *Diagnostic and Statistical Manual. 4th ed. (DSM-IV.)* Washington: American Psychiatric Association; 1994.

[3] World Health Organization. *International Classification of Diseases*. 10th ed. Geneva: WHO; 1992.

[4] Wimo A, Wimblad B, Jonsson L. An estimate of the total world wide societal cost of dementia in 2005. *Alzheimer's & Dementia* 2007;3: pp. 81–91,

[5] Ritchie K, Kildea D. Is senile dementia 'age-related' or 'ageing-related'? Evidence from meta-analysis of dementia prevalence in the oldest old. *Lancet* 1995;346: pp. 931–934.

[6] Hofman AA, Rocca WA, Brayne C, *et al*. The prevalence of dementia in Europe: a collaborative study of 1980-1990 findings. *International Journal of Epidemiology* 1991;20: pp. 736–748.

[7] Jorm AF, Jolley D. The incidence of dementia: a meta-analysis. *Neurology* 1998;51: pp. 728–733.

[8] Hendrie HC, Ogunniyi AO, Hall HS, *et al*. The incidence of dementia in two communities, Yoruba, residing in Ibadan, Nigeria and African Americans in Indianapolis, USA. *JAMA* 2001;285: pp. 739–747.

[9] Chandra V, Pandav R, Dodge HH, *et al*. Incidence of Alzheimer's diseases in a rural community in India: the Indo-US study. *Neurology* 2001;57: pp. 985–987.

[10] Pedersen NL, Gatz M, Berg S, Johansson B. How heritable is Alzheimer's disease late in life? Findings from Swedish twins. *Annals of Neurology* 2004;55: pp.180–185.

[11] Slooter AJ, Cruts M, Kalmijn S, *et al*. Risk estimates of dementia by apolipoprotein E genotypes from a population-based incidence study: the Rotterdam Study. *Archives of Neurology* 1998;55: pp. 964–968.

[12] Folstein MF, Folstein SE, McHugh PR. 'Mini-mental state'. A practical method for grading the cognitive state of patients for the clinician. *Journal of Psychiatric Research* 1975;12: pp. 189–95.

[13] Ganguli M, Ratcliff G, Chandra V, *et al*. A Hindi version of the MMSE: development of a cognitive screening instrument for a largely illiterate rural elderly population in India. *International Journal of Geriatric Psychiatry* 1995;10: pp. 367–377.

[14] Ivnik R, Malec J, Smith G, *et al*. Mayo's Older Americans Normative Studies: WMS-R norms for ages 56 to 97. *Clinical Neuropsychology* 1992;6 (suppl): pp. 49–82.

[15] Stricks L, Pittman J, Jacobs DM, *et al*. Normative data for a brief neuropsychological battery administered to English- and Spanish-speaking community-dwelling elders. *Journal of the International Neuropsychological Society* 1998;4: pp. 311–318.

[16] Hall KS, Gao S, Emsley CL, *et al*. Community Screening Interview for dementia (CSI-D), performance in five desperate sites. *International Journal of Geriatric Psychiatry* 2000;15: pp. 521–531.

[17] Prince M, Acosta D, Chiu H, Scazufca M, Verghese M, for the 10/66 Dementia Research Group. Dementia diagnosis in developing countries: a cross-cultural validation study. *Lancet* 2003;361: pp. 909–917.

[18] Reisberg B, Sartorius N. Diagnostic Criteria in Dementia: A Comparison of Current Criteria. *Journal of Geriatric Psychiatry and Neurology* 2006;19: pp. 137–146.

[19] American Psychiatric Association. *Diagnostic and Statistical Manual. Text Revision. (DSM-IV-TR.)* Washington: American Psychiatric Association; 2000.

[20] Erkinjuntti T, Ostbye T, Steenhuis R, *et al*. The effect of different diagnostic criteria on the prevalence of dementia. *New England Journal of Medicine* 1997;337: pp. 1667–1674.

[21] Rockwood K, Stadnyk K. The prevalence of dementia in the elderly: a review. *Canadian Journal of Psychiatry* 1994;39: pp. 253–257.

[22] American Psychiatric Association. *Diagnostic and Statistical Manual. 3rd ed. Revised. (DSM-III-R.)* Washington: American Psychiatric Association; 1987.

[23] Roth M, Tymm E, Mountjoy C, *et al*. CAMDEX: A standardized instrument for the diagnosis of mental disorder in the elderly, with special reference to the early detection of dementia. *British Journal of Psychiatry* 1986;149: pp. 698–709.

[24] McKhann G, Drachman D, Folstein M, *et al*. Clinical diagnosis of Alzheimer's disease. Report of the NINCDS ADRDA work group under the auspices of the Department of Health and Human Service Task forces on Alzheimer's disease. *Neurology* 1984;34: pp. 939–944.

[25] McKeith IG, Galasko D. Kosaka K, *et al*. Consensus guidelines for the clinical and pathologic diagnosis of dementia with Lewy bodies (DLB). *Neurology* 1996;47: pp. 1113–1124.

[26] Neary D, Snowden JS, Gustafson L, *et al*. Frontotemporal lobar degeneration: a consensus on clinical diagnostic criteria. *Neurology* 1998;51: pp.1546–1554.

[27] Roman GC, Tatemichi T, Erkinjuntti T, *et al*. Vascular dementia: diagnosis criteria for research studies. Report of NINCDS AIRENS International Workshop. *Neurology* 1993;43: pp. 250–260.

[28] Chui HC, Victoroff JI, Margolin D, *et al*. Criteria for the diagnosis of ischaemic vascular dementia proposed by the state of California Alzheimer's Disease Diagnosis and Treatment Centres. *Neurology* 1992;42: pp. 473–480.

[29] Rosen WG, Terry RD, Fuld PA, *et al*. Pathological verification of ischaemic score in the differentiation of dementias. *Annals of Neurology* 1980;7: pp. 485–488.

[30] Green RC. *Diagnosis and management of Alzheimer's Disease and the Dementias, Second Edition*. Professional Communication Inc. 2005; pp. 55–61.

[31] Forstl H. What is Alzheimer's disease. In: Burns A, O'Brien J, Ames D. (eds.) *Dementia*. 3rd ed. London: Hodder Arnold; 2005.

[32] Barker WW, Luis CA, Kashuba A *et al*. Relative frequencies of Alzheimer Disease, Lewy body, vascular and frontotemporal dementia, and hippocampal sclerosis in the state of Florida Brain Bank. *Alzheimer Dis Assoc Discord* 2002;16: pp. 203–212.

[33] Holmes C, Cairns N, Lantos P, Mann A, Validity of current clinical criteria for Alzhimer's disease, vascular dementia, and dementia with Lewy bodies. *Br. J Psychiatory* 174; 45–50.

[34] Blessed G, Tomlinson BE, Roth M. The association between qualitative measures of dementia and senile changes in the cerebral grey matter of elderly subjects. *British Journal of Psychiatry* 1968;114: pp. 797–811.

[35] Terry RD. Alzheimer's disease and the aging brain. *Journal of Geriatric Psychiatry and Neurology* 2006;19: pp. 125–128.

[36] Brun A, Gustafson L. Distribution of cerebral degeneration in Alzheimer's disease - a clinico-pathological study. *Archiv fur Psychiatrie und Nervenkrankheiten* 1979;223: pp.15–23.

[37] Braak H, Braak E. Neuropathological staging of Alzheimer-related changes. *Acta Neuropathologica (Berlin)* 1991;82: pp. 239–259.

[38] Hyman BT, Trojanowski JQ. Editorial on consensus recommendations for post-mortem diagnosis of Alzheimer's disease from the National Institute of Aging and Reagan Institute Working group on diagnostic criteria for the neuropathological assessment of Alzheimer's disease. *Journal of Neuropathology and Experimental Neurology* 1997;56: pp. 1095–1097

[39] Ingelsson M, Fukumoto H, Newell KL, *et al*. Early Abeta accumulation and progressive neuronal loss, gliosis and tangle formation in AD brain. *Neurology* 2004;62: pp. 925–931.

[40] Shoji M. Cerebrospinal fluid Abeta40 and Abeta42: natural course and clinical usefulness. *Front Biosci* 2002;7: pp. 997–1006.

[41] Hulstaert F, Blennow K, Ivanoiu A, *et al*. Improved discrimination of AD patients using beta-amyloid (1-42) and tau levels in CSF. *Neurology* 1999;52: pp.1555–1562.

[42] Schoonenboom NS, Pijnenburg YA, Muler C, *et al.* Amyloid beta(1-42) and phosphorylated tau in CSF as markers for early-onset Alzheimer disease. *Neurology* 2004;62: pp. 1580–1584.

[43] Parnetti L, Lanari A, Amici S, *et al.* CSF phosphorylated tau is a possible marker discriminating Alzheimer's disease from dementia with Lewy bodies. Phospho-Tau International Study Group. *Neurol Sci.* 2001;22: pp. 77–8.

[44] Schipper HM. The role of biologic markers in the diagnosis of Alzheimer's disease. *Alzheimer's & Dementia* 2007;3: pp. 325–332.

[45] Jack CR Jr, Rc Petersen Rc, Xu YC, *et al.* Prediction of AD with MRI-based hippocampal volume in mild cognitive impairment. *Neurology* 1999;52: pp. 1397–1403.

[46] Small GW. Diagnostic Issues in Dementia: Neuroimaging as a Surrogate Marker of Disease. *Journal of Geriatric Psychiatry and Neurology* 2006;19: pp. 180–185.

[47] Silverman DHS, Small GW, Chang CY, *et al.* Position emission tomography in evaluation of dementia: regional brain metabolism and long-term clinical outcome. *JAMA* 2001;286: pp. 2120–2127.

[48] Dougall NJ, Bruggink S, Ebmeier KP. Systemic review of diagnostic accuracy of 99mTc-HMPAO-SPECT in dementia. *American Journal of Geriatric Psychiatry* 2004;12: pp. 554–570.

[49] O'Brien JT, Colloby S, Fenwick J, *et al.* Dopamine transporter loss visualize with FP-CIT SPECT in the differential diagnosis of dementia with Lewy bodies. *Archives of Neurology* 2004;61: pp. 919–925.

[50] Finkel SI, Costa e Silva J, Cohen G, *et al.* Behavioural and psychological signs and symptoms in dementia: a consensus statement on current knowledge and implication for research and treatment. *International Psychogeriatrics* 1996;8 (Suppl 3): pp. 497–500.

[51] Hope T, Keene J, Fairburn C, *et al.* Behaviour changes in dementia. 2: Are there behavioural syndromes? *International Journal of Geriatric Psychiatry* 1997;12: pp. 1074–1078.

[52] Lyketsos CG, Sheppard JM, Steinberg M, *et al.* Neuropsychiatric disturbance in Alzheimer's disease clusters into three groups: Cache County study. *International Journal of Geriatric Psychiatry* 2001;16: pp. 1043–1053.

[53] Reisberg B, Borenstein J, Salob SP, *et al.* Behavioural symptoms in Alzheimer's disease: phenomenology and treatment. *Journal of Clinical Psychiatry* 1987;48(Suppl 5): pp. 9–15.

[54] Cummings JL, Mega M, Gray K, *et al.* The Neuropsychiatric Inventory comprehensive assessment of psychopathology in dementia. *Neurology* 1994;44: pp. 2308–2314.

[55] Lyketsos CG, Steinberg M, Tschanz JT *et al.* Mental and Behavioural Disturbances in Dementia: Findings from the Cache County Study on Memory in Aging. *Am J Psychiatry* 2000;157: 708–714.

[56] O'Brien J, Erkinjuntti T, Reisberg B, *et al.* Vascular cognitive impairment. *Lancet Neurology* 2003;2: pp. 89–98.

[57] Galasko D, Katzman R, Salmon DP, *et al.* Clinical and neuropathological findings in Levy body dementia. *Brain and Cognition* 1996;31: pp. 166–175.

[58] Ballard C, Holmes C, McKeith I, *et al.* Psychiatric morbidity in dementia with Levy bodies: a prospective clinical and neuropathological comparative with Alzheimer's disease. *American Journal of Psychiatry* 1999;156: pp. 1039–1045.

[59] Miller BL, Seeley WW, Mychack P, *et al.* Neuroanatomy of the self. Evidence from patients with frontotemporal dementia. *Neurology* 2001;57: pp. 817–821.

[60] Lee HB, Lyketsos CG. Depression in Alzheimer's disease: heterogeneity and related issues. *Biological Psychiatry* 2003;54: pp. 353–362.

[61] Aalten P, de Vugt ME, Lousberg R, *et al.* Behavioural problems in dementia: a factor analysis of the neuropsychiatric inventory. *Dementia and Geriatric Cognitive Disorders* 2003;15: pp. 99–105.

[62] McCurry SM, Reynolds CF, Ancoli-Israel S, *et al.* Treatment of sleep disturbance in Alzheimer's disease. *Sleep Medicine Reviews* 2000;4: pp. 603–628.

[63] Jeste DV, Finkle SI. Psychosis of Alzhemier's disease and related dementias: Diagnostic criteria for a distinct syndrome. *American Journal of Geriatric Psychiatry* 2000;8: pp. 29–34.

[64] Olin JT, Katz IR, Meyers BS, *et al.* Provisional diagnostic criteria for depression of Alzheimer disease: rationale and background. *American Journal of Geriatric Psychiatry* 2002;10: pp. 129–141.

[65] Jeste DV, Meeks TW, Kim DS, Zubenko GS. Diagnostic category and criteria for neuropsychiatric syndromes in dementia. *Journal of Geriatric Psychiatry and Neurology* 2006;19: pp.160–171.

[66] Barberger-Gateau P, Fubrigoule C, Helmer C, Rouch I, Dartigues JF. Functional Impairment in Instrumental Activities of Daily Living: an early clinical sign of dementia. *Journal of the American Geriatrics Society* 1999;47: pp. 456–62.

[67] Duchek JM, Carr DB, Hunt L, *et al*. Longitudinal driving performance in early stage dementia of the Alzheimer type. *Journal of the American Geriatics Society* 2003;51: pp. 1342–1347.

[68] Nyenhuis DL, Gorelick PB, Freels S, Garron DC. Cognitive and functional decline in African Americans with VaD, AD, and strokes without dementia. *Neurology* 2002;58: pp. 56–61.

[69] Gelians L, Gauthier L, McIntyre M, Gauthier S. Development of a fundamental measure for persons with Alzheimer's disease: the disability assessment for dementia. *American Journal of Occupational Therapy* 1999;53: pp. 471–481.

[70] Petersen RC, O'Brien J. Mild cognitive impairment should be considered for DSM-V. *Journal of Geriatric Psychiatry and Neurology* 2006;19: pp. 147–154.

[71] Morris JC, Storandt M, Miller JP, *et al*. Mild cognitive impairment represents early stage Alzheimer's disease. *Archives of Neurology* 2001;58: pp. 397–405.

[72] Larrieu S, Letenneur L, Orgogozo JM, et al. Incidence and outcome of mild cognitive impairment in a population based prospective cohort. *Neurology* 2002;57: pp.1655–1762.

[73] Unverzagt FW, Gao S, Baiyewu O, *et al*. Prevalence of cognitive impairment: Data from the Indianapolis study of Health and Aging. *Neurology* 2001;57: pp. 1655–1662.

[74] Hughes CP, Berg L, Danziger WL *et al*. A new clinical scale for the staging of dementia. Br. J. Psychiatry 1982;140: 566–572.

[75] Boeve BF, Ferman TJ, Smith GE, *et al*. Mild cognitive impairment preceding dementia Lewy bodies. *Neurology* 2004;62(Supp 5): pp. A86.

[76] Petersen RC, Smith GE, Waring SC, *et al*. Mild cognitive impairment: clinical characterization and outcome. *Archives of Neurology* 1999;56: pp. 303–308.

[77] Bennett DA, Wilson RS, Schneider JA, *et al*. Natural history of mild cognitive impairment in older persons. *Neurology* 2002;59: pp. 198–205.

[78] Petersen RC, Smith GE, Ivnik RJ, *et al*. Apolipoprotein-E status as a predictor of the development of Alzheimer's disease in memory impaired individuals. *JAMA* 1995;273: pp. 1274–1278.

[79] Jack CR, Petersen RC, Xu Y, *et al*. (Rate of hippocampal atrophy correlates with change in clinical status in aging and AD. *Neurology* 2000;55: pp. 484–489.

[80] Jicha GA, Parisi JE, Dickson DW, *et al*. Neuropathological outcome of mild cognitive impairment following progression to clinical dementia. *Archives of Neurology* 2006;63: pp. 674–681.

[81] Hogan DB, Bailey P, Carswell A, *et al*. Management of mild to moderate Alzheimer's disease and dementia. *Alzheimer's & Dementia* 2007;3: pp. 355–384.

[82] Petersen RC, Thomas RG, Grundman M, *et al*. Donepezil and vitamin E in the treatment of mild cognitive impairment. *New England Journal of Medicine* 2005;325; pp. 2379–2388.

[83] Winblad B. Severe Alzheimer's disease: benefit of donepezil therapy. International Psychogeriatrics 2006;18(Suppl 1): pp. S25- S31.

[84] Herrmann N, Gauthier S, Lysy PG. Clinical practice guidelines for severe Alzheimer's disease. Alzheimer's & Dementia 2007;3: pp. 385–397.

[85] Erkinjutti T, Kurz A, Gauthier S, *et al*. Efficacy of galantamine in probable vascular dementia and Alzheimer's disease combined with cerebrovascular disease: a randomized trial. *Lancet* 2002;359: pp. 1283–90.

[86] Black S, Roman GC, Geldmacher DS, *et al*. Efficacy and tolerability of donepezil in vascular dementia: positive result of a 24 week, multi-center, international , randomized, placebo controlled clinical trial. *Stroke* 2003;34: pp. 2323–2330.

[87] Bocti C, Black S, Frank C. Management of dementia with a cerebrovascular component. *Alzheimer's & Dementia* 2007;3: pp. 398–403.

[88] Schneider LS, Dagerman KS, Insel P. Risk of death with atypical antipsychotic drug treatment for dementia: meta-analysis of randomized placebo-controlled trials. *JAMA* 2005;294: pp. 1934–1943.

[89] Herrmann N, Mamdani M, Lanctot KL., A typical antipsychotics and risk of cerebrovascular accidents. *Am J. Psychiatry* 161: 1113–1115.

[90] Raivio MM, Laurila JV, Strandberg TE, *et al.* Psychotropic medication and stroke outcome. *American Journal of Psychiatry* 2005;162: pp. 1027–8.

[91] Suh GH, Shah A. Effect of antipsychotics on mortality in elderly patients with dementia: a 1-year prospective study in a nursing home. *International Psychogeriatrics* 2005;17: pp. 429–41.

[92] Lyketsos CG, DelCampo L, Steinberg M, *et al.* Treating depression in Alzheimer's disease: efficacy and safety of sertraline therapy, and the benefit of depression reduction: the DIADS. *Archives of General Psychiatry* 2003;60: pp. 737–746.

[93] Pollock BG, Mulsant BH, Rosen J *et al.* Comparison of citalopram, perphenazine and placebo for treatment of psychosis and behavioural disturbances in hospital demented patients. *Am J. Psychiatry* 2002;159: pp. 460–465.

[94] Brodaty H, Hadzi-Pavlov D. Psychological effects on categories of living with persons with dementia. *Australian and New Zealand Journal of Psychiatry* 1990;24: pp. 351–61.

[95] Pinquart M, Sorensen S. Differences between caregivers and non caregivers in psychological health and physical health: A meta analysis. *Psychology and Aging* 2003;18: pp. 250–67.

[96] Zarit S, Reever K, Batch-Peterson J. Relatives of impaired elderly: correlates of feeling of burden. *Gerontology* 1980;20: pp. 649–655.

[97] Brodaty H, Green A, Koschera A. Meta-analysis of psychosocial interventions for caregivers of people with dementia. *Journal of the American Geriatrics Society* 2003;48: pp. 268–74.

[98] Fillit HM, Gutterman EM, Brooks RL. Impact of Donezepil on caregiving burden for patients with Alzheimer's disease. *International Psychogeriatrics* 2000;123: pp. 389–401.

[99] Mittelman MS, Haley, WE, Clay OJ, Roth DL. Improving caregiver wellbeing delays nursing home placement of patients with Alzheimer's disease. *Neurology* 2006;67: pp. 1592–1599.

[100] Gureje O, Ogunniyi A, Baiyewu O, *et al.* APOE episolon4 is not associated with Alzheimer's disease in elderly Nigerians. *Annals of Neurology* 2005;59: pp. 182–185.

[101] Baiyewu O, Unverzagt FW, Ogunniyi A, *et al.* Cognitive impairment in community dwelling older Nigerians: clinical correlates and stability of diagnosis. *European Journal of Neurology* 2002;9: pp. 573–580.

CHAPTER 8

Schizophrenia and Related Disorders

Wolfgang Gaebel

Professor & Chair, Department of Psychiatry and Psychotherapy, Heinrich-Heine-University, Rhineland State Clinics, Düsseldorf, Germany; Chair, Section on Schizophrenia, World Psychiatric Association

Jürgen Zielasek

Department of Psychiatry and Psychotherapy, Heinrich-Heine-University, Rhineland State Clinics, Düsseldorf, Germany

8.1 INTRODUCTION

Schizophrenia is a mental disorder with a lifetime prevalence of about 1% and a significant attributable burden of disease due to chronic courses in a majority of patients. While the acute clinical picture is often characterized by the so called 'positive symptoms', i.e. florid delusions and hallucinations, chronic disease states are characterized by the progressive development of incapacitating 'negative symptoms' in both affective and cognitive domains. The chronic disease states, especially, are major causes of disability and impairment. In addition, schizophrenia is associated with an increased mortality rate due to suicidality in about 10% of cases and comorbid mental and somatic disorders. Schizophrenia is a heavily stigmatized disorder, leading to additional negative social and economic consequences besides those caused by the disorder itself.

The etiopathogenesis of schizophrenia is unknown but several lines of evidence indicate that it is a neurodevelopmental disorder occurring on the basis of a genetic predisposition, with considerable influence of learning experiences and social and other environmental factors modulating the phenotyping expression of the disorder. Recent findings about the early stages of schizophrenia indicate that the first manifestation of the disorder is frequently preceded by a prodromal state of several years' duration, in which unspecific symptoms predominate but may indicate incipient schizophrenia. Early antipsychotic pharmacotherapy, once schizophrenia develops, is important for relapse prevention and preserving quality of life [1]. Besides pharmacotherapy with antipsychotic agents, which

Psychiatric Diagnosis: Challenges and Prospects   Edited by I.M. Salloum and J.E. Mezzich
© 2009 John Wiley & Sons, Ltd

are especially effective in treating positive symptoms, psychotherapy and social interventions are mainly used to ameliorate the functional consequences of schizophrenia.

In this chapter, we will first review the current state of the art of the diagnostics of schizophrenia, mainly focusing on issues of psychopathology. We will then describe how the concept of 'schizophrenia' as a mental disorder is currently under investigation in the framework of the revision of the psychiatric classification systems.

8.2   CURRENT DIAGNOSTIC CLASSIFICATION OF SCHIZOPHRENIA

The current diagnostic classification of schizophrenia can be traced back to the German psychiatrist Emil Kraepelin who, about a hundred years ago, divided the endogenous psychoses according to their long-term prognosis into 'dementia praecox' and 'manic depressive insanity'. This distinction is often referred to as 'Kraepelin's dichotomy'. Kraepelin's 'dementia praecox' was later reconceptualized as 'schizophrenia' by Eugen Bleuler (1911), who introduced the term that is still used today. Bleuler chose the term 'schizophrenia' (literally meaning 'split mind') in order to indicate that the disorder was characterized by a dissociation of mental capacities from each other, but not a 'split personality'. Bleuler considered schizophrenia to be a heterogeneous group of disorders with different etiopathogeneses and prognoses. He also distinguished between basic and accessory symptoms, and between primary and secondary dysfunctions. Modern diagnostic categories were heavily influenced by the work of Kurt Schneider, who distinguished between first- and second-rank symptoms in schizophrenia.

With the introduction of modern operationalized, multiaxial and atheoretical (anosological) psychiatric classification systems, these developments were reflected in the conceptualization of schizophrenia in the International Classification of Diseases (ICD) of the World Health Organization (WHO), currently in its tenth revision (ICD-10; [2]). Herein, the characteristic psychopathological findings are grouped similarly to Schneider's first- and second-rank symptoms into two groups with different diagnostic relevance, in that it is sufficient for one symptom of group I or two symptoms of group II to occur to warrant the diagnosis (Table 8.1). Additionally, a time criterion needs to be met (one month's duration), and other organic causes for similar psychopathologic pictures need to have been excluded. This implies that the diagnosis of schizophrenia in ICD-10 largely rests on the psychopathological findings, with the results of technical investigations like laboratory or brain imaging studies only serving to exclude organic disorders.

Furthermore, ICD-10 distinguishes between three clinical types of schizophrenia (paranoid, hebephrenic and catatonic) and offers additional diagnostic categories of the schizophrenic spectrum (Table 8.2). Importantly, ICD-10 also includes an overlap category between schizophrenia and affective disorder (schizoaffective disorder).

In the classification system of the American Psychiatric Association (APA), the Diagnostic and Statistical Manual (DSM, currently in its fourth edition including a text revision, hence DSM-IV-TR; [3]) schizophrenia is defined differently, with some significant overlap to the ICD-10 categories in the core clinical features and the necessity to exclude organic causes, but also major differences such as in the time criterion (Table 8.1). In regard to subtyping schizophrenia, the paranoid type and the undifferentiated types are defined differently in both systems. For research purposes especially, such differences may be of importance.

Table 8.1   Diagnostic criteria for schizophrenia as abridged from ICD-10 [2] and DSM-IV-TR [3].

ICD-10	DSM-IV-TR
Clinical criteria	**Criterion A: Characteristic symptoms**
(a) thought echo, thought insertion or withdrawal, and thought broadcasting	
(b) delusions of control, influence or passivity; delusional perception	(1) delusions
(c) hallucinatory voices giving running commentary on the patient's behaviour, or discussing the patient among themselves, or other types of hallucinatory voices coming from some part of the body	(2) hallucinations
(d) persistent delusions of other kinds that are culturally inappropriate and completely impossible	(3) disorganized speech
(e) persistent hallucinations in any modality when accompanied either by fleeting or half-formed delusions without clear affective content, or by persistent over-valued ideas, or when occurring every day for weeks or months on end	
(f) breaks or interpolations in the trains of thought, resulting in incoherence or irrelevant speech, or neologisms	
(g) catatonic behaviour	(4) grossly disorganized or catatonic behaviour
(h) negative symptoms	(5) negative symptoms
(i) a significant and consistent change in the overall quality of some aspects of personal behaviour	
Evaluation Criterion A minimum of one very clear symptom (and usually two or more if less clear-cut) belonging to any one of the groups (a) to (d) above, or symptoms from at least two of the groups referred to as (e) to (h)	**Evaluation Criteria for Criterion A:** Two (or more) symptoms Only one Criterion A symptom is required if delusions are bizarre or hallucinations consist of a voice keeping up a running commentary on the person's behaviour or thoughts, or two or more voices conversing with each other
	Criterion B Social/occupational dysfunction
Time criterion One month or more	**Time criterion** Criterion C Duration: continuous signs of the disturbance persist for at least six months. This six-month period must include at least one month of symptoms that meet Criterion A

(Continued)

Table 8.1   (Continued).

ICD-10	DSM-IV-TR
Exclusion criteria	**Exclusion criteria**
Extensive depressive or manic symptoms unless it is clear that schizophrenic symptoms antedated the exclusion affective disturbances	Criterion D Schizoaffective and mood disorder
presence of overt brain disease	Criterion E Substance/general medical condition exclusion
states of drug intoxication or withdrawal	Criterion F Relation to a Pervasive Developmental Disorder

Table 8.2   Subtypes of schizophrenia and related disorders as abridged from ICD-10 [2] and DSM-IV-TR [3].

ICD-10	DSM-IV-TR
F20 Schizophrenia	
F20.0 Paranoid schizophrenia	295.30 Paranoid Type
F20.1 Hebephrenic schizophrenia	295.10 Disorganized Type
F20.2 Catatonic schizophrenia	295.30 Catatonic Type
F20.3 Undifferentiated schizophrenia	295.90 Undifferentiated Type
F20.4 Post-schizophrenic depression	
F20.5 Residual schizophrenia	295.60 Residual Type
F20.6 Simple schizophrenia	
F20.8 Other schizophrenia	
F20.9 Schizophrenia, unspecified	
	295.40 Schizophreniform Disorder
F21 Schizotypal disorder	
F22 Persistent delusional disorder	
F23 Acute and transient psychotic disorders	298.8 Brief Psychotic Disorder
F24 Induced delusional disorder	297.1 Delusional Disorder
F25 Schizoaffective disorders	295.70 Schizoaffective Disorder
F28 Other nonorganic psychotic disorders	
F29 Unspecified nonorganic psychosis	298.9 Psychotic Disorder Not Otherwise Specified
	297.3 Shared Psychotic Disorder

Large epidemiological field trials have shown that the inter-rater reliability of a schizophrenia diagnosis obtained using ICD-10 is very high [4]. Also, sensitivity, specificity, and both positive and negative predictive values for a three-year stability of the diagnosis both in ICD-10 and DSM-III-TR are high [5]. While ICD-10 and DSM-IV have become the predominant psychiatric classification systems worldwide, alternative classification systems exist, for example, in China and Latin America, but to review these would be beyond the scope of this article. However, many regional or national traditions exist in the field of schizophrenia classification and this adds to the variability of what psychiatrists in different countries mean when they diagnose schizophrenia. The major advantage of ICD-10 and DSM-IV in the field of schizophrenia research, as well as treatment and care, was that the terminology was largely harmonized and the core psychopathological elements were agreed upon. There was still a major disadvantage in that these classification systems may have lumped mental disorders with putative different pathophysiologies but with a similar 'schizophrenia'-type psychopathology into one disorder category, thus blurring true boundaries between different disorders. Therefore, the diagnostic categories for schizophrenia are currently under review in the framework of developing the new psychiatric classification systems ICD-11 and DSM-V.

8.3 PROSPECTS OF SCHIZOPHRENIA CLASSIFICATION

Kraepelin had already postulated that the signs and symptoms of 'dementia praecox' used for classification at the time when he was writing may not be sufficient to clearly delineate the different mental disorders, but that overlap syndromes may occur [6]. Both schizophrenia and manic depressive disorder frequently manifest in early adulthood and they share some of the risk genes like neuregulin-1, which has recently prompted some authors to announce the 'end of the Kraepelinian dichotomy' [7]. However, the psychopathological findings are sufficiently dissimilar in the majority of cases to warrant two separate disorder categories. Murray and coworkers suggested that the psychopathological consequences of common risk genes may be modulated by different additional genetic or environmental risk factors in schizophrenia and affective disorders [8].

With the revision process of ICD-10 and DSM-IV having been started in the late 1990s, a series of research conferences was jointly sponsored by the APA, the National Institutes of Health and the WHO to review the current state of the art, and to define research questions in preparation of new diagnostic categories. In schizophrenia, the corresponding research conference was entitled 'Deconstructing Psychosis' and was held in Arlington in February 2006.

Main topics were the psychopathological distinction between schizophrenia and affective disorders, especially bipolar affective disorder, and the role of neurobiological findings for the revised classification systems. The participants published their reports in Volume 33 of the *Schizophrenia Bulletin* (2007) with an introductory editorial by Van Os and Tamminga [9]. Two major workgroups were formed and came to somewhat different results. Workgroup I recommended reducing the time criterion to one month in DSM-V and substituting the current dichotomous classification with a General Psychotic Syndrome; and also that dimensional criteria should be introduced and research criteria should be defined for the duration, the time course, and the type of manifestation at onset. Workgroup II recommended a harmonization of the disease duration criteria between ICD-11 and DSM-V and a research focus on overlap syndromes like schizoaffective disorder. Furthermore, the recommendation included defining subtypes like the 'deficit syndrome'. This group also acknowledged the need to introduce dimensional criteria, identifying the selection of dimensions to be used and their assessment as major research topics.

Our review of other findings from this conference shows a need for more epidemiological studies to ascertain the prognostic implications of certain psychopathological findings. No clear picture emerged in the field of endophenotyping schizophrenia. Brain imaging cannot yet yield information beyond the exclusion of organic brain disorders, although important insights into the pathophysiology of some aspects of schizophrenia have been gained by functional neuroimaging [10]. Genetic risk factor analyses showed a large overlap between different diagnostic categories, but only a minor absolute contribution to disease development. There is a multitude of genetic polymorphisms, but their functional consequences and their role in the pathophysiology of schizophrenia are unknown. There are still no 'schizophrenia genes', but certain genotype-phenotype relationships are currently being studied that may result in a closer association between these two domains [11]. Regarding the neurobiology of schizophrenia, a wealth of data is available, but as yet with little if any consequence for the diagnostic process. Importantly, successful treatment was recently achieved using agonists of metabotropic glutamate receptors (mGluR2/3) confirming that dopamine is not the only neurotransmitter involved in the pathophysiology of schizophrenia, although the action of mGluR2/3 agonists may involve the dopamine system [12]. This finding, if reproduced, would still provide a fine example of how an animal model of schizophrenia (phencyclidine 'psychosis' in rodents) and subsequent elucidation of its pathophysiology may result in new therapeutic approaches, which also inform the revision of the diagnostic classification criteria.

Taken together, much more research is needed in neuroimaging and the neurobiology of schizophrenia. Neither field has yet to offer nosologically important information. A radical 'deconstruction' of schizophrenia is not yet warranted since no alternative is available and the construct 'schizophrenia' apparently yields useful prognostic information [5] and information on the therapy that may be helpful. Also, the use of the operationalized diagnostic criteria has led to a better communication between psychiatrists, since the term is now operationalized and thus leaves less space for idiosyncrasies. However, it appears useful to include dimensional categories, endophenotype investigations and a useful clinical subtyping like one focusing on functional consequences for future research purposes [13] in order to circumvent the problem mentioned before that the diagnostic category of 'schizophrenia' may encompass a large range of putatively different nosological disease entities.

Of course, the process of 'deconstructing psychosis' has not ended with the research conference. The focus seems to shift from genetics to neuroimaging and the assessment of the functional correlates of psychopathology. This includes psychophysiological parameters like eye-tracking dysfunction or working memory deficits, which together with other cognitive areas seem to be of central importance for the determination of the long-term prognosis. The MATRICS initiative to develop cognitive test batteries for schizophrenia research is an example for this approach [14, 15]. In April 2007, the participants at the Schizophrenia Research Conference in Colorado Springs discussed the topic of retaining or abandoning the disease category of schizophrenia in revised classification systems. Some argued for a 'General Psychotic Syndrome' considering dimensional features and overlap syndromes, some were in favour of a neurobiological redefinition ('Dopamine Dysregulation Disorder'). On the other hand, some experts voted for retaining 'schizophrenia' as a clinical syndrome or defining subtypes. Both the initial and final votes of the auditorium were split, with half in favour of abolishing the term and half in favour of retaining it. Darrel Regier who, together with David Kupfer, co-leads the task force of the APA for the revision of DSM-IV, has recently listed 'key issues' regarding the development of DSM-V, which may be an indication for the issues also pertaining to the future of the classification of schizophrenia [16]. Among the more important aspects may be the lifetime history of people with mental disorders, the integration of mental disorders into somatic medicine, the question of dimensional classification criteria and the development of core psychopathological features. Finally, gender- and culture-specific issues may be addressed. The APA announced the work groups for the revision of DSM-IV in the summer of 2007, and schizophrenia will be covered in an international group dealing with the more general topic of psychotic disorders. Further information about progress in this area may be found on the Internet (www.dsm5.org and www.psych.org/research/dsm/revision.cfm; both last assessed 12 December 2007).

Regarding the revision of ICD-10, the revision of the mental disorders section will be supervised by a Topic Advisory Group, which will also ensure a harmonization between the ICD process and the DSM process [17]. Special work groups will be established for the major diagnostic groups and will assess the definition of the respective disorders, the identification of key diagnostic features, the role of pathophysiology and genetics, clinical utility and validity, and culture-specific effects. The universality of psychiatric diagnostic categories will be investigated, and user participation will play a role. The role of industry will also be critically analysed, another factor in the DSM process with rigorous examination of 'conflicts of interest' [18]. To assist the WHO in the revision process of the ICD-10 chapter on mental and behavioural disorders, a global network of experts and institutions has been created, the Global Scientific Partnership Coordinating Group (GSP), chaired by Norman Sartorius. The GSP consists of a small group of experts representing special language groups and linking with experts from the respective countries using that language (e.g. for the German speaking countries this task has been attributed to one of us, Wolfgang Gaebel), ensuring the continued involvement and input of scientific evidence and experience from those regions.

A further important issue will be the assessment of the impact of revised diagnostic criteria for forensic issues, economic issues, continuation of epidemiological registries and medical education. An interesting example of the impact on public attitudes of a change in the diagnostic label is the renaming of 'schizophrenia' to 'integration disorder' in Japan in 2002. This was accompanied by informing the public about the treatment options. While the diagnosis of 'schizophrenia' was severely stigmatized, the renaming and the educational activities have resulted in an increased acceptance of the new diagnostic term, reflected by an increased use of the respective diagnostic category [19].

The discussion of the 'deconstruction' of psychotic disorders shows that there is a need for new concepts for the classification of schizophrenia and related disorders. A central issue appears to be a more functional approach, focusing on dysfunctions of psychophysiological functional units of the human brain. There has been renewed interest in Wakefield's 'harmful dysfunction' analysis of mental disorders, which includes a neurobiological (functional) assessment of 'dysfunction' and a value-oriented 'harmfulness' assessment (see [20], and the subsequential commentaries on that article, [21]). Regarding the integration of neurobiological findings, we have proposed to use brain-behaviour modules of the human brain instead of descriptive psychopathology as the substrates of the action of pathogenic factors and genetic polymorphisms [22], with the advantage that modularity is well based in the philosophy of cognition and the mind [23] and the neurosciences [24].

We would suggest including the importance of connections between such modules in such a concept [25]. This would relate well to the current dysconnectivity hypothesis of schizophrenia, which regards schizophrenia as a white matter disease leading to impaired nerve impulse propagation in long tract associative fibres of the human brain, whose function is especially important in the 'binding' of spatially separated functional subunits of the brain (reviewed by Burns [26]). Hallucinations could then be due to spontaneous activity of perceptive modules and delusional ideas would be conceptualized as a lack of accessibility to context information by certain functional modules. Thought disorders could indicate a lack of isolation of modules against influences from other modules, leading to the occurrence of a lack of delineation of the self from the environment, or phenomena like thought withdrawal or thought insertion. Such modular approaches could lead to module specific therapies, which are currently evaluated in the field of facial affect recognition in schizophrenia [27]. While such approaches today appear far away from becoming the foundation of ICD-11 or DSM-V, such research and new concepts bridging the gap between the neurosciences and psychopathological phenomenology may become important for future revisions of the psychiatric classification systems.

It should be noted that a number of other concepts of schizophrenia have been formulated, but a comprehensive review is beyond the scope of this chapter. Evolutionary principles of the origin of psychosis are interesting in that they also bridge several aspects like genetics, the dysconnectivity hypothesis and social cognitive issues [26]. In a similar manner, Tsuang and coworkers have proposed reconceptualizing schizophrenia not as a clinical syndrome defined by the clinical symptoms, but rather as a neurodevelopmental, dimensional disorder incorporating neurobiological and neuropsychological measures occurring prior to the development of psychosis ('schizotaxia' [28]). For readers interested in concepts of schizophrenia beyond the neurobiological/neurodevelopmental models, Chung and coworkers have recently compiled several different views [29].

Considering more practical aspects, the classification criteria of schizophrenia need to be harmonized as far as possible between ICD-11 and DSM-V, and it will be necessary to distinguish between clinically useful and clearly defined subtypes, especially for research purposes. This may include an analysis down to the level of individual psychopathological phenomena, which may all have different pathophysiologies and genetic risk factors. To elucidate such associations and causal relations, it may be necessary to stratify patient cohorts along pathophysiological features accompanied by endophenotype measures. Such an approach may bring schizophrenia research closer to the pathophysiology of psycho-pathological syndromes and may avoid the undue lumping together of putative nosological subunits under the heading of 'schizophrenia'. Even categories like 'paranoid' or 'hebe-phrenic' are too broad. An important aspect will be the definition of early prodromal phenenomena and their respective prospective evaluation, but also of the cognitive impairments that play a central role in the determination of the long-term functional disability in schizophrenia. For these cognitive features of schizophrenia, especially, psychophysiological and neurophysiological tests supplemented by neuroimaging studies may be necessary to elucidate the pathophysiology.

8.4   CONCLUSIONS

In conclusion, with the current limited knowledge about the pathophysiology of schizophrenia, neither a radical revision nor the abandonment of the concept seems to be warranted in the light of the fact that the introduction and operationalized definition of the term have lead to a better communication between psychiatrists and yield useful clinical information regarding prognosis and therapeutic procedures. However, there is a need to harmonize the diagnostic criteria between ICD-11 and DSM-V. Furthermore, new research results in the years to come could provide novel information that may be of classificatory relevance, especially in the fields of genetics and the analysis of functional subsystems of the human brain by psychophysiological methods or human brain imaging, or combinations of these methods.

REFERENCES

[1] Gaebel W, Riesbeck M, Wölwer W, Klimke a, Eickhoff M, van Wilmsdorff M, Jockers-Scherübl MC, Kühn KU, Lemke M, Bechdolf A, Bender S, Degner D, Schlösser R, Schmidt LG, Schmitt A, Jäger M, Buchkremer G, Falkai P, Klingberg S, Köpcke W, Maier W, Häfner H, Ohmann C, Salize HJ, Schneider F, Möller HJ; German Study Group on First-Episode Schizophrenia. Maintenance treatment with risperidone or low-dose haloperidol in first-episode schizophrenia: 1-year-results of a randomized controlled trial within the German research network on schizophrenia. *Journal of Clinical Psychiatry* 2007;68: pp. 1763–1774.

[2] World Health Organization. *The ICD-10 classification of mental and behavioural disorders.* Geneva: World Health Organization;1992.

[3] APA. *Diagnostic and Statistical Manual of Mental Disorders. 4th ed. Text revision. (DSM-IV-TR.)* Arlington: American Psychiatric Association; 2000.

[4] Sartorius N, Üstün TB, Korten A, Cooper JE, van Drimmelen J. Progress toward achieving a common language in psychiatry, II: Results from the international field trials of the ICD-10 diagnostic criteria for mental and behavioral disorders. *American Journal of Psychiatry* 1995;152: pp. 1427–1437.

[5] Amin S, Singh SP, Brewin J, Jones PB, Medley I, Harrison G. Diagnostic stability of first-episode psychosis. Comparison of ICD-10 and DSM-III-R systems. *British Journal of Psychiatry* 1999;175: pp. 537–543.

[6] Kraepelin E. Die Erscheinungsformen des Irreseins. *Z ges Neurol Psychiatr* 1920;62: pp. 1–29.

[7] Craddock N, Owen MJ. Rethinking psychosis: the disadvantage of a dichotomous classification now outweigh the advantages. *World Psychiatry* 2007;6: pp. 20–27.

[8] Murray RM, Sham P, Van Os J, Zanelli J, Cannon M, McDonald C. A developmental model for similarities and dissimilarities between schizophrenia and bipolar disorder. *Schizophrenia Research* 2004;71: pp. 405–419.

[9] Van Os J, Tamminga C. Deconstructing Psychosis. *Schizophrenia Bulletin* 2007; 33: pp. 861–862.

[10] Gur RE, Keshavan MS, Lawrie SL. Deconstructing Psychosis with Human Brain Imaging. *Schizophrenia Bulletin* 2007;33: pp. 921–931.

[11] Owen MJ, Craddock N, Jablensky A. The Genetic Deconstruction of Psychosis. *Schizophrenia Bulletin* 2007;33: pp. 905–911.

[12] Patil ST, Zhang L, Martenyi F, Lowe SL, Jackson KA, Andreev BV, Avedisova AS, Bardenstein LM, Gurovich IY, Morozova MA, Mosolov SN, Neznanov NG, Reznik AM, Smulevich AB, Tochilov VA, Johnson BG, Monn JA, Schoepp DD. Activation of mGlu2/3 receptors as a new approach to treat schizophrenia: a randomized Phase 2 clinical trial. *Nature Medicine* 2007;13: pp. 1102–1107.

[13] Allardyce J, Gaebel W, Zielasek J, Van Os J. Deconstructing Psychosis Conference 2006: The validity of schizophrenia and alternative approaches to the classification of psychosis. *Schizophrenia Bulletin* 2007;33: pp. 863–867.

[14] Green MF, Nuechterlein KH, Gold JM, Barch DM, Cohen J, Essock S, Fenton WS, Frese F, Goldberg TE, Heaton RK, Keefe RSE, Kern RS, Kraemer H, Stover E, Weinberger DR, Zalcman S, Marder SR. Approaching a consensus cognitive battery for clinical trials in schizophrenia: The NIMH-MATRICS conference to select cognitive domains and test criteria. *Biological Psychiatry* 2004;56: pp. 301–307.

[15] Green MF, Penn D, Bentall R, Carpenter W, Gaebel W, Gur R, Kring A, Park S, Silverstein S, Heinssen R. Social cognition in schizophrenia: NIMH Consensus Meeting on Definitions, Assessment, and Research Opportunities. *Schizophrenia Bulletin*. Forthcoming 2008.

[16] Regier DA. Time for a fresh start? Rethinking psychosis in DSM-V. *Schizophrenia Bulletin* 2007;33: pp. 843–845.

[17] Üstün TB, Jakob R. Die Entwicklung der 11. Revision der Internationalen Klassifikation der Krankheiten (ICD-11). *Die Psychiatrie* 2007; 4: pp. 77–85.

[18] Saraceno B, Saxena S. Fragen zur Klassifizierung von psychischen und Verhaltensstörungen als Aufgabe der WHO. *Die Psychiatrie* 2007; 4: pp. 86–90.

[19] Sato M. Renaming schizophrenia: A Japanese perspective. *World Psychiatry* 2006;6: pp. 53–55.

[20] Wakefield JC. The concept of mental disorder: diagnostic implications of the harmful dysfunction concept. *World Psychiatry* 2007;6: pp. 149–156.

[21] First MB. Potential implications of the harmful dysfunction analysis for the development of DSM-V and ICD-11. *World Psychiatry* 2007;6: pp. 158–159.

[22] Gaebel W, Wölwer W, Zielasek J. Von der deskriptiven zur funktionalen Psychiatrie. Auf dem Weg zu einer modularen Psychiatrie. *Die Psychiatrie* 2006;4: pp. 221–232.

[23] Fodor J. *The modularity of mind*. Cambridge: MIT Press; 1983.

[24] Frégnac Y, Blatow M, Changeux JP, DeFelipe J, Lansner A, Maass W, McCormick DA, Michel CM, Monyer H, Szathmary E, Yuste R. Group Report: Neocortical Microcircuits. UPs and DOWNs in Cortical Computation. In: Grillner S, Graybiel AM. (eds.) *Microcircuits. The Interface between Neurons and Global Brain Function*. Cambridge: MIT Press; 2006. pp. 393–433.

[25] Calabretta R, Parisi D. Evolutionary Connectionism and Mind/Brain Modularity. In: Callebaut W, Rasskin-Gutmann D (eds.) *Modularity. Understanding the Development and Evolution of Natural Complex Systems*. Cambridge: MIT Press; 2005. pp. 309–330.

[26] Burns J. *The Descent of Madness. Evolutionary Origins of Psychosis and the Social Brain*. Hove: Routledge; 2007.

[27] Wölwer W, Frommann N, Halfmann S, Piaszek A, Streit M, Gaebel W. Remediation of impairments in facial affect recognition in schizophrenia: Efficacy and specificity of a new training program. *Schizophrenia Research* 2005;80: pp. 295–303.

[28] Tsuang MT. Schizotaxia and the Prevention of Schizophrenia. In: Helzer JE and Hudziak JJ (eds.): *Defining Psychopathology in the 21st Century*. Washington: American Psychiatric Publishing; 2002. pp. 249–260.

[29] Chung MC, Fulford KWM and Graham G (eds.) *Reconceiving Schizophrenia*. Oxford: Oxford Medical Publications; 2007.

CHAPTER 9

Mood Disorders

Marna S. Barrett

*Department of Psychiatry, University of Pennsylvania School of Medicine,
Philadelphia, PA, USA*

Michael E. Thase

*Professor of Psychiatry, University of Pennsylvania School of
Medicine, Philadelphia, PA, USA*

9.1 INTRODUCTION

Early efforts to create a classification system for mood disorders were influenced by a mixture of psychoanalytic and descriptive observations of human behaviour. Although some of these entities remain in the nomenclature under different names, others have disappeared and even the best-validated diagnoses were described so superficially in the first two editions of the American Psychiatric Association Diagnostic and Statistical Manual (DSM), which were published in 1952 and 1968, that there was an unacceptably low level of agreement, even among researchers. Revisions to the approach to psychiatric diagnosis in the late 1960s and 1970s sought to address these problems and better validate the diagnostic criteria used for classification of psychiatric disorders, culminating with publication of DSM-III in 1980. What the DSM-III lacked in theoretical richness in its approach to classification of mood disorders (e.g., the diagnoses of neurotic depression and involutional melancholia were abandoned), it more than compensated for with careful description and specification, making it possible for the first time for clinicians to make reliable diagnoses of the major forms of mood disorders. Since 1980, the DSM has undergone several additional revisions, resulting in refinements in the diagnostic criteria based on both new research and changes in expert consensus.

9.2 CURRENT DIAGNOSTIC CLASSIFICATIONS

There currently exist two, widely accepted systems for the classification and diagnosis of mood disorders – the Diagnostic and Statistical Manual of Mental Disorders, Fourth Edition (DSM-IV-TR [1]) and the International Classification of Diseases and related Health Problems, Tenth Edition (ICD-10 [2]). Both diagnostic systems are symptom-based,

Psychiatric Diagnosis: Challenges and Prospects   Edited by I.M. Salloum and J.E. Mezzich
© 2009 John Wiley & Sons, Ltd

and clinicians can utilize both systems for diagnosis, treatment planning and third party payment. The ICD, which developed from the work of Jacques Bertillon in 1893 and began to include a section on mental disorders starting with the sixth edition in 1949, is relatively broader in its attempt to offer comparisons of mortality and morbidity across cultures, countries, and time. The DSM-IV-TR, by contrast, aims to be more specific in defining diagnostic criteria that would allow for investigations of underlying pathophysiology. Although the two systems overlap substantially, they are not strictly interchangeable and employing one system over the other can and does result in differences in prevalence rates, prognoses, and research findings.

9.2.1 Major Depressive Disorder

Both ICD-10 and DSM-IV-TR use the term major depressive disorder (MDD) to describe the state of nonbipolar (or unipolar) depression and agree that the defining symptoms include persistently depressed mood, anhedonia, decreased energy, psychomotor retardation, worthlessness and guilt, sleep and appetite disturbances, and reduced concentration. Beyond these key features of depression, differences in diagnostic criteria are evident. For instance, ICD-10 allows for brief episodes of hypomania in the context of MDD, whereas DSM-IV-TR excludes evidence of hypomania within a major depressive episode. DSM-IV-TR is similarly restrictive in requiring the presence of at least one of two essential criteria for diagnosis of MDD (anhedonia and depressed mood) regardless of other presenting symptoms. Perhaps the largest difference between the two systems is that ICD-10 offers only mild, moderate or severe specifiers of the depressive episode, without an indication of presentation (i.e., atypical or melancholic features) or manner of onset (i.e., post-partum) as the DSM-IV-TR does. These subcategories of MDD become particularly important in light of research demonstrating symptomatic overlap between MDD and bipolar disorder (particularly with the bipolar II and bipolar Not Otherwise Specified diagnoses), gender differences in symptomatic profile and risk, and treatment response.

9.2.2 Dysthymia

According to the ICD-10, dysthymia is defined as a chronic depressed mood not severe enough to warrant an MDD diagnosis and lasting for several years. The expansiveness of this definition affords clinicians a wide berth in determining the severity and duration of the disorder, yet hinders the diagnostic specificity necessary for research. A prime example of this difficulty is the symptomatic overlap between dysthymia and depressive personality disorder ([3, 4]). Consistent with dysthymia, depressive personality disorder (DPD) is characterized by pervasive and persistent depressive symptoms with negativity and pessimism pre-eminent. Differentiating the two, research has also shown greater Axis I and II co-morbidity in DPD [4]. Debate remains, however, as to whether these few differences warrant the distinction of a new diagnostic entity.

In contrast to the overly broad diagnostic criteria of ICD-10, DSM-IV TR has a more restrictive definition of dysthymia. Characterized by the presence of two or more depressive symptoms lasting at least two years, there must also be no inter-episode recovery and no evidence of MDD during the two-year period. The DSM further requires that the depressed mood causes 'clinically significant distress or impairment' in various aspects of functioning. This requirement of impairment in functioning is unique to the DSM and is included for a number of diagnostic categories. While useful in encouraging attention to the social and occupational difficulties that accompany these disorders, it does little to enhance diagnostic accuracy or improve treatment.

The validity of dysthymia as a unique diagnosis is challenged by the fact that, during longitudinal follow-up, the vast majority of individuals will develop major depressive episodes. Referred to by some as 'double depression', to others the almost inherent comorbidity between dysthymia and MDD simply represents a common variation in the natural history of depression [5]. Moreover, studies examining various forms of chronic depression have found few differences between dysthymia and chronic episodes of MDD or recurrent episodes of MDD with incomplete inter-episode recovery (see, for example, McCullough et al. [6]).

9.2.3   Bipolar Affective Disorder

As is true for MDD and dysthymia, the ICD classification system is overly broad in defining bipolar affective disorder, whereas the DSM is quite specific. For instance, ICD-10 states that episodes of both elevated mood/increased activity (i.e., hypomanic or manic) and depressed mood/decreased activity must occur to warrant a diagnosis of bipolar disorder. (Also noted are cases with only episodes of elevated mood/increased activity.) DSM-IV-TR, on the other hand, requires one or more specific manic or mixed episodes with at least one major depressive episode. The DSM does not allow for the presence of hypomanic symptoms as the sole evidence of elevated mood. However, the DSM does not hold to the ICD requirement of changes in mood as well as activity level.

A further distinction of bipolar affectivity made by DSM-IV-TR is the less severe bipolar II. ICD-10 offers no diagnostic criteria for bipolar II disorder, whereas DSM-IV-TR stipulates the absence of any manic or mixed episodes in the presence of mood variability. Further differentiation about the etiology or presentation of bipolar symptoms is noticeably absent from the ICD-10 classification. The DSM-IV-TR, in contrast, lists diagnostic specifiers that include patterns of rapid cycling between depressed and manic states, periods in which no depressive episodes occur, and the presence of mood variability in conjunction with delusional disorder or residual schizophrenia.

The considerable heterogeneity of symptoms in bipolar disorder has led to the current shift toward a dimensional or spectrum classification of this group of disorders. Referred to as bipolar spectrum disorders, the term consists of two dimensions: variability in severity (e.g., hypomania, bipolar dysthymia, cyclothymia) and variability in mood (encompassing both mania and depression) [7]. Although research is just beginning to offer support for this concept [8], it has the potential to facilitate greater differentiation of diagnoses and develop more specialized treatments.

9.2.4   Cyclothymia

Both the DSM and ICD classification systems agree that cyclothymia represents a persistent state of mild mood variability in which the symptoms are never severe enough to warrant either a MDD or bipolar II diagnosis. Although DSM acknowledges the possibility of a change in diagnosis to bipolar II after two years of cyclothymia, no clear distinction is provided. Thus, it is not surprising that researchers have long debated the usefulness of cyclothymia as a distinct diagnostic category. Instead, many have proposed a bipolar spectrum of which cyclothymia is a part.

Akiskal [9] first suggested such a dimension based on evidence in which 44% of cyclothymic patients experienced brief hypomanic episodes while taking tricyclic drugs, and 35% developed hypomanic, manic or depressive episodes during drug-free follow-up. Today, cyclothymia is considered a part of the bipolar spectrum and has been suggested by some to result from the same underlying genetic liability as bipolar I and II [10].

9.2.5   Summary of Current Diagnostic Classifications

Comparing the ICD-10 and DSM-IV-TR classifications of mood disorders, we have noted the generally broad inclusion criteria of the ICD-10 versus the more specific requirements of the DSM. Of course, the most striking difference is the absence of bipolar II disorder in ICD-10. In addition to its greater specificity, DSM-IV-TR also provides information about prevalence, familial patterns, course, prognosis, potential predisposing factors, and differential diagnoses for each of the mood disorders. However, drawing attention to the specificity of the DSM is not meant to suggest it as a better, more valid, diagnostic system. In fact, the greater specificity of the DSM has not led to significant differences in diagnostic accuracy between the DSM and ICD systems.

9.3   FUTURE DIRECTIONS FOR CLASSIFICATION

When considering future directions for the classification of mood disorders, it seems prudent to reflect on the fundamental purpose of a classification system. Is there a need for clearer communication about disorders? Do we need more precise classification for epidemiological studies? Is research imprecise because of diagnostic ambiguity? Will it be possible to develop more specific diagnoses that facilitate better matching of patients to particular treatment protocols? For these reasons and more, improvements in the current classification systems are needed, although there is considerable debate about what changes to make and how to do so. Three major issues are at the centre of the debate: the high rate of comorbidity and symptomatic overlap between disorders; the usefulness of categorical versus dimensional approaches to diagnosis; and whether systematic revisions improve diagnostic validity and treatment.

9.3.1   Comorbidity and Symptomatic Overlap

Of all the barriers hindering the development of a valid and reliable diagnostic system for mood disorders, diagnostic comorbidity and symptomatic overlap between disorders are among the greatest challenges. In order to classify a set of symptoms or features as a unique disorder, we must be able to empirically delineate one disorder from another and, as previously discussed, considerable overlap exists between the various mood disorders.

For instance, irritability, psychomotor agitation, and distractibility are features of mania and hypomania, yet can also be found in MDD and attention deficit hyperactivity disorder. Racing thoughts and obsessive worry are evident in MDD, mania, and OCD [11]. In regard to the distinction between mania and hypomania there is considerable controversy about the number and nature of the symptoms as well as the episode duration [12].

If we cannot clearly differentiate one cluster of symptoms from another, the validity of the disorder as a discrete entity is brought into question and resulting conclusions suspect. Likewise, such overlap no doubt precludes identification of truly selective treatments. A symptom-based classification system is not the answer, however, as we would lose the overall Gestalt of the disorder and, as may be true for many disorders, there may not be 'pure' categories to distinguish.

9.3.2 Categorical Versus Dimensional Approaches

With the introduction of DSM-III in 1980, classification of disorders shifted from an etiological or theoretically guided approach to one that was categorical and criteria-based in nature. Designed to improve the uniformity of diagnosis and standardize diagnostic practices [13], in which it was successful, DSM-III and its descendents failed to address the degree to which the variability of depressive symptoms impact diagnostic specificity [14]. For example, whereas one person with MDD may exhibit symptoms of depressed mood, guilt, worthlessness and suicidal ideation, another person can show a quite different pattern characterized by anhedonia, decreased appetite, poor concentration and low energy. And, as noted earlier for cyclothymia and bipolar II disorder, exactly the same symptoms and history can be present in two supposedly distinct disorders, with 'accurate' diagnosis hinging on a matter of days' duration or the intensity of the depressive episodes.

In response to these limitations, researchers have argued for the use of a dimensional system for classification that attends to the variation in symptomatic severity [14] and comorbidity [15]. Whereas a categorical system requires qualitative differences between groups of people, dimensional approaches assess characteristics of people along a continuum of quantitative differences. One difficulty in holding to either a categorical or dimensional approach is that the underlying structure may not correspond [16]. For example, clinician-rated assessments of mania, such as the Young Mania Rating Scale, provide a quantitative measure of symptomatic severity that may or may not correspond to hypomanic or manic qualifications or the larger bipolar I or II distinctions. Thus, ICD-11 and DSM-V working groups have begun to consider the usefulness of a combined approach in which dimensional assessments of severity are but one feature comprising a categorical entity. One example of the combined approach is data from a study of MDD in which some symptoms were better predictors of a depressed state than others, although all symptoms had empirical support for defining MDD [17].

9.3.3 Improvement in Diagnostic Validity

A third issue to consider in revising diagnostic classifications is that of the validity of diagnostic categories. Already discussed are issues of symptom and diagnostic overlap, but there also exists considerable variability in presentation due to factors such as personality and gender. For instance, individuals with a dependent personality pattern often experience depression in terms of loneliness, loss and isolation. In contrast, more independent, self-critical individuals evidence depression with symptoms of defeat, self-blame and with-drawal ([18] Blatt & Zuroff, 1992; [19] Widiger, Trull, Clarkin, Sanderson, & Costa, 1994). These findings have led to suggestions to revive one of the older ways of viewing the 'nature' of depression, namely that the condition now called MDD consists of two general subtypes – endogenous and nonendogenous (reactive, situational, or neurotic) forms of depression.

Across a number of countries and cultures, gender differences in depression have been found for symptomatic profile, prevalence and risk factors [20]. MDD consistently shows higher prevalence rates in women, with the difference typically ranging between 1.5:1 and 2:1. The preponderance of affected females, which emerges in early adolescence, has been shown to increase with increasing numbers of symptoms. Differing symptomatic profiles have also been suggested, with women reporting more somatic and atypical symptoms whereas men evidence more irritability. Although the evidence is not as strong or consis-tent, women may also be at greater risk for chronicity and have higher rates of relapse or recurrence. Interestingly, exactly the same gender differences are evident in bipolar II disorder but not consistently found in bipolar I disorder. Recent studies are examining links between estrogen, serotoninergic function and responses to stress as possible differing risk factors for depression in women than men.

Stemming from questions about diagnostic validity, some researchers have argued for a complete transformation of the DSM multiaxial system. Rather than focusing on diagnosis and psychological development, they propose a biologically informed system in which genotype, phenotype and environmental factors are described. Although there is no doubt about the potential and promise of this approach, it is a long way from being a clinical reality and, although a number of alleles have been linked to risk of mood disorder, there are not yet any genetic markers for mood disorders that can be used in practice. The variability and instability of depressive symptoms over time create additional challenges for this type of approach.

9.4 CONCLUSION

The current state of classification of mood disorders represents a field in transition. On the one hand, the principal diagnoses now used in DSM-IVTR and ICD-10 have adequate reliability and some degree of validity. On the other hand, there is a sense that the descriptive, criteria-based approach has reached a maximum possible level of utility and that additional, comple-mentary approaches are needed in order to reach the next level of precision.

REFERENCES

[1] American Psychiatric Association. *Diagnostic and statistical manual of mental disorders.* 4th ed. Text Revision. (DSM-IV-TR). Washington, DC: American Psychiatric Association; 2000.

[2] World Health Organization. *International Classification of Diseases and Related Health Problems.* Tenth Revision. (ICD-10). Volume 1. Geneva: WHO; 1992.

[3] Klein DN. Depressive Personality: Reliability, validity, and relation to Dysthymia. *Journal of Abnormal Psychology* 1990;99: pp. 412–421.

[4] McDermut W, Zimmerman M, Chelminski I. The construct validity of depressive personality disorder. *Journal of Abnormal Psychology* 2003;112: pp. 49–60.

[5] Gelenberg AJ, Kocsis JH, McCullough JP Jr, Ninan PT, Thase ME. The state of knowledge of chronic depression. *Journal of Clinical Psychiatry* 2006;67(2): pp.179–184.

[6] McCullough JP Jr, Klein DN, Keller MB, Holzer CE, Davis SM, Kornstein SG, Howland RH, Thase ME, Harrison WM. Comparison of DSM-III-R chronic major depression and major depression superimposed on dysthymia (double depression): validity of the distinction. *Journal of Abnormal Psychology* 2000;109(3): pp. 419–427.

[7] Akiskal HS. The Emergence of the Bipolar Spectrum: Validation along Clinical-Epidemiologic and Familial-Genetic Lines. *Psychopharmacology Bulletin* 2007;40(4): pp. 99–115.

[8] Judd LL, Akiskal HS, Schettler PJ, *et al.* A prospective investigation of the natural history of the long-term weekly symptomatic status of bipolar II disorder. *Archives of General Psychiatry* 2003;60: pp. 261–269.

[9] Akiskal HS. Cyclothymic disorder: validating criteria for inclusion in the bipolar affective group. *American Journal of Psychiatry* 1997;134: pp. 1227–1233.

[10] Edvardsen J, Torgersen S, Roysamb E, Lygren S, Skre I, Onstad S, Oien P. Heritability of bipolar spectrum disorders. Unity or heterogeneity? *Journal of Affective Disorders* 2008;106: pp. 229–240.

[11] Benazzi F. Is there a continuity between bipolar and depressive disorders? *Psychotherapy and Psychosomatics* 2007;76: pp. 70–76.

[12] Angst J. The bipolar spectrum. *British Journal of Psychiatry* 2007;190: pp. 189–191.

[13] Mayes R, Horwitz AV. DSM-III and the revolution in the classification of mental illness. *Journal of the History of the Behavioral Sciences* 2005;41: pp. 249–267.

[14] Andrews G, Brugha T, Thase ME, Duffy FF, Rucci P, Slade T. Dimensionality and the category of major depressive episode. *International Journal of Methods in Psychiatric Research* 2007;16 (Suppl 1): pp. S41–51.

[15] McGlinchey JB, Zimmerman M. Examining a dimensional representation of depression and anxiety disorders' comorbidity in psychiatric outpatients with item response modeling. *Journal of Abnormal Psychology* 2007;116(3): pp.464–474.

[16] Ruscio J, Ruscio AM. Categories and dimensions: Advancing psychological science through the study of latent structure. *Current Directions in Psychological Science* 2008;17: pp. 203–207.

[17] Ruscio J, Zimmerman M, McGlinchey JB, Chelminski I, Young D. Diagnosing major depressive disorder XI: a taxometric investigation of the structure underlying DSM-IV symptoms. *Journal of Nervous and Mental Disease* 2007;195(1): pp. 10-9.

[18] Blatt SJ, Zuroff DC. Interpersonal relatedness and self-definition: two prototypes for depression. *Clinical Psychology Review* 1992;12(5): pp. 527–562.

[19] Widiger TA, Trull TJ, Clarkin JF, Sanderson C, Costa PT. A description of the DSM-III-R and DSM-IV personality disorders with the five-factor model of personality. In: Costa PT, Jr., Widiger TA (1994). *Personality disorders and the five-factor model of personality.* (pp. 41–56). Washington, DC, US: American Psychological Association. viii, 364 pp.

[20] Kuehner C. Gender differences in unipolar depression: an update of epidemiological findings and possible explanations. *Acta Psychiatrica Scandinavica* 2003;108: pp. 163–174.

CHAPTER 10

Anxiety and Obsessive-Compulsive Disorders

Juan J. López-Ibor, Jr

Chairman, Institute of Psychiatry and Mental Health, San Carlos Hospital,
Complutense University, Madrid, Spain

María Inés López-Ibor

Professor of Psychiatry, Department of Psychiatry and Medical Psychology,
Complutense University, Madrid, Spain

10.1 INTRODUCTION

10.1.1 Anxiety and Stress

The psychological reaction to a stressful situation is anxiety. Anxiety is the emotional experience that appears when confronting a non-identified threat [1] and that sets in motion unspecific coping mechanisms. Emotions are always accompanied by bodily phenomena. For the philosopher Sartre [2], these vegetative correlates are the serious side of emotions, since without them they would be a fraud. The vegetative correlate of anxiety is stress. Both represent unspecific reactions of the individual organism when its internal balance (homeostasis) is endangered by potentially insuperable variations of the external milieu challenging the adaptation capacity of the individual. When confronting external threats, the organism sets in motion specific mechanisms (increased blood flow through the muscles, a reaction of alertness and the inhibition of functions not immediately necessary for survival) to face any type of danger. After some time, when the threat has been identified, these unspecific reactions of anxiety and stress are substituted by other much more specific reactions, like fight, escape, adaptation or immunological mechanisms.

Under some circumstances, these essential mechanisms for the survival of the individual become threats themselves, and the reaction is considered pathological. This is the case when they are released by trivial stimuli, when they are of exaggerated intensity or when

Psychiatric Diagnosis: Challenges and Prospects   Edited by I.M. Salloum and J.E. Mezzich
© 2009 John Wiley & Sons, Ltd

they persist longer than needed. In fact, physicians more often treat the response to an external threat than the threat itself. Corticoids, which slow down the reaction of adaptation to stress, act as 'cellular tranquilizers' and anxiolytics have been described as 'corticoids for the mind'. Both drug groups raise the same problems of long-term dependence, precisely by interfering in important physiological mechanisms for the survival of the individual.

10.1.2 Anxiety and Stress-Related Disorders

Anxiety disorders, obsessive compulsive disorder (OCD) and post-traumatic stress disorder (PTSD) are among the most prevalent psychiatric conditions. A considerable burden is associated to these illnesses, not only for the individual sufferer but also for health care systems. Patients with anxiety disorders are frequent users of medical services, especially emergency services [3], are at a high risk for suicide attempts [4] and are at risk for substance abuse [5]. Costs associated with anxiety disorders represent approximately one third of the total attributed to mental health, and anxiety disorders are often underdiagnosed [6] or recognized only years after onset. Many patients who might benefit from treatment are not diagnosed, and even less treated, as clinicians fail to take advantage of available effective treatment strategies [7, 8]. All of this may be due in part to lack of sufficient awareness of anxiety disorders in primary health care and in non-psychiatric facilities. In addition, there is still stigma associated with mental illnesses, and the perception that anxiety disorders are 'minor' diseases that are subject to the goodwill or the manipulation of the sufferers. Patients are often perceived to be feeble persons who 'give in' when confronted by the ordinary stresses of life. All of these facts increase the need for a proper definition and correct diagnosis of anxiety and stress-related disorders.

10.1.3 ICD-10 and DSM-IV-TR Main Principles

The present classifications do not help to solve the issues mentioned above. Both ICD-10 (Table 10.1) and DSM-IV (Table 10.2) establish the diagnosis of diseases mainly on the symptoms present and not on the pathophysiology or other features. Symptom-based classifications have many advantages: they lead to arrangements that are atheoretical, close to clinical reality, easy to grasp and less prone to be contaminated by untested hypothesis. They also have a 'cleansing' effect, leading to a return to the sources of the description of the disorders and above all, they allow a common language worldwide throughout the different schools and perspectives that have dominated psychiatry for decades. This symptom-based approach was introduced by Pinel [9] and his disciple Esquirol [10] two hundred years ago, leading to the birth of scientific psychiatry, although over the decades it was replaced with other methods based on the pathology, the patho-physiology, or the course and outcome.

But classifications based on symptoms also have some drawbacks. They allow a great inter-rater validity, but they may have a low internal validity. For instance, the same patient may get the same diagnosis in different facilities all over the world, but the psychiatrists or even raters of a diagnostic instrument may ignore what the disease in question really is. Classifications based on symptoms do not state what diseases are and, furthermore, the concept of symptom in psychiatry can only be properly applied to organic and symptomatic

Table 10.1   Anxiety disorders in ICD-10. Summarized from [54].

F40-F48 Neurotic, Stress-Related and Somatoform Disorders

F40 Phobic anxiety disorders
    F40.0   Agoraphobia
    F40.1   Social phobias
    F40.2   Specific (isolated) phobias
    F40.8   Other phobic anxiety disorders

F41 Other anxiety disorders
    F41.0   Panic disorder [episodic paroxysmal anxiety]
    F41.1   Generalized anxiety disorder
    F41.2   Mixed anxiety and depressive disorder
    F41.3   Other mixed anxiety disorders
    F41.8   Other specified anxiety disorders Anxiety hysteria

F42 Obsessive-compulsive disorder
    F42.0   Predominantly obsessional thoughts or ruminations
    F42.1   Predominantly compulsive acts [obsessional rituals]
    F42.2   Mixed obsessional thoughts and acts
    F42.8   Other obsessive-compulsive disorders

F43 Reaction to severe stress, and adjustment disorder
    F43.0   Acute stress reaction
    F43.1   Post-traumatic stress disorder
    F43.2   Adjustment disorders
    F43.8   Other reactions to severe stress (culture shock, grief reaction, hospitalism in
           children)

F44 Dissociative [conversion] disorder
    F44.0   Dissociative amnesia
    F44.1   Dissociative fugue
    F44.2   Dissociative stupor
    F44.3   Trance and possession disorders
    F44.4   Dissociative motor disorders
    F44.5   Dissociative convulsions
    F44.6   Dissociative anaesthesia and sensory loss
    F44.7   Mixed dissociative [conversion] disorders
    F44.8   Other dissociative [conversion] disorders (Ganser's syndrome, multiple
           personality)

F45 Somatization disorder
    F45.1   Undifferentiated somatoform disorder
    F45.2   Hypochondriacal disorder
    F45.3   Somatoform autonomic dysfunction
    F45.4   Persistent somatoform pain disorder
    F45.8   Other somatoform disorders (psychogenic: dysmenorrhoea, dysphagia, including
           'globus hystericus', pruritus, torticollis, teeth-grinding)

F48 Other neurotic disorders
    F48.0   Neurasthenia
    F48.1   Depersonalization-derealization syndrome
    F48.8   Other specified neurotic disorders (Dhat syndrome, occupational neurosis,
           including writer's cramp, psychasthenia, psychasthenic neurosis, psychogenic
           syncope)

Table 10.2 Anxiety and other disorders in DSM-IV-TR. Summarized from [55].

ANXIETY DISORDERS	
300.02	Generalized anxiety disorder
Panic disorder	
300.21	With agoraphobia
300.01	Without agoraphobia
300.22	Agoraphobia without history of panic disorder
300.29	Specific phobia
300.23	Social phobia
300.3	Obsessive-compulsive disorder
309.81	Posttraumatic stress disorder
308.3	Acute stress disorder
Anxiety disorder	
293.89	Anxiety disorder due to a general medical condition
SOMATOFORM DISORDERS	
300.81	Somatization disorder
300.81	Undifferentiated somatoform disorder
300.11	Conversion disorder
Pain disorder	
307.89	Associated with both psychological factors and a general medical condition
307.80	Associated with psychological factors
300.7	Hypochondriasis
300.7	Body dysmorphic disorder
FACTITIOUS DISORDERS	
Factitious disorder	
300.19	With combined psychological and physical signs and symptoms
300.19	With predominantly physical signs and symptoms
300.16	With predominantly psychological signs and symptoms
DISSOCIATIVE DISORDERS	
300.6	Depersonalization disorder
300.12	Dissociative amnesia
300.13	Dissociative fugue
300.14	Dissociative identity disorder

psychoses [11]. As a consequence, this kind of approach may generate confusion and disappointment. As we will see, ICD-10 and DSM-IV-TR are not identical and, in the case of anxiety disorders, they use different names and different subtyping.

The titles of the chapters on anxiety disorders are different in ICD-10 and DSM-IV-TR. The WHO classification refers to 'Neurotic, Stress-Related and Somatoform Disorders'. 'Neurotic' is not always a descriptive term and therefore it was not accepted in DSM-III. The ICD-10 advisory members decided to use it for two reasons. First, the psychoanalytic semantic loading of the word is significant in the USA during a particular period of history, but not elsewhere, where the term has a descriptive connotation. Second, there are not many alternative terms. One of them is 'emotional disorders', but this would have led to the embarrassment of having to explain the differences between these and the group of affective disorders. Nevertheless, as we will see later, it may be that there are not such profound differences between the two groups of disorders.

Under the heading 'F40-F48 Neurotic, Stress-Related and Somatoform Disorders', ICD-10 includes anxiety, obsessive-compulsive, reaction to severe stress and adjustment, dissociative (conversion) and somatization disorders; while DSM-IV-TR, under the heading of 'Anxiety Disorders' does not include somatoform, factitious or dissociative disorders. Besides the fact that there are differences in the placement of some disorders (i.e, body dysmorphic disorder) in the names given to others, and the fact that there is no place for neurasthenia in DSM-IV-TR, the lack of consistency between the two systems is due to the fact that DSM-IV-TR follows the principles of symptom-based classifications more strictly.

Here, we will analyse four concrete points: the two approaches to considering and classifying anxiety disorders; some new ways of interpreting clinical evidence; and the case of obsessive-compulsive disorder and stress-related disorders.

10.2   THE TWO APPROACHES TO CONSIDERING AND CLASSIFYING ANXIETY DISORDERS

There are two approaches to considering and classifying anxiety disorders. The first one is guided by lumping, the second by splitting.

William Cullen introduced the term and concept of 'neurosis' in 1777 to describe a group of illnesses being 'preternatural affections of sense or motion' ('preternatural' meaning 'exaggerated' or, in modern terms, 'beyond statistical normality'). The same idea reappears in Kurt Schneider's [11] '*abnorme Persönlichkeiten*', where it is the suffering that makes the abnormality a medical concern.

Freud [12] took a step forward by articulating the neuroses around anxiety. This standpoint opens two questions: first, what is the origin of anxiety and what are the differences between it and 'normal' anxiety; and second, what (secondary) facts are the reasons for the different neuroses. The traditional approach of considering neuroses as psychogenic disorders confuses the boundaries with normality, and is at the core of the stigma mentioned above. In 1950, López Ibor [13] proposed for the first time that at least a significant part of neuroses had a biological origin. This 'medicalization' of the concept based on brain dysfunction and not only on suffering (as in Schneider) is today well accepted.

The experience of anxiety can be so overwhelming that the individual puts in motion psychological mechanisms to cope with it. Some are considered as defence mechanisms, others as coping strategies or styles, and they led to the different clinical pictures of the neuroses.

This 'lumping' perspective is based on some hypotheses, not all of them sufficiently explored; but this fact in itself opens the door for future research. The problem of the 'splitting' atheoretical perspective is that it conveys the message that, by sticking to clinical reality, there is no need for further research. Any layperson can make reliable psychiatric diagnoses for epidemiological studies if correctly trained in the use of diagnostic instruments. This brings great comfort to clinicians who, for the first time in history, can speak a common language worldwide. But this does not mean that the disease is only a set of criteria. The DSM-IV-TR approach has been criticized because it leads to a vicious circle research approach.

Behaviour psychology is based on a splitting perspective. Each neurotic disorder is characterized by a different psychological ill-learned mechanism, which requires a different therapeutic approach. In vivo exposure with response prevention is a technique that works with obsessive patients but not with phobic ones, while the opposite is the case for systematic desensitization. Behaviour therapy does not require so many hypothetical assumptions and DSM-IV-TR anxiety disorders can therefore be seen as a triumph of behaviourism.

10.3 NEW WAYS OF INTERPRETING CLINICAL EVIDENCE

We believe that there is sufficient clinical evidence today for reconsidering the splitting of neurotic-anxiety disorders, to find common features between them and to look for more unitary pathophysiologic mechanisms or phenotypes. The evidence is both in longitudinal and in transversal studies.

10.3.1 The Long-term Evolution of Anxiety Disorders

We have recently published the results of a follow-up, after almost 50 years, of 370 patients diagnosed with anxiety disorder between 1950 and 1961, by López Ibor Sr. [14, 15]. About two thirds of them were re-diagnosed with DSM-III-R criteria as suffering from panic disorder, and the rest from generalized anxiety. On the whole, there is a common pattern of evolution, starting with school phobia in childhood (more prevalent in panic disorder patients), followed by anxiety in the 20s and 30s, depression in the 40s and 50s and somatization disorders at later ages. Interestingly enough, this same pattern is present in one of Freud's patients, the Wolfman [16, 17, 18], although in that case it was tainted by the strong obsessional personality of this character.

Another significant finding is that half of patients with panic disorder ended up having agoraphobia a decade later, while none of those who initially had panic and agoraphobia

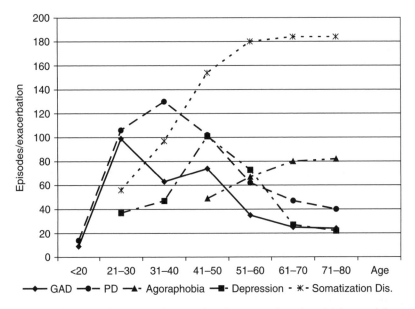

Figure 10.1 Follow-up of panic and generalized anxiety disorders (elaborated from Rubio *et al.*, [14, 15]).

(14% of all PD patients) was relieved of the phobic avoidance symptoms. We found no case of agoraphobia without panic at any point during the five decades. This is strong support for the DSM-IV-TR approach, where phobic avoidance is presented as a consequence of panic; and is in disagreement to ICD-10, where agoraphobia is presented as a self-standing condition (Figure 10.1).

On the same lines of thought, clinicians in the mid-19th century, especially in France, were confronted with cases that presented different symptom configurations at different times. They considered that, although the symptoms of different episodes were dissimilar, they should all be considered as expressions of the same illness. This led to the description of diseases that were characterized by these particular mutations of symptoms, challenging the principles of Pinel [9] and Esquirol [10]. These were the cases of Falret's *folie a double forme* and Broussais' *folie circulaire*, both described in 1854. With our data in hand, GAD, PD, major depression and somatization disorder could be considered as a *folie a quadruple forme*, and agoraphobia as a complication of PD.

10.3.2   Internalizing Disorders

Externalizing behaviours is a concept introduced in child psychiatry several decades ago to consider behaviours that were described by parents or teachers, not by the children themselves. They were present in children in different settings, and the children themselves minimized their problems. As a consequence, the primary informants were parents and teachers. A study by Krueger [19] has brought renewed attention to the concept. The study consisted on factor analyses of patterns of DSM-III-R comorbidity among ten common mental disorders in the National Comorbidity Survey. The ten disorders were: major depressive disorder; dysthymia; generalized anxiety disorder; social phobia; simple phobia; agoraphobia; panic disorder; alcohol dependence; drug dependence; and antisocial personality disorder. Four statistical models were compared:

1. one factor;
2. two factors: internalizing problems (major depressive disorder, dysthymia, GAD, social phobia, simple phobia, agoraphobia and PD) vs externalizing problems (alcohol dependence, drug dependence and antisocial personality disorder);
3. three factors, internalizing problems being divided in two subfactors: anxious-misery (major depressive disorder, dysthymia and GAD) and fear (social phobia, simple phobia, agoraphobia and PD);
4. four factors (affective, anxiety, substance dependence, and antisocial factors).

The three-factor model provided the best fit in the entire sample although, for treatment purposes, the two-factor model provided the best fit.

Several others studies have produced concordant results in clinical and non clinical samples, and demonstrated continuity between childhood and adult problems.

Therefore, taking into account longitudinal as well as transversal studies, there is a need to reconceptualise anxiety and neurotic disorders by:

1. grouping them together in a large cluster; and
2. looking for phenotypes that put emphasis on common pathophysiology and corresponding therapeutic interventions.

10.4   THE CASE OF OBSESSIVE-COMPULSIVE DISORDER

The symptoms of obsessive-compulsive disorders (OCD) consist in different kinds of obsessions and compulsions with rituals, sensory abnormalities, doubts, overvalued ideas, speech abnormalities, emotional abnormalities (depression, anxiety), immediate memory alterations and minor (soft) neurological signs. Obsessions are intrusive, unwanted mental events, usually evoking anxiety or discomfort, and compulsions are behaviours that are experienced with a sense of pressure that is usually reduced once completed. The patient attributes both obsessions and compulsions to an internal source, and both are resisted and lead to significant interference in functioning.

In the DSM-IV-TR, OCD is classified as an anxiety disorder. DSM-IV-TR considers anxiety's principal role in OCD. The obsessions associated with OCD contribute to escalating anxiety, and the compulsive behaviours are often performed to try to reduce this anxiety. In ICD-10, OCD is separated from anxiety disorders. This is consistent with several findings, such as age of onset, prevalence in men and women, and family studies of comorbidity. Pharmacological challenges in some (but not all) studies show exacerbation of symptoms to 5-HT receptor agonists (i.e., mCPP, sumatriptan), but not to other anxyogenic challenges, such as yohimbine, sodium lactate, caffeine, CO_2, cholecystokinin (CCK) and pentagastrin, known to elicit anxiety symptoms in anxiety disorders. On the other hand, as opposed to anxiety disorders and depression, in which there is a return of symptoms following a tryptophan-depletion diet in remitted patients or an augmentation of anxiety during a challenge test, OCD patients seem unaffected. OCD is clearly different from major depression and panic disorder, at least in terms of the involvement in 5HT 1a receptors [20, 21].

OCD patients are unique in regard to their specific response to serotonin reuptake inhibitors, but the pattern of response is different from the response usually seen in depressed patients [22]. On the other hand, noradrenergic medications, which are effective in anxiety and mood disorders, are largely ineffective in OCD. Treatment response to benzodiazepines, which are ineffective in OCD but can be effective in anxiety disorders, is a third pharmacological discriminator. Furthermore, patients with OCD usually do not abuse alcohol or GABA-related drugs, as opposed to patients with anxiety.

Brain circuitry also differentiates OCD from anxiety disorders. Neuroimaging studies have shown hyperactivity of the fronto-striatal circuits with specific and state-dependent increases in the orbital frontal cortex (OFC) of patients with OCD. This hyperactivity is not present when there is comorbid depression [23], a fact that can explain some conflicting results in different studies. The hyperactivity disappears after effective drug or behavioural treatment [24]. Hyperactivity, although not consistently, has also been found in the anterior cingulate cortex (ACC). Electrophysiological studies have shown significantly greater error-related activation of the ACC in OCD patients. Hence, the particular brain circuitry that mediates in OCD appears to be different from that involved in fear, stress-related and mood disorders. Clinical and neuropsychological data attribute most of these symptoms to a frontal lobe dysfunction [25, 26, 27].

OCD is not a homogeneous disorder. Rauch *et al.* [28] have been able to distinguish three symptomatic dimensions, which they have correlated with neuronal abnormalities. These dimensions are:

1. checking behaviour and religious and sexual obsessions;
2. symmetry
3. cleaning obsessions and washing compulsions.

OCD includes subtypes that overlap with both anxiety, mood, motor and other disorders. On the other hand, Leckman *et al.* [29] found four dimensions of OCD:

1. obsessions/checking;
2. symmetry/ordering;
3. contamination/cleaning
4. hoarding.

The first dimension is characterized by obsessions of aggression, sex, religion or about the body and checking behaviours; the second dimension involves preoccupations with order, symmetry or exactness, and/or compulsions of counting, rearranging or ritualistic repetitions; the third dimension involves obsessions about contamination and compulsive washing and cleaning; and the fourth dimension includes hoarding obsessions and compulsions. Correlates have been found between symmetry/hoarding factors and comorbid chronic tics and obsessive-compulsive personality disorder [30]. Individuals diagnosed with Tourette's syndrome or chronic tic disorder scored significantly higher on obsessions/checking and symmetry/ordering factors [29] and hoarding is also associated with pathological grooming behaviours seen in trichotillomania, skin picking and nail biting [31].

Clinicians have long noted an association between obsessive-compulsive disorder and neurological disorders. There are reports of OCD symptoms in seizure disorder, head trauma, cerebral infarction, brain tumours, developmental disorders and other neurological diseases. Research on neurological disorders associated with OCD provides further evidence for a link between OCD and movement disorders due to basal ganglia dysfunction. Symptoms of OCD have been reported in Hungtington's disease, Parkinson's disease, and spasmodic torticollis. Early studies suggested a link between Sydenham's chorea and OCD symptoms and a study by Swedo *et al.* [32] demonstrated that rheumatic fever patients with Sydenham's chorea had significantly greater scores on Leyton Obsessional Inventory than those without chorea. This has led to the inclusion of OCD as a candidate among the Paediatric Autoimmune Neuropsychiatric Disorders Associated with Streptococcal infections (PANDAS). Long ago, Schilder [33] suggested that subtle neurological abnormalities were present in about one third of OCD cases, while Conde *et al.* [34] and Hollander *et al.* [35] described soft neurological soft signs in OCD.

The Cape Town OCD Consensus Group [36] has put forward the proposal for a reclassification of OCD into an obsessive compulsive-spectrum disorder (OCSD) cluster. Similarities in symptomatology, course of illness, patient population and neurocircuitry of OCD and OCSD are supported by co-morbidity, family and neurological studies, which also offer a critical re-evaluation into the relationship between OCD and anxiety disorders. Because of shared obsessive-compulsive features, co-morbidity, lifetime course, neurocircuitry, patient demographics, lifetime course and treatment response, OCD may be reconceptualized as an element of an OCD spectrum disorder (Table 10.3) alongside body dysmorphic disorder, pathological gambling, eating disorders and autism [37, 38, 39, 40].

In conclusion, OCD is associated with symptoms that involve several neuropsychiatric functions: thought, sense, language, memory and movement. Furthermore, OCD patients have perception disorders, doubts, over-valued ideas, speech disorders and emotion disorders, immediate memory deficits, and neurological soft signs. Therefore, in the pathophysiology of this disorder, many brain regions must be affected. These regions are also involved in other neuropsychiatric disorders and as a consequence it seems reasonable to withdraw OCD from the anxiety disorders group and to create a new cluster of OCD spectrum disorders.

Table 10.3 Suggested obsessive-compulsive related disorders.

Currently not classified as OCDs	Currently classified as OCD
Tourette's syndrome	Hoarding
Trichotillomania	OCD plus tics
Body dysmorphic disorder	Sydenham's chorea/PANDAS
Hypochondriasis	
Eating disorders	
Impulse control disorders – NOS	
Paraphilia	
Behavioural addiction (e.g. pathological gambling)	

10.5   THE CASE OF STRESS-RELATED DISORDERS

The classification of stress-related disorders is an exception in ICD-10 and DSM-IV-TR because the basic criterion for diagnosis is not the clinical manifestations but the pathogenesis of the disorder. Therefore, the section on stress related disorders is not articulated around symptoms. This fact is more pronounced in ICD-10 than in DSM-IV-TR, which still considers some peculiarities in the clinical manifestations of stress-related disorders. This exception in the differences between both systems is due to a more elaborated proposal by DSM (Table 10.4).

Stress-related disorders include only those disorders that appear in extremely stressing situations. The notion is that it should be an overwhelming event. Most of the individuals, when confronted with such an event, may give way. Ordinary life events are not considered here. The underlying concept is that so-called life events, although important for the unchaining of many diseases, have an unspecific effect (they may unchain different diseases in different individuals), while, here, we are dealing with specific effects and specific disorders.

Only the chapter on schizophrenia stress has relevance due to the presence of brief psychotic disorder in DSM-TR and a series of acute and transient psychotic disorders

Table 10.4 Stress-related disorders in ICD-10 and DSM-IV-TR. Summarized from [54, 55].

ICD-10	DSM-IV
Neurotic, stress-related and somatoform disorders	Anxiety Disorders
F43 Reaction to severe stress, and adjustment disorders	
F43.0 Acute stress reaction	308.3 Acute stress disorder
F43.1 Post-traumatic stress disorder	309.81 Postraumatic stress disosder
F43.2 Adjustment disorders	ADJUSTMENT DISORDERS
	309.0 With depressed mood
	309.24 With anxiety
	309.28 With mixed anxiety and depressed mood
	309.3 With disturbance of conduct
	309.4 With mixed disturbance of emotions and conduct
F43.8 Other reactions to severe stress	

with marked stressors (brief reactive psychoses) in ICD-10 (F23.01 Acute polymorphic psychotic disorder without symptoms of schizophrenia, due to acute stress; F23.11 Acute polymorphic psychotic disorder with symptoms of schizophrenia, due to acute stress; F23.21 Acute schizophrenia like psychotic disorder, due to acute stress; F23.31 Other acute predominantly delusional psychotic disorder, due to acute stress and F23.81 Other acute and transient psychotic disorders, due to acute stress). Nevertheless, there are other kinds of psychotic disorder that appear after being exposed to a disaster, which are not include neither in ICD-10 nor in DSM-IV [41]. On the other hand, the personality changes following exposure to trauma that were described by Venzlaff [42] do not appear in DSM-IV-TR, and in ICD-10 they are mentioned in the chapter on personality disorders (F62.0 Enduring personality change after catastrophic experience).

The clinical manifestations of stress-related disorders overlap considerably with those of mood, anxiety and personality disorders, although post-traumatic stress disorder (PTSD) has some particular features. Sometimes the criteria for differentiation of those manifestations seem to be arbitrary and provisional, mainly when timeframes are considered. For instance, the duration of brief depressive reaction is up to one month, and the time span for adaptative depressive reaction is from one month to two years. What if the patient is still ill beyond this limit? The answer is that the diagnosis should be changed to dysthymia, a diagnosis that requires a minimum of two years of evolution. In this example, from one day to the next, the basic criterion of diagnosis (stress) is suddenly shifted to another (the presence of depressive symptoms of a minimum duration). This fact puts forward the limits of current classification systems. The main criteria, symptoms, course, aetiology and pathophysiology are not independent. The diagnosis of brief depressive reaction, adaptative depressive reaction and dysthymia shows a combination of the three criteria. Stress is the aetiopathogenic factor in brief and adaptative reactions, while the clinical manifestations and the course get priority at latter stages.

10.5.1 The Psychiatric Responses to Disasters

The anxiety-stress model mentioned above also applies to disasters. Here the stressor is an event that threatens the social 'homeostasis', that is, the mechanisms that operate to maintain the structure and functions of social groups. Disasters have been defined in many ways [43], among them one that underlines the fact that disasters overcome the possibilities of adaptation of a social group [44]. That is why disasters require external help. The issue is not the intensity of the stressor, but the fact that a disaster is an unexpected or unwanted misfortune (dis-aster, lit. is something wrong with the stars). A disaster challenges the foundations of a society and urges it to look for new explanations and give a meaning to the misfortune.

These social aspects of stress are not sufficiently explicit in ICD-10 or DSM-IV. They should be, because social dimensions are essential to cope with disasters and implement interventions that are useful for preventing and treating individual reactions.

Another aspect that is not sufficiently considered in ICD-10 nor in DSM-IV-TR is the fact that reactions to stress develop in stages. These were initially described by Glass [45] in war related disasters and are constantly observed in everyone: (1) the pre-impact phase; (2) impact; (3) post-impact; and (4) recovery. They correspond with the stages of development of stress according to Selye [46, 47]. This time dimension is also useful for clinical intervention, including prevention and rehabilitation. The consequences of a disaster are not over until some kind of reconciliation is reached [48, 49], in which all the agents involved assume the meaning and responsibility of the adversity, for which the stars are not to be blamed. This is clear for man-made disasters but in every natural disaster there are some human implications: natural disasters always hit and have the worst consequences in the most deprived zones of the globe.

In any case, the description of the psychiatric consequences of exposure to disasters of mass violence in ICD-10 and DSM-IV-TR does not always cover the reality or the needs of the rescue teams [50, 51, 52].

10.5.2   Diagnostic Criteria for Acute Stress Disorder in ICD-10 and DSM-IV-TR

In ICD-10, acute stress disorder is immediate and disappears in two days. It is characterized by one or both of two groups of symptoms:

1. the reduction of awareness, difficulty in understanding, disorientation, isolation, depression and desperation;
2. flight, anxiety, irritability and vegetative hyperexcitability.

ICD-10 follows the model that Kretschmer [53] proposed for hysteria, arranged around primitive defence mechanisms, the *Totstellung reflex* (death feigning reflex, death feint) manifested in the mimetic behaviour of an animal trying to disappear at the sight of a predator and the *Bewegungssturm* (movement storm or tempest, instinct flurry) of the poultry in the henhouse when they fly around madly, frightened by some danger. López Ibor Sr. [13] extended this description to all neurotic phenomena and called them *'sobre-cogimiento'* and *'sobresalto'* (lit. terrifying and startle reactions).

DSM-IV describes a different picture. Acute stress disorder lasts from two days to four weeks but it can start later, until the end of the four first weeks. The picture includes dissociative symptoms (subjective sense of numbing, detachment, absence of emotional responsiveness), reduction of awareness, de-realization, de-personalization and dissociate amnesia. It may also present symptoms of PTSD and if it lasts more than four weeks, then this last condition is the diagnosis.

10.5.3   Diagnostic Criteria for Post-Traumatic Stress Disorder (PTSD) in ICD-10 and DSM-IV-TR

Both ICD-10 and DSM-IV require the presence of a stressor, but ICD-10 puts an emphasis on the event itself while DSM-IV puts an emphasis on the person affected.

In ICD-10, a stressor is an event or situation of exceptionally threatening or catastrophic nature, and is likely to cause pervasive distress in almost anyone. In DSM-IV-TR, the criteria are:

1. The person experienced, witnessed or was confronted with an event or events that involved actual or threatened death or serious injury, or a threat to the physical integrity of self or other.
2. The person's response involves intense fear, helplessness or horror (or unorganized or agitated behaviour in children).

Following this, both systems require the presence of particular symptoms. The first necessary symptom is similar in both, but formulated in different ways: repetitive intrusive recollection or re-enactment of the event in memories, daytime imagery or dreams; persistent remembering or 're-living' of the stressors in intrusive 'flashbacks', vivid memories or recurring dreams; and experiencing distress when exposed to circumstances resembling or associated with the stressor.

The traumatic event is persistently re-experienced in one (or more) of the following ways: recurrent and intrusive distressing recollection of the event; recurrent distressing dreams of the event; acting or feeling as if the traumatic event was recurring; intense psychological distress at exposure to internal or external clues that symbolize or resemble an aspect of the traumatic event; and psychological reactivation at exposure to internal or external clues that symbolize or resemble an aspect of the traumatic event.

ICD-10 Diagnostic Guidelines (ICD-10-DG) do not add any other necessary symptoms, but adds a few that are either typical or common, which are necessary symptoms in ICD-Research Diagnostic Criteria (ICD-10-RDC) and in DSM-IV, such as avoidance and actual or preferred avoidance of circumstances resembling or associated with the stressor, which was not present before the exposure to the stressor. ICD-10-RDC does not mention numbness. DSM-IV-TR includes persistent avoidance of stimuli associated with the trauma and numbing of general responsiveness (not present before trauma), as indicated by three (or more) of the following: (1) efforts to avoid thoughts, feelings, or conversations associated with the trauma; (2) efforts to avoid activities, places or people that arouse recollections of the trauma; (3) inability to recall an important aspect of the trauma; (4) markedly diminished interest or participation in significant activities; (5) feelings of detachment or estrangement from others; (6) restricted range of affect and (7) a sense of foreshortened future.

Autonomic hyperarousal is an important diagnostic feature in ICD-10 and in DSM-IV-TR. ICD-10 mentions autonomic hyperarousal with hypervigilance, enhanced startle reaction, insomnia, persistent symptoms of increased psychological sensitivity and arousal (not present before exposure to stressor), shown by any two of the following: difficulty in falling or staying asleep; irritability or outbursts of anger; difficulty in concentrating, hypervigilance and exaggerated startle response. In DSM-IV-TR, hyperarousal is defined as persistent symptoms of increased psychological sensitivity and arousal (not present before exposure to stressor), shown by any two of the following: difficulty in falling or staying asleep; irritability or outbursts of anger; difficulty in concentrating, hypervigilance and exaggerated startle response.

ICD-10-DG, although less strict for the diagnosis, adds a series of typical, common or rare symptoms not present in ICD-10-RDC or DSM-IV-TR, such as: a sense of 'numbness' and emotional blunting; detachment from others; unresponsiveness to surroundings; anhedonia; anxiety and depression; and dramatic acute bursts of fear, panic or aggression triggered by reminders. The symptom set of inability to recall is only present in ICD-10-RDC.

In summary, the presence of a stressor and the re-experience of the event are the two criteria present in all the diagnostic systems. ICD-10-RDC and DSM-IV, being stricter, add two more criteria: avoidance and increased physiological arousal. ICD-10-RDC allows this to be substituted by inability to recall, while ICD-10 Guidelines add a few more symptoms that are not necessary for the diagnosis but may be typical (numbness), common (anxiety and depression) or rare (acute bursts of fear or aggression).

REFERENCES

[1] Baeyer W von. Angst als erlebtes Bedrohtsein. *Der Nervenarzt* 1984;55: pp. 349–357.

[2] Sartre JP. Esquisse d'une Théorie des Emotions. Paris: Hermann; 1939.

[3] Wang PS, Berglund P, Olfson M, Pincus HA, Wells KB, Kessler RC. Failure and delay in initial treatment contact after first onset of mental disorders in the National Comorbidity Survey Replication. *Archives of General Psychiatry* 2005;62(6): pp. 603–613.

[4] Weissman MM, Bland RC, Camino GJ, Greenwald S, Hwu HG, Lee CK. The cross national epidemiology of obsessive compulsive disorder. The Cross National Collaborative Group. *Journal of Clinical Psychiatry* 1994;55: (Suppl) pp. 5–10.

[5] Brady KT, Lydiard RB: The association of alcoholism and anxiety. *Psychiatric Quarterly* 1993;64(2): pp. 135–149.

[6] Sartorius N, Üstün TB, Lecrubier Y, Wittchen HU. Depression comorbid with anxiety: results from the WHO study on psychological disorders in primary health care. *British Journal of Psychiatry*. 1996(30): Suppl pp.38–43.

[7] Bandelow B, Sievert K, Röthemeyer M, Hajak G, Broocks A, Rüther E. Panic disorder and agoraphobia: what is effective? *Fortschritte der Neurologie-Psychiatrie* 1995;63(11): pp. 451–464.

[8] Cowley DS, Ha EH, Roy-Byrne PP. Determinants of pharmacologic treatment failure in panic disorder. *Journal of Clinical Psychiatry* 1997;58(12): pp. 555–561; quiz pp. 562–563.

[9] Pinel P. *Traité médico-philosophique sur l'alienation mentale.* (1809) Paris: Brosson; 1842.

[10] Esquirol E. *Des maladies mentales considerées sous les rapports médical, hygiénique et médico-légal.* París: JB Baillière et fils; 1864.

[11] Schneider K. *Clinical Psychopathology.* New York: Grune and Stratton; 1959.

[12] Freud S. *Hemmung, Symptom und Angst.* Leipzig-Vienna-Zurich: Internationaler Psychoanalytischer Verlag; 1926. GW, 14: pp. 111–205; Inhibitions, symptoms, and anxiety. SE, 20: pp. 77–172.

[13] López Ibor JJ. *La angustia vital.* Madrid: Paz Montalvo; 1950.

[14] Rubio G, López-Ibor JJ. Generalized anxiety disorder: a 40-year follow-up study. *Acta Psychiatrica Scandinavica* 2007;115(5): pp. 372–379.

[15] Rubio G, López-Ibor JJ. What can be learnt from the natural history of anxiety disorders? *European Psychiatry* 2007;22(2): pp. 80–86.

[16] Gardiner M. *The Wolf-Man and Sigmund Freud.* Hardmondsworth: Penguin; 1973.

[17] López-Ibor Aliño JJ. Sergio, el Hombre de los Lobos. ¿Un espejismo de psicoanálisis? *Actas Luso-Españolas de Neurología, Psiquiatría y Ciencias Afines* 1973;1 (1): pp. 127–151.

[18] Obholzer K. *The Wolf-Man: conversations with Freud's patient sixty years later.* 1982. Continuum, New York, 1982.

[19] Krueger RF. The structure of common mental disorders. *Archives of General Psychiatry* 1999;56(10): pp. 921–926.

[20] Lesch KP. Modulation of receptor G-Protein complex function by psychotropic drugs and glucocorticoids: implications for anxiety disorders and depresión. *European Neuropsychopharmacology* 1991;3: pp. 340–343.

[21] Zohar AH, Kindler S. Serotoninergic probes in obsessive-compulsive disorder. *International Clinical Psychopharmacology* 1992:7: pp. 39–40. 1992.

[22] Fernández Córdoba E, López-Ibor JJ. Monochlorimipramine in the treatment of psychiatric patients resistant to other teraphies. *Actas Luso-Españolas de Neurología, Psiquiatría y Ciencias Afines* 1967;26: pp. 119–147.

[23] Crespo Facorro B, Cabranes JA, López-Ibor Alcocer MI, Paya B, Fernández Perez C, encinas M, Ayuso Mateos JL, López-Ibor JJ. Regional cerebral blood flow in obsessive-compulsive patients with and without cronic tic disorder. A SPECT study. *European Archives of General Psychiatry and Clinical Neuroscience* 1999;249: pp. 156–161.

[24] Baxter LR, Scwartz JM, Bergman KS *et al.* Caudate glucose metabolic rate changes with both drug and behaviour therapy for obsessive-compulsive disorder. *Archives of General Psychiatry* 1992;49: pp. 681–689.

[25] Behar BM, Rapoport JL, Berg CJ. Computerized tomography and neuropsychological measures in adolescents with obsessive-compulsive disorder. *American Journal of Psychiatry* 1984;141: pp. 363–369.

[26] Flor-Henry P, Yeudall LT, Koles ZJ, Howarth B. Neuropsychological and power spectral EEG investigations of the obsessive-compulsive syndrome. *Biological Psychiatry* 1979;14: pp. 119–130.

[27] Khama S. Obsessive-compulsive disorder: Is there a frontal lobe dysfunction? *Biological Psychiatry* 1988;24: pp. 602–613.

[28] Rauch S, Dougherty D, Shin L, Alpert N, Manzo P, Fiscman A, Jenike M, Baer L. Neuronal correlates of factor analyzed OCD symptom dimensions: a PET study. *CNS Spectrums* 1998;3 (7): pp. 37–43.

[29] Leckman JF, Zhang H, Alsobrook JP, Pauls DL. Symptom dimensions in obsessive-compulsive disoder Toward Quantitative phenotypes. *American Journal of Medical Genetics* 2001;105: pp. 28–30.

[30] Baer L. Factor analysis of symptom subtypes of obsessive-compulsive disorder and their relation to personality and tic disorders. *Journal of Clinical Psychiatry* 1994;55: pp. 18–23.

[31] Bienvenu OJ, Samuels JF, Riddle MA, Hoehn-Saric R, Liang KY, Cullen BA. The relationship of obsessive–compulsive disorder to possible spectrum disorders: results from a family study. *Biological Psychiatry* 2000;48: pp. 287–293.

[32] Swedo SE, Rapoport JL, Cheslow DL *et al*. High prevalence of obsessive-compulsive symptoms in patients with Sydenham's chorea. *American Journal of Psychiatry* 1989;146: pp. 246–249.

[33] Schilder P. The organic background of obsessions and compulsions. *American Journal of Psychiatry* 1983;94: pp. 1397–1414.

[34] Conde López V, de la Gándara Martín JJ, Blanco Lozano ML, Cerezo Rodríguez P, Martínez Roig M, de Dios Francos A. Minor neurologic signs in obsessive-compulsive disorders. *Actas Luso-Españolas de Neurología, Psiquiatría y Ciencias Afines* 1991;19(1): pp. 1–21.

[35] Hollander E, De Caria CM, Saud JB, Klein DF, Liebowitz MR. Neurological soft signs in OCD. *Archives of General Psychiatry* 1991;48: pp. 278–279.

[36] Cape Town OCD Consensus Group (Eric Hollander E, Stein DJ, Westenberg HGM, Baldwin DS, Bandelow B, Black DW, Blier P, Fineberg NA, Flament MM, Geller D, Khanna S, López-Ibor JJ, Pallantini S, Zohar J.) *CNS Spectrum* 2007;12(3): Suppl Feb.

[37] Hollander E, Friedberg JP, Wasserman S, Yeh CC, Iyengar R. The case for the OCD spectrum. In: Abramowitz JS, Houts AC. (eds.) *Handbook of controversial issues in obsessive–compulsive disorder*. New York: Kluwer Academic Press; 2005.

[38] Jenike MA. Illnesses related to obsessive–compulsive disorder. In: Jenike MA, Baer LB, Minichiello WE. (eds.) *Obsessive compulsive disorders: theory and management*. 2nd ed. Year Book Medical; 1990. pp. 39–60.

[39] McElroy SL, Phillips KA, Keck PE. Obsessive compulsive spectrum disorder. *Journal of Clinical Psychiatry* 1994;55: pp.33–51 (Suppl. 10).

[40] Stein DJ. Neurobiology of the obsessive–compulsive spectrum disorders. *Biological Psychiatry* 2002;47: pp. 296–304.

[41] Crocq L, Doutheau C, Louville P, Cremniter D. Psychiatrie de catastrophe. Réactions immédiates et différées, troubles séquellaires. Paniques et psychopathologie collective. Encyclopédie Médico-Chirurgicale. (Paris: Elsevier.) *Psychiatrie* 1998;37–113-D-10: p. 8.

[42] Venzlaff U. *Die psychoreaktiver Störungen nach entschädingungspflichten Ereignissen*. Berlin: Springer Verlag; 1958.

[43] Quarantelli EL. *The consequences of disasters for mental health: conflicting views*. Preliminary paper no. 62. Ohio State University, Columbus; 1979.

[44] Benyakar M, Kutz I, Dasberg H, Stern M. The Collapse of a Structure: A Structural Approach to Trauma. *Journal of Traumatic Stress* 1989;2 (4): pp. 431–449.

[45] Glass AJ. Psychological aspects of disasters. *Journal of the American Medical Association* 1959;171: pp. 188–191.

[46] Selye H. *The Stress of Life*. New York: McGraw-Hill; 1956.

[47] Selye H. The Stress Concept Today. In: Kutash IL, Schlesinger LB *et al*. (eds.) *Handbook of Stress and Anxiety*. San Francisco: Jossey-Bass; 1980.

[48] López-Ibor Aliño JJ. Psychopathological aspects of the Toxic Oil Syndrome Catastrophe. *British Journal of Psychiatry* 1985;147: pp. 352–365.

[49] López-Ibor Aliño JJ, Jiménez Arriero MA. Psychosocial Rehabilitation in Disasters: The Experience of the Spanish Toxic Oil Syndrome. *International Disability Studies* 1987;9: pp. 78–80.

[50] Crocq L, Doutheau C, Salham, M. Les réactions emotionnelles dans les catastrophes. In: *Encyclopédie Médico-Chirurgicale*. Éditions Techniques. Paris; 1987.
[51] Crocq L. Le trauma et ses mythes. *Psychologie Medicale* 1993;25(10): pp. 992–999.
[52] Crocq L, 1999. Les traumatismes psychiques de guerre. Paris, Jacob.
[53] Kretschmer E. *Hysterie, Reflex und Instinkt*. Stuttgart: Georg Thieme Verlag; 1948.
[54] World Health Organization. *International Statistical Classification of Diseases and Related Health Problems, Tenth Revision (ICD-10)*. Geneva: WHO; 1992.
[55] American Psychiatric Association. *Diagnostic and statistical manual of mental disorders, Fourth Edition. Text Revision. (DSM-IV-TR)*. Washington, DC: American Psychiatric Association; 2000.

CHAPTER 11

Substance-Use Disorders

Christian Haasen
Professor, Zentrum für interdisziplinäre Suchtforschung, Hamburg, Germany
Nady el-Guebaly
Addiction Division, University of Calgary, Canada; Chair, Section on Addiction Psychiatry, World Psychiatric Association
Ihsan M. Salloum
Professor of Psychiatry and Director, Division of Alcohol and Substance Abuse: Treatment and Research, University of Miami Miller School of Medicine, FL, USA; Section on Classification, Diagnostic Assessment and Nomenclature, World Psychiatric Association

11.1 INTRODUCTION: SUBSTANCE USE ASSESSMENT

The identification of an individual with an addiction disorder begins by observing indicators of impairment, the presence of signs, symptoms or aberrant behaviour. The presence of such an indicator may point toward a diagnosis of an addiction disorder, but does not by itself determine such a diagnosis. It is essential that an accurate diagnosis be obtained by further evaluation.

A comprehensive evaluation consists of the following:

1. interview by a physician experienced in the treatment of addictive disorders;
2. accumulation of data from collateral sources, such as family members, friends, partners or others;
3. a physical examination and laboratory studies.

The interview should be completed by a physician experienced in performing careful assessment of substance abuse history and potential psychiatric comorbidity. It is helpful to conceptualize drug or alcohol use history as progressing through four stages:

a. Experimental: This refers to the first use of a substance and is limited to the initial substance-use experiences.
b. Occasional: The individual is a passive occasional user of a substance (one to three times a month), using it only when offered or made available, but without actively seeking it.

Psychiatric Diagnosis: Challenges and Prospects   Edited by I.M. Salloum and J.E. Mezzich
© 2009 John Wiley & Sons, Ltd

c. Regular: The user actively pursues the substance and spends money on it. Frequency of use increases to several times a week.
d. Substance abuse or dependence.

Important for the assessment of the substance abuse history is the age at which each of these stages occurred, as well as information on the pattern of use, as reflected by route of administration, frequency of use, duration of use, and circumstances of use. A similar history should be assessed for all substances ever used. It is also important to determine the consequences of each substance used, including possible accidents, conflicts with others, and health or legal problems. Abstinence periods also need to be assessed, including information on how abstinence was achieved, whether other substances were used in that period and where the motivation to abstinence or treatment is derived from. The function of substance use with respect to gender-specific aspects should also be assessed.

Laboratory tests that are useful for the diagnostic evaluation include the following:

1. urine screen for drugs of abuse: opiates, cocaine, marijuana (cannabis), amphetamines, benzodiazepines, phencyclidine, and barbiturates;
2. complete blood count (CBC);
3. blood chemistry profile including Gamma Glutamyl Transpeptidase (GGT), Aspartate Amino Transferase (AST), and Alanine Amino Transferase (ALT);
4. hepatitis antigen and antibody tests, possibly also HIV test (with patient's permission).

Furthermore, there are other possible laboratory indicators of an alcohol use disorder that can be used. These include Carbohydrate Deficient Transferrin (CDT), Ethyl Glucoronide (EtG), and Phosphatidyl Ethanol (PEth), which are much more specific for alcohol use compared to the traditional biomarkers reflecting liver damage (GGT, AST, ALT).

Accurate diagnosis of a substance-use disorder is often made more difficult by the characteristic defences of patients with these disorders (e.g., minimization, denial, projection, grandiosity) and the reluctance of the patient's family, friends or co-workers to confront the patient or disclose information about these sensitive issues. Covert and overt attitudes of physicians about substance use, such as reluctance to recognize the harmful effects because of the physician's own pattern of substance use, a tendency to view these disorders as moral shortcomings rather than valid psychiatric disorders, or concerns about 'labelling' and the patient's potential angry response, may also interfere with timely diagnosis and treatment. Far from stigmatizing the patient, however, accurately diagnosing a substance-use disorder and clearly delineating the patient's problems as a result of substance use are critical steps in motivating behavioural change and commitment to treatment.

11.2   DIAGNOSTIC INSTRUMENTS

A number of short, self-report questionnaires are available to aid in the routine detection of substance-use disorders. Once a disorder has been detected, structured interviews can provide a reliable method to elicit diagnostic information and decrease the chance of omitting questions about significant signs or symptoms. Among the short questionnaires to detect alcohol use disorders, two merit special mention: the CAGE and the AUDIT. The four-question CAGE questionnaire has been found to improve routine detection rates in primary care. The Alcohol Use Disorder Identification Test (AUDIT) was developed by the WHO as a simple, 10-question method of screening for excessive drinking and to assist in brief assessment. With respect to drug abuse, similar short questionnaires have been developed, such as the 20-question Drug Abuse Screening Test (DAST), but are not as widely used in primary care as the counterparts for alcohol use. An attempt to screen for all major substance groups is made with the Alcohol, Smoking, Substance Involvement Screening Test (ASSIST), an eight-item questionnaire recently developed by the WHO.

One of the most widely used structured interviews for substance-use disorders is the Addiction Severity Index (ASI). The ASI facilitates a multidimensional assessment by evaluating the severity of problems experienced by the patient on seven domains including alcohol and drug abuse, and medical, psychiatric, social, legal and occupational problems. Initial ASI ratings of problem severity are highly correlated with treatment outcome and can be used to guide treatment selection such as specialized psychiatric interventions or hospital-based treatment. The Structured Clinical Interview for DSM-IV (SCID) and the Psychiatric Research Interview for Substance and Mental Disorders for DSM-IV (PRISM) are clinician administered interviews primarily used in research settings, which provide a systematic assessment of psychopathology designed to obtain a DSM-IV diagnosis of substance use and other psychiatric disorders, and are therefore useful tools to diagnosing comorbid psychiatric disorders.

11.3   DIAGNOSTIC CRITERIA OF SUBSTANCE-USE DISORDERS

Of the many proposed systems for diagnosing and classifying substance-use disorders, two are most widely used across the world: the International Classification of Diseases (ICD) published by the World Health Organization (WHO), presently in its tenth revision (ICD-10), with most international use for clinical care, and the Diagnostic and Statistical Manual of Mental Disorders (DSM) issued by the American Psychiatric Association (APA), currently in its fourth edition (DSM-IV), with most wide international use, especially for research purposes . Both systems were strongly influenced by the dependence syndrome concept caused by the repetitive use of psychoactive substances, with subsequent development of adverse consequences. Therefore, the concept of substance dependence in DSM-IV is very similar to that in ICD-10 (see Table 11.1). However, the diagnoses of harmful substance use (ICD-10) and substance abuse (DSM-IV) substantially differ and probably address different conditions.

Only one of the criteria truly differs between DSM and ICD: the inclusion of subjective compulsion in ICD-10 and not in DSM-IV. Furthermore, the DSM-IV gives more weight to the elements of preoccupation with substances and impaired control of substance use by including two criteria for each of these concepts where the ICD-10 includes pairs of DSM-IV criteria in a single symptom. In clinical practice, the difference between the diagnoses of substance dependence is marginal between the two classification systems – agreement is high across classes of drugs and across different settings and countries.

Agreement between the diagnosis of a substance-related disorder below the threshold of substance dependence in the two classification systems DSM and ICD is very low. For

Table 11.1 Comparison of criteria for substance use disorders in DSM-IV and ICD-10 [10, 11].

DSM-IV	ICD-10
Substance dependence:	*Substance dependence:*
At least three of the following, occurring at any time in the same 12-month period:	At least three of the following, occurring at any time in the same 12-month period:
• Tolerance • Withdrawal • Use in larger amounts or longer periods than intended • Wish to cut down use • Time spent to obtain substance • Other activities are given up • Use despite physical or psychological problems	• Tolerance • Withdrawal • Impaired control with respect to amount or length of period using substance, or wish to cut down use Preoccupation with substance use, giving up other activities, spending much time to obtain substance • Use despite harmful consequences • Compulsion (craving)
Substance abuse:	
Any of the following within a 12-month period: • Failure of role obligations • Hazardous use (e.g. driving under the influence) • Substance-related legal problems • Use despite social problems	
	Harmful use: • Substance-induced psychological or physical harm

ICD-10, the category 'harmful use' is defined by clear-cut medical or psychological consequences of substance use in the absence of dependence. In DSM-IV, the category 'substance abuse' emphasizes social and legal consequences in the absence of dependence. The lack of inclusion of social consequences in the ICD-10 concept of harmful use reflects the aim to develop criteria that can be applied uniformly across different countries and cultures, as social and legal consequences of substance use are likely to vary widely across cultures and across time. Cross-cultural concerns were less important for DSM-IV, which was designed principally for the use in the USA. Furthermore, the development of social consequences most often predates physical and psychological consequences in the natural history of pathological substance-use disorders, so that the inclusion of social consequences as one of the criteria allows treatment providers to document a substance-related diagnosis as the target of their treatment at an early stage.

11.4   OTHER SUBSTANCE-INDUCED DISORDERS

There are a number of other diagnoses, in both DSM-IV and ICD-10, covering syndromes that result from acute or chronic substance use. For both systems, the greatest number of syndromes is associated with alcohol use, and there are only few differences

Table 11.2 Comparison of substance-induced disorders in DSM-IV and ICD-10 [10, 11].

DSM-IV	ICD-10
Intoxication	Acute intoxication
Intoxication delirium	With delirium
Withdrawal	Withdrawal
(no longer included)	Pathological intoxication
Alcohol-induced persisting dementia	Residual and late-onset psychotic disorder
Alcohol-induced persisting amnestic disorder	Amnestic syndrome
Substance-induced psychotic disorder with hallucinations	Organic delusional disorder, organic hallucinosis, residual or late-onset psychotic disorder
Substance-induced mood disorder	Organic mood (affective) disorder or residual and late onset psychotic disorder
Substance-induced anxiety disorder	Organic anxiety disorder
Substance-induced sexual dysfunction	–
Substance-induced sleep disorder	–
Substance-related disorder NOS	Other disorder; unspecified mental or behavioural disorder

between DSM-IV and ICD-10 (see Table 11.2). The three exceptions – exclusion of pathological intoxication and inclusion of substance-induced sexual and sleep disorders in DSM-IV – were based on results of literature reviews suggesting the absence of a unique syndrome of pathological intoxication and the presence of substance-induced sexual and sleep disorders.

11.5 FUTURE DIRECTIONS OF DIAGNOSING ADDICTION DISORDERS

As all diagnostic systems strive to be of optimal use in the clinic and for the needs of epidemiology and public health planning, diagnostic concepts undergo continuous evaluation, looking at whether criteria is both valid and straightforward, and reviewing new evidence relevant to the diagnosis and classification of substance-use disorders. Workgroups have been set up to spearhead this review process in preparation for the development of DSM-V and ICD-11. The issues that need to be covered by future diagnostic systems reflect the shortcomings of past and present diagnostic concepts on the one hand, as well as a change in the understanding of disorders on the other.

11.6 CATEGORICAL VS DIMENSIONAL

One of the most important issues being discussed with respect to substance-use disorders (SUDs) is the question of whether SUDs should be considered as categorical or dimensional. The choice between categorical and dimensional views of disorders has created a long-standing debate, not only for SUDs but also in psychiatry in general. In the context of present diagnostic concepts, the categorical view dominates because it meets clinical needs, especially in the light of reporting to insurance companies. The interest in dimensional approaches, where a quantitative score is measured, has mainly been a focus for research purposes. The questions raised are which of the two approaches is most suitable for which particular purpose, and how we can translate between categorical and dimensional representations. Categorical distinctions are essential to clinical decision-making [1], while dimensional assessments are superior for predicting treatment needs and clinical outcome [2]. Furthermore, comorbidity among SUDs represents a major challenge for a strictly categorical approach, with multiple diagnoses being very common – a quantitative taxonomic model may reflect comorbidity among SUDs more adequately [3].

Extensive research has been undertaken to develop a dimensional model, which has resulted in the development of dimensional tools regularly used in the identification and quantification of various aspects of substance use. By including a dimensional component, even on a symptom level, the clinical database would not only be enriched, but the patient response burden is also reduced as patients are not forced to choose between two response extremes of present or absent. Helzer *et al.* (2006) [4] suggest that a dimensional approach should be offered in future revisions of the classification systems, but that these dimensional approaches be linked to an amplified categorical definition.

11.7   INCLUSION OF NEUROBIOLOGICAL FEATURES IN DIAGNOSING ADDICTIVE DISORDERS

Much progress in neurobiology has provided a heuristic neurocircuitry framework with which to identify mechanisms involved in the development of addictive disorders (see also Koob [5]). The brain reward system implicated in the development of addictive disorders is comprised of key elements of a basal forebrain macrostructure, termed the extended amygdala, and its connections. Studies have provided evidence for the dysregulation of specific neurochemical mechanisms in specific brain reward neurochemical systems in the extended amygdale (dopamine, opioid peptides, GABA and endocannabinoids). There is also recruitment of brain stress systems and dysregulation of brain antistress systems that provide the negative motivational state associated with abstinence. Additional neurobiological and neurochemical systems in the prefrontal cortex and basolateral amygdala have been implicated in drug- and cue-induced relapse. Genetic studies suggest roles for the genes encoding the neurochemical elements involved in the brain reward and stress systems in the vulnerability of addiction, and molecular studies have identified transduction and transcription factors that may mediate the dependence-induced reward dysregulation and chronic-vulnerability changes in neurocircuitry associated with the development and maintenance of addiction. Human imaging studies reveal similar neurocircuits involved in addiction. Although there are no neurobiological markers of addictive disorders on the immediate horizon, the progress in understanding the neurobiological features of addictive disorders may eventually aid in the specific diagnoses of use, misuse and dependence.

11.8   COMORBIDITY VS SUBSTANCE-INDUCED DISORDERS

Considerable attention has been focused on the issue of dual diagnosis of substance-use disorders and other co-occurring psychiatric disorders, with a high rate having been described in numerous epidemiological studies. Increased clarity of diagnostic criteria and improvements in diagnostic methods have enhanced the assessment process, which is essential in the search for the etiology and pathogenesis of both disorders. However, potential problems arise in the diagnostic process: if the two disorders are seen as independent conditions, they may influence the course of each disorder, or they may both be a consequence of actions of the same predisposing factors (e.g. stress, childhood environment). The psychiatric disorder can lead to the development of a substance-use disorder or vice versa, leading clinicians to distinguish between a primary and secondary condition. And some psychiatric syndromes may be seen as temporary psychiatric pictures, being considered a consequence of intoxication of specific substances (e.g. psychosis) or withdrawal conditions (e.g. depressive syndromes).

In the future, there will be a need to establish and standardize definitions of comorbidity along with clearer definitions of criterion items for substance-induced disorders that are not presently well defined. These substance-induced disorders include such common syndromes such as cannabinoid-induced psychoses or those induced by stimulant substances, as well as depressive syndromes induced by an alcohol use disorder. These substance-induced conditions have important implications with respect to prognosis, as well as specific consequences with respect to unique treatment. The variations in results of antidepressants across studies on the treatment of depressive syndromes among alcoholics might reflect the fact that these studies insufficiently differentiated between a comorbidity of alcohol use and depressive disorder, and alcohol-induced depressive episodes, the latter being cases where passage of time may have the same effect as antidepressants.

11.9   SUBTYPES OF SUBSTANCE-USE DISORDERS

Recognition of the heterogeneity of alcoholics has led to attempts to identify subgroups of persons with substance-related problems according to a variety of defining indicators, such as onset age, chronicity of problems, patterns of use, antecedent psychopathology and childhood vulnerability factors. Despite a long tradition of research in this field, the research suggests that no consensus has emerged about the nature, much less the number, of subtypes that could be used to characterize the clinical heterogeneity among those with substance-use disorders. Nevertheless, two subtypes of alcoholics have been consistently identified. These divide into a low-severity, low-vulnerability subgroup (similar to type A [6]) and a high-severity, high-vulnerability subgroup (similar to type B). The former is characterized by later onset of problematic drinking, few childhood vulnerability factors, a relative absence of alcohol problems in family history, a low level of antecedent psychopathology and a less severe drinking pattern. The latter subtype is characterized by early onset of alcohol problems, greater number of childhood vulnerability factors and a family history of alcohol problems, a variety of antecedent and concomitant psychopathology and a pattern characterized by excessive drinking, severe dependence and serious alcohol-related problems. Unfortunately, there have been few cross-national replications for alcohol typologies, and there is only limited evidence that the binary classification applies to other psychoactive substances. Therefore, it is considered premature to recommend the adoption of a subtyping scheme in the DSM or ICD classification systems, but future research is likely to eventually contribute to a more specific diagnostic classification of addictive disorders.

11.10   INCLUSION OF NON-SUBSTANCE-RELATED CONDITIONS AMONG ADDICTIVE DISORDERS

The nomenclature system within the classification systems DSM and ICD do not use the term addiction, using the terms substance-use disorders (SUDs); and the subgroups abuse, harmful use, dependence, withdrawal and intoxication. The question arises of whether addiction should extend beyond SUD, as the importance of impaired control over a specific behaviour has become more of a central element in defining addiction. Pathological gambling is one of the main conditions, which has fuelled the debate on the inclusion of non-substance-related conditions among addictive disorders. Pathological gambling is presently diagnosed and categorized under the impulse control disorders (ICDs). Other ICDs where an inclusion among addictive disorders has been discussed are compulsive shopping, compulsive computer use (with the special case of Internet use) and compulsive sexual behaviour.

Non-substance-related conditions such as pathological gambling (PG) share many features with those for substance dependence, yet interest in research has been more recent, so that substantial gaps of knowledge still exist in the biological, phenomenological and clinical characteristics of these conditions. Nonetheless, the natural histories of PG and SUDs suggest that many people recover on their own, following peaks of problem behaviours in adolescence and early adulthood. Individuals with PG and SUDs have been shown to perform similarly on personality and neurocognitive assessments of impulsivity. Multiple transmitter systems have been similarly implicated in PG and SUDs. Emerging brain imaging data suggest that similar components of the mesolimbic pathway are involved in PG and SUDs, while other neuroimaging data suggest differences between PG and OCD [7]. This common link between PG (as well as other ICDs) and SUDs needs to be considered in possibly expanding the classification system to include pathological gambling and other non-substance-related conditions within the context of addictive disorders.

11.11   PERSON-CENTRED INTEGRATIVE DIAGNOSIS AND SUBSTANCE-USE DISORDERS

Psychiatry for the person and the Person-Centred Integrative Diagnosis (PID) proposes the whole person in context as the centre and goal of clinical care and public health. Thus, in PID, the totality of health in context is considered. This includes ill health (a traditional focus of medical practice), but it also includes positive aspects of health, essential for the recovery process and health restoration, as the two cardinal domains of assessment. Substance-use disorders are perhaps among the most emblematic examples of the dynamic link between the disorder, the totality of the person's health, and the context. It is also very telling that patient- or user-generated self-help approaches consider recovery as a central focus of attention, with primary emphasis on restorative aspects of health and on contextual factors. Primary examples of that approach are the steps and traditions of Alcoholics Anonymous (AA). AA emerged during the first half of the 20th century as an independent self-help movement within the community of persons suffering from alcoholism [8]. This tradition emphasized social support and elements related to recovery, such as promoting wellness behaviour, spirituality and personal growth. PID articulates the assessment of the totality of health as informational bases for clinical care and public health. In addition to standardized assessments, it also highlights the subjective experiences of illness and of health. Another feature of the PID is its emphasis on the protagonists of the clinical evaluation, which would include a partnership approach between the clinician, the person seeking care, and families and other carers (see Mezzich & Salloum, Chapter 30 in this book). Although empirical testing has not been undertaken yet, PID conceptually appears to offer an added advantage over traditional, pathology-focused assessment models, especially when considering complex conditions such as substance-use disorders.

11.12 CONCLUSIONS

There are several other issues that will have to be considered in future revisions of diagnostic classification systems. Cultural/ethnic issues limit the applicability of certain criteria of substance-use disorders in some societies, and meaningful cultural annotations and a glossary of cultural terms that are applicable in daily clinical practice and not limited to less frequently encountered syndromes (culture-bound) may have to be considered in future revisions. Considering the great difference between the non-dependence diagnoses in DSM-IV and ICD-10, a new non-dependence diagnosis is required, as well as a subthreshold diagnosis of hazardous or risky substance use.

Another issue is whether future diagnostic systems should also include positive aspects of health and protective factors, as proposed in the PID model. When looking at substance-use disorders in different age groups, the high differences in prevalence rates suggest that these may be inflated because of measurement error, mainly among young adults. Modifications in diagnostic classification of early substance use may be necessary, such as the development of a form of 'adolescent alcohol dependence', which may represent a less severe form of alcohol use disorder than that observed in adults [9]. Evidence is still inclusive whether specific dependence criteria for different substances represent an advantage to more sophisticated generic criteria, but a modification seems necessary in order to account for cross-substance differences in the general dependence severity level and specific symptom profiles.

Nonetheless, the process of diagnosing addictive disorders has considerably improved in the last decades and will continue to do so in the near future, as theory-driven research as well as blind empiricism help us to better understand the underlying mechanisms of the development of addictive disorders. There are many open questions, some of which can be addressed immediately by analyzing existing data sets, others that require more consensual discussions among experts, and others where more research is needed. The more accurate the diagnosis of addictive disorders, the better will be the clinicians' ability to determine the need for specific treatment and therefore the potential for the patient to overcome (or mature out of) the addictive disorder.

REFERENCES

[1] Kraemer HC, Noda A, O'Hara R. Categorical versus dimensional approaches too diagnosis: methodological challenges. *Journal of Psychiatric Research* 2004;38: pp. 17–25.

[2] van Os J, Gilvarry C, Bale R, van Horn E, Tattan T, White I, Murray R. A comparison of utility of dimensional and categorical representations of psychosis. UK700 Group. *Psychological Medicine* 1999;29: pp. 595–606.

[3] Krueger RF, Markon KE. Reinterpreting comorbidity: a model-based approach to understanding and classifying psychopathy. *Annual Review of Clinical Psychology* 2006;2: pp. 111–133.

[4] Helzer JE, van den Brink W, Guth SE. *Addiction* 2006; 101 (Suppl.1) pp. 17–22.

[5] Koob GF. The neurobiology of addiction: a neuroadaptational view relevant for diagnosis. *Addiction* 2006;101 (Suppl.1): pp. 23–30.

[6] Babor TF, Hofmann M, DelBocca F, Hesselbrock V, Meyer R, Dolinsky Z, Rounsaville B. Types of alcoholics. I. Evidence for an empirically-derived typology based on indicators of vulnerability and severity. *Archives of General Psychiatry* 1992;49: pp. 599–608.

[7] Potenza MN, Steinberg MA, Skudlarski P, Fullbright RK, Lacadie CM, Wilber MK, Rounsaville BJ, Gore JC, Wexler BE. Gambling urges in pathological gamblers: an fMRI study. *Archives of General Psychiatry* 2003;60: pp. 828–836.

[8] William W. The society of Alcoholics Anonymous. *American Journal of Psychiatry* 1949;105(5): pp. 370–375.

[9] Caetano R, Babor TF. *Diagnosis of alcohol dependence in epidemiological surveys: an epidemic of youthful alcohol dependence or a case of measurement error? Addiction*, 2006;101(Suppl.1): pp. 111–114.

[10] American Psychiatric Association. *Diagnostic and statistical manual of mental disorders, Fourth Edition. Text Revision.* (DSM-IV-TR). Washington, DC: American Psychiatric Association; 2000.

[11] World Health Organization. *International Statistical Classification of Diseases and Related Health Problems, Tenth Revision (ICD-10).* Geneva: WHO; 1992.

CHAPTER 12

Advances in Diagnosis and Classification of Sexual Disorders

Rubén Hernández Serrano
Universidad Central de Venezuela, Caracas, Venezuela
Antonio Pacheco Palha
Hospital San Joao, University of Porto, Portugal
Said Abdel Azim
Emeritus Professor of Psychiatry, Cairo University, Egypt
Chiara Simonelli
Professor, Institute of Sessuologia Clinica, University of La Sapienza, Rome, Italy
Felipe Navarro Cremades
Universidad Miguel Hernandez, Alicante, Spain
Aminta Parra
Universidad Central de Venezuela, Caracas, Venezuela

12.1 INTRODUCTION

Medical sexology is growing up very quickly. After the launch of new vasoactive drugs (sildenafil in 1998, and tadalafil and vardenafil in 2002), the field is now very extensive. Avanafil, dapoxetine and testosterone patches for women are soon to be available.

Both men and women are now losing their fears about consulting their physicians for effective and secure ways of treatment, and there has been a successful WPA initiative, the Sexual Health Educational Program (SHEP), consistent with the WPA Institutional Program on Psychiatry for the Person (Mezzich 2007 [1]).

Despite this, many myths and false beliefs still remain in the collective unconsciousness. We have a lot to do in terms of disseminating information and creating a paradigm change

Psychiatric Diagnosis: Challenges and Prospects Edited by I.M. Salloum and J.E. Mezzich
© 2009 John Wiley & Sons, Ltd

related to the bad aspects of sex and promoting 'the good of sex' [2] as also looking into the positive aspects of sexual health.

The main tools for a good diagnosis are perhaps the first step in a good approach. Schematically, we may say these are:

1. A comprehensive medical and sex history. The clinician must have good expertise to do that in a patient and complete manner. A scheme from UTES, Caracas was published in *Psiquiatria* [3]. It is important in today's globalised world to interview patients carefully, and to respect their values

2. Instructing the patient to prepare an autobiographic list of events. Usually, when patients do this recovery exercise, some traumas are present and they will get insight into their sexual complaints.

3. Laboratory tests are extremely important because sexual dysfunctions are usually the first sign of a complex metabolic syndrome that includes diabetes, hypertension, hyperlipidemia, morbid obesity and many endocrinological or genetic problems.

4. Psychological evaluation of the couple is also important, and the use of scales is now very common. The APA *Handbook of Psychiatric Measures* [4] and the Davis and Yarber *Handbook of Sexuality* [5] are good examples of an extensive way to conduct protocols and research studies with a comprehensive and reliable method. More than 500 scales were presented and validated. It is also crucial to check the views of the person's partner, because many false beliefs are viewed in this format. It is invaluable to check questionnaires individually and assess the couple afterwards, keeping controversial issues like infidelity or occasional extramarital relationships confidential, a theme which is not touched in scientific research. The investigation of erotic fantasies and imageries is extremely important for the evaluation of disorders relating to desire.

5. Phalodinamic study of the penis, with the use of intracavernous drugs, mainly papaverine, prostaglandin E1, and a combination with phentolamine, may be useful in the diagnosis of predominantly organic or psychological causes of erectile dysfunction. We believe in a continuum, with organic and psychological causes at each end and the majority of cases falling on the line accordingly. Of course, good training is needed in order to do this, as complications may arise, like priapism, infections, pain, etc. In some specific cases, an eco-Doppler and PET scan may be indicated.

   In women, a gynecological examination must be made. It is practical to have a team that includes a urologist and a gynecologist, because this will be more familiar and practical for the examiner and the patient.

6. A case referral pathway must be available in order to evaluate psychiatric, neurological, endocrinological, genetic and sociocultural determining factors.

7. It is also advisable to conduct medical joint discussions to establish a consensus pathway to treat each case. It is difficult to design a fixed algorithm for the sexual dysfunctions. There are so many variables to consider properly.

8. Quality of life scales and life habits scales must be considered. Human sexuality is so complex that these usually interfere, affecting each person positively or negatively. The same applies to the couple and their relationships with their family and society. The WHO changed the definitions of sex, sexuality and sexual health in 2004 (www.worldsexology.org), updating the definitions from 1974.

9. The WPA (2003) [6] International Guidelines for Diagnostic Assessment have at their core a comprehensive diagnostic model. It includes first a Standardized Multiaxial Formulation composed of the following axes:

    (i)   Clinical problems;
    (ii) Disabilities;
    (iii) Contextual Factors;
    (iv) Quality of Life.

    Second, it includes a Personalized Idiographic Formulation with the following elements:

    (i)   Contextualized Clinical problems;
    (ii) Patient's positive factors;
    (iii) Expectations for restoration and promotion of health.

    In *Psychiatry and Sexual Health* [7], illustrative cases were presented through Tables 2.4.1, 3.1.2, and 3.1.3.

10. Today, the old human response cycle from Masters and Johnson (1966) [8] has been substituted by a six-phase cycle, which is different in men and women. A circular pathway reinforcing model, of desire, excitement, plateau, orgasm, resolution and, more important, sexual satisfaction, has been presented by Basson [9], Whipple [10], Berganza [11] and Hernández Serrano [12].

11. The relevance of human sexual rights is also important in the area of diagnosis. This can be seen in the 1997 Valencia Declaration from the World Association for Sexology (WAS) [12], later approved unanimously at the Hong Kong World Congress in 1999 [13].

We are aware of difficulties regarding religious, spiritual and sociocultural values. Our recommendation is not to impose this, but to discuss these issues openly in order to fulfil a global and respectful view.

The importance must also be pointed out of the many comorbidities that usually obscure the real problem. This is frequent in chronic illnesses and disabilities. The same occurs when you deal with sexuality along the life-cycle stages.

Classifications have been made in relation to other views:

(a) Primary/secondary
(b) General/situational/selective
(c) Total/partial
(d) 3P factors: predispose, precipitating and perpetuating [25]
(e) dysfunctional and dysadaptive consequences.

12.2   NEW CATEGORIES FOR CLASSIFICATION

Segraves, Balon and Clayton [14] proposed new changes in the diagnostic criteria for sexual dysfunctions in a very comprehensive and descriptive paper in 2007. We agree with them for the majority of these criteria.

We will add the following categories for discussion:

1. *Discronaxia*. A term created by Gindin [15], or Discronia (Dyschronia), according with Mezzich review, referring to time and frequency disparity in the couple, a very common

situation in clinical practice. Usually it is women who have complaints in this new category, and who ask for a consultation despite the neglect from their male partners. As sexologists, from the clinical point of view of rapid ejaculation, we do not agree with the two-minute time proposed by Waldinger [16]. Sex is too complicated to use a chronometer during the marvellous and ceremonial sexual act. It can be useful for research purposes, however.

2. *Postcoital dysphoria.* This term was added by Berganza, in order to describe mood changes, generally in a high position after coitus. Singing opera arias or highly pitched conversations are frequently seen in these cases.

3. *Postcoital headache.* Also from Berganza, this is seen as a characteristic symptom occurring in refractory periods of men.

4. *Sexual monotony.* Hernandez described this category for couples, who have generally been together for a long time, who always do the same thing in the same place at the same time, with no variations in their sexual lives, which is usually felt in separation, divorce, infidelity and so on.

5. *Paraphilias.* This is a family of persistent, intense fantasies and behaviours involving sexual arousal from non socially accepted stimulus. This is an open field that varies from time to time. John Money [17] presented 40 categories at the 1981 World Congress of Sexology in Israel. Later, Brenda Love [18] described 400 unusual sexual practices, and presented these at the Sexology World Congress in Brazil in 1993. Later, long lists of these cases were presented. Culture and religion have a very important role in the scientific classification of paraphilias. The discussion of what is a paraphilia and what is not, will cover many areas and, of course, will be very controversial because of changes in behavioural models [26].

6. *Desire disorders.* These are also a frequent cause for consultation. Sexologists are aware of hypoactive desire dysfunctions, defined as persistent lack of responsive desire, usually in women. Post-traumatic stress disorder is often associated with this. Here, we have a clear distinction between sexual addictions and compulsive sexual behaviour, taking into account the pathway that addictions follow in general, with clear sporadic and intermittent sexual acts that respond to a particular stimulus in a specific situation. There has been a long discussion between two groups in Minnesota, USA, without a clear consensus that can result in definitive conclusions. There are several books dealing with this issue [19, 20].

7. *Sex Internet dependence.* This relates to pornography or particular sexual groups. It is incredible how many people, usually isolated, are in this extremely time consuming category, in which persons with social anxiety disorders or obsessive compulsive personalities try to solve their loneliness with the computer.

8. *Late-onset hypogonadism (LOH).* This syndrome is different from the well-known ADAM syndrome, characterized by clinical and biochemical changes with age and low levels of testosterone.

9. *Sexual post-traumatic disorders.* These are also frequently associated with several sexual disorders. It is very important to review true or false accusations carefully, with any specific purpose. An insight into these pathologies is very useful in sex therapy.

10. *Anaejaculation.* Persons who have prostatic surgical intervention are in this category, as a consequence of the seminal vesicles desaparition, as are patients taking psychotropic drugs, but we see some cases without these two clear explanations. Fear of pregnancy is also associated with it [27].

11. *Homophobia.* This is a very controversial issue, as reconversion therapy proposed by Spitzer [21]. Discussion of these issues needs a long and specific paper. The same occurs with gender dysphorias, a field that is also expanding quickly. Holly Devor [22] has written a book on this.

12. *Relational sexual dysfunction.* Presented by Simonelli *et al.* [23], this refers to conditions in which a sexual disorder in one partner induces a sexual disorder in the other (Schnarch, 2000 [24]).

13. *Chronic sexual pain disorders,* with a clear distinction from dyspareunias, are also important to differentiate.

We are quite sure that these ideas need a long and fruitful process of discussion and, later on, consensus agreement.

REFERENCES

[1] Mezzich JE. Psychiatry for the person: articulating medicine's science and humanism. *World Psychiatry* 2007;6: pp. 1–3.

[2] Hernández Serrano R. Parra A. The Good of Sex. XI CLASES. Margarita Is.2002.

[3] Alarcón R, Mazzoti G, Nicolini H. (eds.) *Psiquiatria.* 2nd ed. PAHO/Manual Moderno; 2005.

[4] American Psychiatric Association. *Handbook of Psychiatric Measures.* Washington: APA Press; 2000.

[5] Davis CM, Yarber WL, Bauserman R, Schreer G, Davis SL. (eds.) *Handbook of sexuality-related measures.* London: Sage; 1998.

[6] WPA. Essentials of the world psychiatric association's international guidelines for diagnostic assessment. *British Journal of Psychiatry* 2003;182 (45 Suppl).

[7] Mezzich JE, Hernandez-Serrano R, *et al. Psychiatry and Sexual Health.* New York, London: Jason-Aronson; 2005.

[8] Masters W and Johnson V. Human Sexual Response. Boston. Little Brown. (1966)

[9] Basson R. Human Sexual Response. *Journal of Sex and Marital Therapy* 2001;27: pp. 33–43.

[10] Whipple B. International Consensus development conference on female sexual dysfunction. Definitions and Classification. *Journal of Urology* 2000;16: pp. 888–893.

[11] Berganza C. *SHEP Panel Discussions.* 1999–2005.

[12] World Association for Sexology (WAS). Valencia World Congress, 1997. (www.worldsexology.org).

[13] World Association for Sexology (WAS). Hong Kong World Congress, 1999. (www.worldsexology.org).

[14] Segraves, Balon, Clayton. *Journal of Sexual Medicine* 2007;4: pp. 567–580.

[15] Gindin LR. *La Nueva Sexualidad del Varon.* Paidos Ed.;1985.

[16] Waldinger M. Changing paradigms from a historical DSM III and DSM IV view toward and evidence based definition of PE. *Journal of Sexual Medicine* 2006;3: pp. 682–692, 693–705.

[17] Money J, Muspah H. *Encyclopedia of Sex.* Elsevier Ed; 1977.

[18] Love B. *Encyclopedia of unusual sexual practices.* New Jersey: Barricade Books; 1992.

[19] Goodman A. *Sexual Addiction.* Madison, CT: International Universities Press, Inc; 1998.

[20] Coleman E. Sexual compulsion vs. sexual addiction. *SIECUS Report* 1986;14(6) pp. 7–10.

[21] Spitzer R. *APA Annual Meeting NY.* USA: Book of Abstracts; 2004.

[22] Devor H. *FTM: Female to male transsexuals in society.* Bloomington, IN: Indiana University Press; 1999.

[23] Simonelli C, *et al. International Conference on Paraphilias.* Rome, Italy; 2001.

[24] Schnarch. The Passionate marriage. *The Journal of the Professional Pastoral Counseling Institute*; 2000.
[25] Navarro Cremades F. WPA Sexual Health Course. WPA World Congress Prague, Czech.; 2008.
[26] Hernandez Serrano R. Parra A. *Proceeding Int. Symposium Education Sexual*. Ed UCV WAS FNUAP. Caracas, Venezuela; 1995.
[27] Academia Internacional de Sexologia Medica. Consensus. Ed El Colegio. Caracas, Venezuela; 2002.

CHAPTER 13

Personality Disorders

Giles Newton-Howes
Peter Tyrer
Division of Neurosciences and Mental Health, Imperial College London,
London, UK

This chapter summarises current diagnostic practice in the field of personality disorders and complements a much fuller account in the WPA book series [1]. In carrying out this review, it will be clear that the classification of personality disorder in both major classification systems is in a state of flux and is liable to be transformed dramatically. What is summarized below is therefore best described as an interim report with a best guess on likely developments.

13.1   INTRODUCTION

Despite the current difficulties of diagnosis in personality disorder, the importance of this group of disorders is increasingly recognized as fundamental to psychiatric practice [2]. It is also increasingly recognized that personality disorders play a significant part in the overall morbidity of patients with comorbid mental disorders [3, 4] and are disabling. Everyone has a personality, and its quirks and idiosyncrasies, particularly when pathological, alter the presentation and influence of almost all other psychopathology, even if the conditions concerned are considered to be quite independent of personality disorder.

Despite this growing recognition, debate remains about the most scientifically accurate methodology for diagnosing personality pathology whilst retaining its clinical utility. This debate is long-running and still not resolved, although much has been done to lay the foundations for this emerging speciality. An overview of the historical context of personality diagnosis allows for a clear understanding of the current classification and its inherent strengths and weaknesses. This system both encourages research and promotes debate as to the future direction of personality disorder classification.

13.2   THE HISTORICAL CONTEXT

The notion of classifying personality has always been considered odd to many people, because it is self-evident that each personality is unique and so a classification system that

Psychiatric Diagnosis: Challenges and Prospects   Edited by I.M. Salloum and J.E. Mezzich
© 2009 John Wiley & Sons, Ltd

will accommodate all abnormality is unattainable. It is fortunate in many ways that when the international classification of disease was first developed (initially as the International List of Causes of Death) in 1900, that mental health was not completely forgotten, so we have had the advantage of over a century of practice. Mental health disorders first entered the classification in 1938 with the fifth edition, and personality disorders appeared in both the sixth edition of the International Classification of Disease (ICD) and the first edition of the Diagnostic and Statistical Manual of Mental Disorder (DSM-I).

The most significant change with regard to personality disorders (and indeed with regard to most mental disorders) came in 1980 with the publication of DSM-III [5]. The success of DSM-III was primarily due to the monumental efforts of one man, Robert Spitzer, whose place in the panoply of achievement in nosology is still not determined but is likely to be a very high one. Although the classification of DSM-III was one based on the senses among experts, it was guided very cleverly by Robert Spitzer, and most of the diagnoses introduced there have been retained because Spitzer considered both the political and scientific aspects of their inclusion. The personality disorders described in both the latest edition of the Diagnostic and Statistical Manual of Mental Disorders (DSM-IV) and the International Classification of Diseases (ICD-10) use almost similar labels to those described 28 years ago in DSM-III.

But none of this was new. Speculation as to the foundations of personality disorder and its impact on patients' health have existed almost as long as Western medicine. Hippocrates hypothesized that illness was caused by an imbalance of the four humours that in turn were represented by Galen as constituting four personality types. Choleric personality was represented by yellow bile, melancholic by black bile, phlegmatic by phlegm and sanguine by blood. Although we would not now attach these humours to particular personality types, these four major grouping have been repeatedly reappeared in various forms as equivalent personality groups. The grouping was expanded by Schneider [6] in 1923 into ten categories of personality disorder: hyperthymic, depressive, insecure, fanatical, attention-seeking, labile, explosive, affectionless, weak-willed and asthenic. This focused the psychiatric world on the problem of personality and its effects on other disorders. It also served to separate the influence of personality from that of other 'major' mental disorders and as such encouraged its investigation and diagnostic applicability in its own right.

13.3 CURRENT DIAGNOSTIC STRUCTURE

The revisions of Schneider led to the most significant diagnostic separation of personality in psychiatry by separating it from other mental disorders. The DSM-III placed personality disorders on Axis II, thereby separating them from major mental disorders (on Axis I). In a similar fashion, the 10th International Classification of Diseases (ICD-10) sub-classified personality (F60) as 'Disorders of Adult Personality and Behaviour' although this section also includes impulse and gender based disorder [7].

Both systems also followed the standard model, well served in other parts of psychiatry, of using operationally defined criteria to base diagnosis. This system required a set number of particular features to be present as well as general criteria to allow a diagnosis to be made (Table 13.1). Although this type of system functions smoothly for the many diagnoses of depressive, bipolar and schizophrenic disorders, it does badly with personality disorder and almost all authorities agree it is seriously flawed [8]. Only the diagnoses of borderline and

Table 13.1 Summary of current classification of personality disorder in ICD-10 and DSM-IV.

Cluster	ICD-10	DSM-IV
A (odd eccentric cluster)	Paranoid Schizoid	Paranoid Schizoid Schizotypal
B (flamboyant dramatic cluster)	Dissocial Emotionally unstable, borderline-type Emotionally unstable, impulsive-type Histrionic No equivalent	Antisocial Borderline No equivalent Histrionic Narcissistic
C (anxious fearful cluster)	No equivalent Anxious Dependent Anankastic Personality change (enduring) after catastrophic experience Personality change (enduring) after psychiatric illness (Organic personality disorder) Personality change due to general medical condition	Depressive (not a fully accepted disorder) Avoidant Dependent Obsessive compulsive No equivalent No equivalent Other specific personality disorders Personality disorder not otherwise specified (PD-NOS)

antisocial personality are reasonably well used, even though antisocial personality disorder has not been able to embrace the notion of psychopathy adequately [9], and the failure of the system is illustrated by the very frequent use of personality disorder not otherwise specified (PDNOS) in practice [10]. Although diagnoses are often made with enthusiasm, they are unreliable, unwieldy and used only in parentheses in everyday clinical practice because their attribution is so stigmatizing. There is an additional problem of extensive co-occurrence of several personality disorders at the same time, as the simplest explanation of this co-occurrence is that it is likely to mean consanguinity rather than genuine comorbidity [11]. In order to combat this problem, there has been a move towards clustering the ten/eleven diagnostic categories in three or four clusters. This clustering simplifies the process of diagnosis, reduces multiple personality diagnoses and more closely mirrors the research findings to the underlying trait structure of human personality. The four clusters are the schizoid/avoidant cluster, the flamboyant cluster, the anxious/dependent cluster and the obsessive cluster, which is currently part of Cluster C but is sufficiently separate to be examined on its own [12].

13.4 DIMENSIONAL APPROACHES TO PERSONALITY DIAGNOSIS

The most commonly and scientifically based alternative to the operational categorical structure currently used to diagnose personality is the implementation of a dimensional, trait based system. This idea is not new. Such a structure of classification would allow for the severity or impact of a number of general personality traits to be measured on a dimensional scale, and then used to assess overall impact. The number of core traits range from three to five and remain an area of debate [13]; however, four traits probably have the most historical and research weight. These traits can be summarized as the four A's; asocial (odd-eccentric), antisocial (dissocial), anxious (avoidant) and anankastic (obsessive-compulsive), equivalent to the four clusters described above [14]. This system has significant advantages, including: being more closely aligned to the empirical research on personality; factoring in the degree of deviance from normal for well established personality traits; and better establishing the severity of personality pathology – an important clinical marker of morbidity. The major drawback is the lack of distinction between disorder/no disorder, making it difficult for clinicians to implement and use to inform treatment and management. It further blurs the questions as to how best assess personality and come to a stable diagnosis.

13.5   ASSESSMENT AND DIAGNOSIS OF PERSONALITY DISORDER

Following the publication of the DSM-III, research into personality, its morbidity and interactions with other mental disorders has flourished. A myriad of tools has also been developed, predominantly peer-reviewed with good face and internal validity, to ensure uniformity of diagnosis within the field. Unfortunately, although each tool may function to measure 'personality' itself, there is generally poor reliability across tools and poor inter-rater reliability. This position is handicapped further by the difficulty of finding a gold standard against which to contrast and compare. Much of the difficulty lies in what is measured by each instrument; some focus on symptoms, others on outcomes and others on social or interpersonal disability. This makes sensible collation of the data available to support a single diagnostic instrument next to impossible to achieve at the current time. Despite these major difficulties, it is clear that research assessments have become significantly more accurate, with the use of such tools and studies that take a general approach; dividing diagnosis into personality disorder/no personality disorder further improves the research diagnosis.

The application of some research remains difficult, however, as there is a gulf between the research diagnosis of personality disorder and its clinical use. This is perhaps best highlighted by the repeated finding that research tools consistently diagnose personality disorder more frequently than clinical assessment [15]. Clearly clinicians and researchers are examining different diagnostic entities. The reasons for this divide remain unclear, although there is some anecdotal evidence that the complexity of the current system renders it clinically cumbersome to the point of paralysis.

The issue of stigma is also significant. Much work has been undertaken on an international level to reduce the stigma surrounding mental disorder. The Royal Colleges of Britain and Australia and New Zealand, among others, have run extensive campaigns using a combination of celebrity, education and promotion to normalize mental disorder in the community. It is noticeable that these campaigns tend to ignore or marginalize personality disorder. As such, it is a sub-speciality of psychiatry that remains relatively stigmatized, not only in the public domain but also within the profession itself [16]. It would seem likely that this stigmatization influences clinical decision making, further widening the diagnostic gap between research and clinical practice.

13.6   THE FUTURE OF PERSONALITY DISORDER DIAGNOSIS

What is known about personality disorder and its diagnosis is that for it to be useful to clinicians and patients it needs to: be easy to understand and explain; be useful in clinical settings; have meaning for patients in the real world; and be scientifically robust. Such a diagnosis would not only act to guide both prognosis and management but would also allow repeatable research to guide such treatment. The current system of personality disorder diagnosis found in both major psychiatric classifications struggles to attain these goals. It is likely that a system that would accommodate such standards would have a dual structure. Firstly, it would set out basic criteria against which a general diagnosis of personality disorder could be made. These criteria would need to reflect the instability of the diagnosis as currently used, and the significant social and inter-personal morbidity associated with such a disorder. The second, or specific tier, would then be used to explain the general diagnosis of personality disorder, most probably using a dimensional trait based system to identify the domains of dysfunction more accurately to guide further management. Such a diagnostic structure allows not only for an accurate and valid general diagnosis, useful in both a research and a clinical setting, but clarification of the diagnosis such that helpful management strategies can be clinically trialled and implemented in practice. Furthermore, it would align with our current understanding of the basic structure of personality developed in all people.

DSM-V and ICD-11 are likely to be published in 2012. The form these will take for personality disorders is not yet known but, reflecting this, it is likely to include the following:

(a) a better description of the core features of generic personality disorder and the expectation that this will take precedence in assessment;
(b) an acknowledgement that dimensional traits should appear in the classification, as they are the core persistent features of personality;
(c) recognition that personality deviance alone is not diagnostic of personality disorder and that degree of social dysfunction is also critical;
(d) that severity of disorder also needs to be addressed [17].

Thus, in such a system, a patient may receive a diagnosis of 'moderate personality disorder with significant introverted and eccentric traits', identifying the major areas causing impairment (introversion and eccentricity) and that the impairment is sufficient to cause morbidity that amounts to a disorder. Such a diagnostic system is perhaps more similar to other psychiatric classifications, where a broad diagnostic classification is used (e.g. schizophrenia) and then subtyped (e.g. disorganized) to aid in clinical management. What is imperative is that, for personality disorder to become useful to clinicians, the gross deficiencies in the current system need to be addressed. With a scientifically robust and applicable system, clinical management of personality dysfunction and prediction of its outcome should be able to be addressed with confidence.

REFERENCES

[1] Maj M, Akiskal HS, Mezzich JE, Okasha A. *Personality Disorders. Evidence and Experience in Psychiatry* Volume 8 in the WPA series. Chichester: John Wiley & Sons, Ltd; 2005.

[2] National Institute of Mental Health (England) *Personality Disorder: No longer a diagnosis of exclusion*. Department of Health: London; 2003.

[3] Newton-Howes G, Tyrer P, Johnson T. Personality disorder and the outcome of depression: a meta-analysis of published studies. *British Journal of Psychiatry* 2006;188: pp. 13–20.

[4] Massion A, Dyck I, Shea T, *et al*. Personality disorders and time to remission in generalized anxiety disorder, social phobia and panic disorder. *Archives of General Psychiatry* 2002;59: pp. 434–440.

[5] American Psychiatric Association. *Diagnostic and Statistical Manual of Mental Disorders, Third Revision*. Washington DC: American Psychiatric Association; 1980.

[6] Schneider, K. *Die Psychopathischen Personlikeiten*. Berlin: Springer; 1923.

[7] World Health Organization. *Classification of Mental and Behavioural Disorders. International Classification of Disease and Related Health Problems. 10th Revision*. (ICD-10) Geneva: WHO; 1992.

[8] Livesley W. Classifying personality disorders: ideal types, prototypes or dimensions? *Journal of Personality Disorders* 1991;5: pp. 52–59.

[9] Tyrer P. New approaches to the diagnosis of psychopathy and personality disorder. *Journal of the Royal Society of Medicine* 2004;97: pp. 371–374.

[10] Verheul R, Bartak A, Widiger T. Prevalence and construct validity of Personality Disorder Not Otherwise Specified (PDNOS). *Journal of Personality Disorders* 2007;21: pp. 359–370.

[11] Tyrer P. Consanguinity or comorbidity? *British Journal of Psychiatry* 1996;168: pp. 669–671.

[12] Tyrer P, Coombs N, Ibrahimi F, Mathilakath A, Bajaj P, Ranger M, Rao B, Din R. Critical developments in the assessment of personality disorder. *British Journal of Psychiatry* 2007;suppl 49: pp. 51–59.

[13] Widiger T, Simonsen E. Alternative dimensional models of personality disorder: finding a common ground. *Journal of Personality Disorders* 2005;19: pp. 586–593.

[14] Mulder R, Joyce P. Temperament and the structure of personality disorder symptoms. *Psychological Medicine* 1997;27: pp. 99–106.

[15] Westen D. Divergences between clinical and research methods for assessing personality disorders: implications for research and the evolution of axis II. *American Journal of Psychiatry* 1997;154: pp. 895–903.

[16] Newton-Howes G, Tyrer P, Weaver T. Stigmatic perceptions of staff towards patients with personality disorder in community mental health teams. *Australian and New Zealand Journal of Psychiatry* 2008 (in press).

[17] Tyrer P, Johnson T. Establishing the severity of personality disorder. *American Journal of Psychiatry* 1996;153: pp. 1593–1597.

CHAPTER 14

Intellectual Disabilities

Sally-Ann Cooper

Professor of Learning Disabilities, Section of Psychological Medicine, Division of Community Based Sciences, Faculty of Medicine, University of Glasgow, Gartnavel Royal Hospital, Glasgow, UK

Luis Salvador-Carulla

Professor of Psychiatry, University of Cadiz (Spain); Section on Psychiatry of Intellectual Disability, World Psychiatric Association

14.1 INTRODUCTION: CLASSIFICATION OF INTELLECTUAL DISABILITIES

Intellectual quotient (IQ) is often used to indicate a person's level of intellectual ability or impairment, i.e. their ability and speed in processing and learning new information. Test instruments have limitations in the extent to which they can accurately measure IQ, and the extent to which they are appropriate across cultures. However, if IQ can be accurately measured, and was normally distributed in the population, with a mean of 100 and standard deviation of 15, then about 2% of the population would significantly differ from the mean, with an IQ below 70. However, reported rates of intellectual disabilities (ID) are typically lower than this, and vary widely, from 2-85/1000 general population in developed countries, with few robust studies in developing countries. Recent data point to a decreasing rate of ID in Western societies, whereas an opposite trend appears in very low income countries, where rates of ID may reach 4% according to some estimates [1].

Given the variation, it is inappropriate to provide average figures from across the studies. The variability is dependent upon several factors, with the definition of intellectual disabilities used being important, along with the country and region of study, the time of the study, the age range and ethnicity of the population, and the method of population ascertainment [2, 3, 4].

Reasons for a higher prevalence in low and medium income countries include socio-economic factors, the fact that iodine deficiency is indigenous in some regions of Asia and Africa, exposure to heavy metals and toxins lowering IQ by a few points, regions with a high level of consanguineous marriages, and the availability and sophistication of antenatal, perinatal and neonatal care. Some studies show differences between ethnic groups, although the cultural suitability of the measures used may have contributed to these findings. Prevalence also varies with time, due to preventative measures and social developments, e.g. antenatal and neonatal screening, and developments in neonatal care. Prevalence is higher in child than adult cohorts, and lower in older than younger adult cohorts, with the highest prevalence at around age 10 years. This is due to intellectual disabilities having been identified by this age, combined with an earlier age of death for persons with intellectual disabilities compared with the general population, and some children with intellectual disabilities no longer meeting the ICD-10 or DSM-IV-TR criteria in adulthood.

The term 'mental retardation' has been changed to 'intellectual disability' by main national and international organizations in this field. The name of the WPA section on this topic was changed to 'Psychiatry of Intellectual Disability' in 2006 [5]. WHO has implicitly accepted this new term in its recent *Atlas-ID* [6]. ICD-10 and DSM-IV-TR both still use the term 'mental retardation'.

The three criteria used in DSM and ICD to code intellectual disability are similar:

- significantly sub-average intellectual functioning (IQ below 70 {ICD-10} or 70–75 {DSM-IV-TR}; mental age less than approximately 12 years);
- concurrent impairments in present adaptive functioning; diminished ability to adapt to the daily demands of the social environment;
- onset before the age of 18 years.

These criteria have remained largely unchanged during the last 30 years and they do not fit current knowledge and developments in this field. ICD-10 and DSM-IV-TR definitions of intellectual disabilities are not statistical constructs; the requirement of impaired adaptive functioning may halve estimated prevalence rates compared with a statistical definition. Furthermore, different methods to assess intelligence and adaptive behaviour can lead to different prevalence rates. Children with the mildest intellectual disabilities are likely to benefit from additional support for learning at school, but will develop skills and experience over time, such that some no longer meet criteria for intellectual disabilities in adulthood. It is important to consider these classification issues when interpreting results from published studies, particularly regarding prevalence rates, and when conducting needs assessments and planning services.

From a nosological point of view, ID may be regarded not as a disease or as a disability but as a syndrome grouping (metasyndrome) similar to the construct of dementia. It includes a heterogeneous group of clinical conditions, ranging from genetic to nutritional, infectious, metabolic or neurotoxic conditions. The ID metasyndrome is characterized by a deficit in cognitive functioning prior to the acquisition of skills through learning. The intensity of the deficit is such that it interferes in a significant way with individual normal functioning as expressed in limitations in activities and restriction in participation (disabilities). The name 'developmental cognitive impairment' has been suggested to coexist with ID for naming the metasyndrome previously called mental retardation following a polysemic-polynomious approach [5].

14.2 ACCURATE ASSESSMENT OF SYMPTOMS OF MENTAL ILL-HEALTH PRECEDES CLASSIFICATION

Mental ill-health is more prevalent and has higher incidence in the population with intellectual disabilities than in the general population for children and adolescents [7] and adults [8, 9]. This is particularly due to the higher prevalence of problem behaviours and autism, but also due to higher rates of other types of mental ill-health, including attention deficit hyperactivity disorder, psychosis, and bipolar disorder. Some genetic causes of intellectual disabilities have specific behavioural phenotypes, such as Down syndrome with dementia, and Prader-Willi syndrome with affective psychosis. However, these alone do not account for the higher rates of mental ill-health overall in the population with intellectual disabilities, and there appear to be other biological, psychological, social and developmental factors that contribute and are as yet not well investigated or understood. Detection of the higher rate is dependent upon accurate diagnosis, including both the assessment methods used to measure psychopathology and the diagnostic criteria that are used to classify the psychopathology.

Hidden psychiatric morbidity is over 50%, even in vocational settings with psychological support [10]. The phrase 'diagnostic overshadowing' has been coined for the phenomenon whereby 'some debilitating emotional problems appear less important than they actually are, when viewed in the context of the debilitating effects of intellectual disabilities' [11, 12]. Several scientific studies have demonstrated that the presence of intellectual disabilities reduces professionals' opinion regarding the diagnostic significance of an accompanying behaviour problem. This is of considerable importance to the person with intellectual disabilities, as diagnostic overshadowing by professionals and carers will contribute an additional barrier to the person accessing appropriate treatment. A structured approach to the assessment of psychopathology may be helpful in preventing overshadowing.

Questions need to be asked in a developmentally aware manner, using language and communication appropriate to the person's ability levels. More time will be needed to complete an assessment compared to the amount of time needed for assessments with the general population. The health professional must be aware of the possibility of suggestibility. Informant histories are always an important part of any psychiatric assessment, as it can be difficult to elicit psychopathology if a person has limited verbal communication skills. Even persons with only mild intellectual disabilities are likely to experience some difficulties providing a full account, e.g. regarding temporal sequencing. The assessor must take account of how well the carer knows the person with intellectual disabilities, for how long, and how well teams of carers share information. Sometimes it is necessary to interview several carers. In order to determine any changes (i.e. symptoms) that have occurred, it is essential to access information on the person's longstanding personality and traits. Some symptoms of mental ill-health may actually present as a reduction in long standing traits e.g. lethargy may result in a reduction in long-standing problem behaviours, or increased sleep in a person with trait sleep disturbance. More typically, though, existing psychopathology is exacerbated by superimposed psychiatric illness. The assessor needs to be aware that the carers may volunteer information about problems presenting the most severe management challenges (e.g. problem behaviours), rather than symptoms that may be distressing for the person with intellectual disabilities (e.g. social withdrawal, loss of interest). Hence, it is always necessary to enquire about the full range of all possible psychopathology when assessing a person with intellectual disabilities for mental ill-health.

Assessment of psychopathology must also take into account the effect that developmental level and previous life experiences may have on the *content* of psychopathology. Sovner and DesNoyers Hurley described some of the pathoplastic effects of intellectual disabilities upon psychopathology [13, 14]. 'Psycho-social masking' refers to the concrete content/lack of imagination in symptom presentations; i.e., some significant abnormal *forms* of thought and perception may present with a childlike quality, reflecting the person's mental age and experiences. Despite this, hallucinations and delusions are almost always abnormal and indicative of serious mental ill-health, regardless of their content; i.e., symptoms should not be dismissed on the grounds that they appear childlike in content.

14.3 ICD-10 AND DSM-IV-TR, INTELLECTUAL DISABILITIES, AND CLASSIFICATION OF MENTAL ILL-HEALTH

Several researchers have previously commented upon the specific and general conceptual difficulties of diagnostic criteria designed for use with the general population, when applied with adults with intellectual disabilities. Researchers have usually modified the DSM and ICD diagnostic systems, with modifications tending to be ad hoc and not clearly operationalized [15, 16]. This is particularly so the more severe the intellectual disabilities of the study participants, and hinders future interpretation and replication of study results. Some of these issues are now discussed.

General population criteria contain numerous sub-categorizations. However, for persons who are non-verbal, there are limitations in the reliability of the assessed psychopathology, suggesting that extensive sub-classification lacks validity.

There has been much study and debate about the role of 'behavioural equivalents' in place of language-based symptoms, particularly for persons who do not have verbal communication skills (e.g. irritability/screaming in place of low mood in depressive episodes). Several items in the standard criteria require self-report, whereas they could be detected by observation if they were included in the criteria, which they are not (e.g. fear). For the same group, there is difficulty in applying general population criteria for schizophrenia and psychotic disorders.

There are inconsistencies and confusion in the DSM and ICD manuals regarding the use of the organic disorder categories, the status of behavioural phenotypes, and problem behaviours. The organic categories within ICD-10 'Personality and Behavioural Disorders and Other Mental Disorders due to Brain Disease, Damage and Dysfunction' are frequently interpreted in the literature to suggest that if a person has a psychiatric disorder together with epilepsy, or even just intellectual disabilities, then the organic category should be used. Such an approach leads to incomplete assessment and treatment, and therapeutic nihilism. The person's intellectual disabilities or epilepsy may be caused by an underlying brain damage that predisposes them to additional mental ill-health, or may be associated with a behavioural phenotype, but other contributory causes may be present and should always be sought. Diagnostic criteria designed for use with the general population make no reference to classification where there are known behavioural phenotypes, and this has led to much variability and confusion in the published literature.

Some items require sophisticated intellectual skills, e.g. concepts of body image distortion, guilt, death, hopelessness. A full understanding of concepts such as guilt and death may require a developmental level of about seven years to have been achieved, and hence is unlikely ever to be achieved by a person with severe or profound intellectual disabilities. Hence, these symptoms will not occur during episodes of mental ill-health in this group, and there is a distortion or pathoplastic effect on the way that psychopathology is manifest. Sovner and DesNoyes Hurley called these phenomena 'intellectual distortions' [14].

Some categories require a minimal chronological/mental age that describes when a presentation is considered developmentally inappropriate (e.g. elimination disorders). However, as Sturmey pointed out, it cannot be assumed that the development of a person with intellectual disabilities is the same as that for a person of average intelligence, but delayed, as development may not only be delayed, but may also be different [15]. This then complicates the judgement of what is 'developmentally appropriate'.

Problem behaviours are the most common type of mental ill-health experienced by people with intellectual disabilities [8]. ICD-10 adopts a confusing approach to the classification of problem behaviours. Some can be coded in up to three separate places in ICD-10 with no clear instructions on which is most appropriate. The ICD-10 mental retardation codes allow specifiers for problem behaviours, but fail to distinguish between problem behaviours secondary to psychiatric/physical illness, and longer standing traits. Such differentiation does have important treatment implications. DSM-IV-TR includes categories dependent on the person's underlying intent, which often cannot be determined in this group, and largely does not otherwise include problem behaviours within its system.

14.4   DC-LD AND DM-ID, INTELLECTUAL DISABILITIES, AND CLASSIFICATION OF MENTAL ILL-HEALTH

DC-LD was published in 2001 [17]. It was developed to be complementary to ICD-10, for use with persons with more severe levels of intellectual disabilities for whom the issues described in the previous section are relevant. The impetus for its development came from a desire to foster diagnostic standardization in research work, and hence allow study findings to be comparable. There was also a desire to raise awareness of diagnostic issues and so work towards more standard and improved clinical diagnostic practice. It drew on the evidence base as far as there was one, and also consensus opinion. The field trials were conducted in UK and the Republic of Ireland. DC-LD provides a hierarchical framework, which accommodates behavioural phenotypes and problem behaviours. It also adjusts items within criteria to account for the pathoplastic effect of intellectual disabilities on psychopathology. All criteria are fully operationalized. It is currently being revised for a second edition.

DM-ID was published in 2007 [18]. It was developed using an expert consensus process and is a diagnostic manual designed to be an adaptation of the DSM-IV-TR. Its field trials were conducted internationally. Rather than adjusting the items within criteria, it aims to interpret them to be of greater relevance for use with people with more severe intellectual disabilities. It provides detailed information to facilitate classification of mental ill-health by both inexperienced and experienced practitioners, particularly for use with persons with more severe intellectual disabilities. Unlike DC-LD, DM-ID does not introduce a section on problem behaviours, reflecting ongoing debate regarding the nosological status of these disorders.

Even though a significant advance in the recognition and the assessment of psychiatric disorders in ID has been made in recent years, the newness of these two manuals renders it difficult to judge the impact and utility they will have, and the extent to which they do achieve their aim of addressing the problems in classification of mental ill-health in people with intellectual disabilities.

REFERENCES

[1] Durkin M. The epidemiology of developmental disabilities in low-income countries. *Mental Retardation Developmental Disability Research Reviews* 2002;8: pp. 206–11.

[2] Leonard H, Wen X. The epidemiology of mental retardation: challenges and opportunities in the new millennium. *Mental Retardation and Developmental Disabilities* 2002;8: pp. 117–134.

[3] Roeleveld N, Zielhuis GA, Gabreëls F. The prevalence of mental retardation: a critical review of recent literature. *Developmental Medicine & Child Neurology* 1997;39: pp. 125–32.

[4] Leonard H, Petterson B, Bower C, Sanders R. Prevalence of intellectual disability in Western Australia. *Paediatric and Perinatal Epidemiology* 2003;17: pp. 58–67.

[5] Salvador-Carulla L, Bertelli M. 'Mental retardation' or 'intellectual disability': time for a conceptual change. *Psychopathology* 2008;41: pp. 10–16.

[6] World Health Organization. *Atlas on Country Resources in Intellectual Disabilities (Atlas-ID)*. Geneva: WHO; 2007. www.who.int/mental_health/evidence/atlas_id_2007.pdf (Last accessed July 20th, 2008).

[7] Einfeld SL, Hofer SM, Taffe J, Gray KM, Bontempo DE, Hoffman LR, Parmenter T, Tonge BJ. Psychopathology in young people with intellectual disability. *Journal of the American Medical Association*, 2006; 296: pp. 1981–1989.

[8] Cooper S-A, Smiley E, Morrison J, Allan L, Williamson A. Prevalence of and associations with mental ill-health in adults with intellectual disabilities. *British Journal of Psychiatry*, 2007; 190: pp. 27–35.

[9] Smiley E, Cooper S-A, Finlayson J, Jackson A, Allan L, Mantry D, McGrother C, McConnachie A, Morrison J. The incidence, and predictors of mental ill-health in adults with intellectual disabilities. Prospective study. *British Journal of Psychiatry* 2007;191: pp. 313–319.

[10] Salvador-Carulla L, Rodríguez-Blázquez C, Rodríguezde Molina M, Pérez-Marín J, Velázquez R. Hidden psychiatric morbidity in a vocational programme for people with intellectual disability. *Journal of Intellectual Disability Research* 2000;44: pp. 147–154.

[11] Reiss S, Levitan GW, Szyszko J. Emotional disturbance and mental retardation: diagnostic overshadowing. *American Journal of Mental Deficiency* 1982;86: pp. 567–574.

[12] Reiss S, Szyszko J. Diagnostic overshadowing and professional experience with mentally retarded persons. *American Journal of Mental Deficiency* 1983;87: pp. 396–402.

[13] Sovner R. Limiting factors in the use of DSM-111 criteria with mentally ill/mentally retarded persons. *Psychopharmacology Bulletin* 1986;22: pp. 1055–1059.

[14] Sovner R, DesNoyers Hurley A. Four factors affecting the diagnosis of psychiatric disorders in mentally retarded persons. *Psychiatric Aspects of Mental Retardation Reviews* 1986;5: pp. 45–48.

[15] Sturmey P. DSM-IIIR and persons with dual diagnoses: conceptual issues and strategies for future research. *Journal of Intellectual Disability Research* 1995:39: pp. 357–364.

[16] Sturmey P. Diagnostic-based pharmacological treatment of behaviour disorders in persons with developmental disabilities: a review and a decision-making typology. *Research on Developmental Disabilities*, 1995;16: pp. 235–252.

[17] Royal College of Psychiatrists. *DC-LD [Diagnostic criteria for psychiatric disorders for use with adults with learning disabilities/mental retardation]*. Occasional Paper OP 48. London: Gaskell; 2001.

[18] Fletcher R, Loschen E, Stavrakaki C, *et al*. *Diagnostic manual – intellectual disability: A clinical guide for diagnosis of mental disorders in persons with intellectual disability (DM-ID)*. Kingston, NY: NADD Press; 2007.

CHAPTER 15

Specificities of Diagnosis and Classification in Child and Adolescent Psychiatry

Michel Botbol

*World Psychiatric Association Zonal Representative for Western Europe;
Member of the Steering committee of the Institutional Program
on Psychiatry for the Person; Section on Psychoanalysis in Psychiatry,
World Psychiatric Association*

Carlos E. Berganza

*Professor of Child Psychiatry, San Carlos University School of Medicine, Guatemala;
Past President, Executive Committee on the Latin American Guide for Psychiatric
Diagnosis*

15.1   INTRODUCTION

Whether or not the diagnosis and classification of psychiatric disorders need to attend to specific perspectives of child and adolescent psychiatry remains, to a certain extent, an open question. Current diagnostic and classification system seem to assume they do, by proposing specific categories for children and adolescents on Axis I (such as F93, emotional disorders with onset specific to childhood [1]) or when they condition the use of Axis II personality disorders categories. For instance, the American Psychiatric Association's Diagnostic and Statistical Manual [2] states that:

> 'To diagnose a Personality Disorder in an individual under age 18 years, the features must have been present for at least 1 year. The one exception to this is Antisocial Personality Disorder, which cannot be diagnosed in individuals under age 18 years'. ([2] p. 687).

These exceptions notwithstanding, the specificities considered so far for the child and adolescent psychiatric practice are still quite limited, with only a small number of these specific categories being included, and a notable lack of alternatives to replace

Psychiatric Diagnosis: Challenges and Prospects   Edited by I.M. Salloum and J.E. Mezzich
© 2009 John Wiley & Sons, Ltd

those Axis II conditions already being developed in the child or adolescent patient. Moreover, in spite of the differences these classifications are implicitly recognizing for child and adolescent psychiatry, the diagnostic process is supposed to remain strictly the same as in adult psychiatry, that is to say, based on descriptive items to type the disorders, and the use of comorbidity to correct the ill-effect of this model of the diagnostic process and to bring diagnostic categories closer to real clinical situations. These limited adaptations of the current classificatory systems to the needs of the child and adolescent psychiatric practice contrast remarkably with the multiple specificities involved concerning diagnosis in child and adolescent psychiatry. Such specificities can be considered from at least four relevant perspectives: (1) symptomatic; (2) developmental; (3) environmental; and (4) prognostic.

15.2   SYMPTOMATIC SPECIFICITIES

In childhood and adolescence, there are specific limitations in the type of externalized manifestations, as well as in the possibility to have insight-dependant symptoms. The relation between observed symptoms and underlying psychological organization is then particular in child and adolescent psychiatry. More frequently than in adult psychiatry, a specific set of behavioural descriptive symptoms may be related to quite different underlying psychopathological organizations. Thus, at this age, consideration given to dynamic defence mechanisms and structural organizations underlying the behavioural symptoms frequently leads to profound modification in the diagnostic evaluation and in the therapeutic indications. This perspective can lead, for example, to consider some obsessive compulsive disorder (OCD) patients to be much closer to schizophrenic or narcissistic patients than to those suffering from other anxiety disorders. Although this perspective may not generally call for a change in the pharmacological prescription, the rest of the treatment strategy, so important at this age, will be more adapted to the patient's specific needs when taking into account the underlying psychopathological organization rather than the sole OCD symptoms. In some cases, this may lead to a therapeutic programme that is much closer to what would be proposed to a schizophrenic patient [3] than to the one we would generally offer to other anxiety disorder patients.

Conversely, a particular psychopathological constellation may have very different symptomatic expressions. Depression in adolescence, for instance, can be expressed in very different ways; for example, it can be expressed through acting-out or psychotic symptoms more often than in adult psychiatry. For many authors, this should be taken into account for the pharmacological prescriptions at this age. [4].

15.3   DEVELOPMENTAL SPECIFICITIES

Developmental considerations are of more importance in child and adolescent psychiatry than they are in adults'. They are crucial to differentiate pathological symptoms and developmental conflicts, to appreciate developmental breakdowns, regressions or fixations, to recognize disharmonies on the different developmental lines, to integrate biological and environmental dimensions of development and, finally, to adapt therapeutic responses. Taking into account this developmental dimension allowed a team of French child psychiatrists, nearly thirty years ago, to describe a clinical condition they include in the French classification of child and adolescent mental disorders [5] under the name of 'Psychotic Disharmony'; this disorder appeared to be very similar to what Donald Cohen proposed 15 years later under the name 'Multiplex Developmental Disorders' to differentiate them from other Pervasive Developmental Disorders (PDD) Not Otherwise Specified (NOS) [6].

15.4 ENVIRONMENTAL SPECIFICITIES

There is obviously, in childhood, a specific dependency upon current and past environmental conditions; this implies that relational aspects have a bigger impact on the expression of mental disorders at this age. In child and adolescent psychiatry, there are therefore greater risks that a number of diagnostic labels might be nothing more than a psychiatric reformulation of a social impairment (e.g., the 'Conduct Disorders' category could merely be a psychiatric formulation of delinquency), when diagnostic labelling does not bring any added value to the social construct.

Conversely, psychopathological disorders are ignored or denied when covered by hyper adaptation to local or global social norms, even when this hyper adaptation is mainly a way to deal with underlying psychological distress (as shown in some stabilized high functioning PDD or in some childhood undiagnosed OCD) that may be hidden to the child or adolescent him- or herself. It may also be observed in behavioural disorders fitting well social definitions and social responses in specific circumstances. For instance, learning difficulties at school or delinquency in educational or judicial settings have less chance of being seen as symptoms of psychological distress unless specifically addressed from a psychopathological perspective. Social norms are, thus, one of the main determinants of the diagnostic labelling in childhood.

Finally, in everyday practice, there is a great risk in child and adolescent psychiatry that the choice between a social or a psychiatric definition of a disorder, and the assistance it will generate, would not be based as much on the disorder characteristics as it is on its social context and on the type of interaction between the child and his environment.

There is, then, in child and adolescent psychiatry, a specific need to avoid diagnostic processes that are strictly limited to individual approaches, as much as those focusing only on the adaptation to the environment; instead, child psychiatry requires diagnostic processes taking into account the subjective aspects resulting from the interaction of individual and environmental dimensions. In other words, there is at this age a specific need for diagnostics to consider the psychic functioning and not to limit itself to the description of social symptoms. Moreover, this approach constitutes a useful basis for the multi-focal approaches always required to deal with such psychopathological social expressions at this age.

15.5 PROGNOSTIC SPECIFICITIES

Prognosis has a specific value in child and adolescent psychiatry, where the main concern is not only the current status of the disorder but also its continuity into adulthood.

From this viewpoint, data show the lack of reliability of Axis I categories alone for adolescents, and a significant increase in the prognostic reliability when Axis II categories are added [7], even if they are not supposed to be used at this age. From this perspective, too, child and adolescent psychiatry shows a specific need to take into account the underlying psychological functioning of the individual patient, and not to rely solely on descriptions of externalised symptomatic expressions on which current classifications base their categorical definitions.

In summary, most of the specific needs of child and adolescent psychiatry are not addressed by current classifications and diagnostic systems; the main issue is not their lack of specific categories but the diagnostic process they adopt that does not take into account what seems crucial in child and adolescent mental disorders classification: an overall evaluation of the mental functioning of the child, and not only a description of his/her symptoms. To a smaller extent, this difficulty is also found in adult psychiatry, but it has more serious consequences in child and adolescent psychiatry. For instance, big differences of prevalence of attention deficit hyperactivity disorder (ADHD) in different parts of the world cannot be explained only as cultural or biological variations, but rather as resulting from variations in the social use of psychiatric nosographical labelling [8].

To address these issues, classifications and diagnostic processes require conceptual modifications, such as: (a) better integration of individual, relational and environmental dimensions; (b) stronger references to developmental dimensions and longitudinal aspects of disorders; and (c) a bigger need to take into account psychic functioning and defence mechanisms to define the personality patterns as much as the process leading to the symptom.

There is, then, a need to introduce more complexity into the current classification systems to allow them to get closer to the clinical situations we face in child and adolescent psychiatry. The problem is that the introduction of more complexity necessarily implies more room for the psychiatrist interpretation (that is to say, to its theoretical background) while we also need to maintain common references to a universal nosographical frame.

15.6   ALTERNATIVE NOSOLOGICAL PROPOSALS IN CHILD AND ADOLESCENT PSYCHIATRY

Faced with the above-mentioned limitations of the most visible diagnostic and classification systems for the child psychiatric practice, child psychiatrist across the world have proposed alternative nosological schemas. Of interest for this review are the British multiaxial classification of child and adolescent psychiatric disorder [9], the third Cuban glossary of psychiatry [10]), The Latin American guide for psychiatric diagnosis [11], the French classification of child and adolescent mental disorders [5] and the Psychodynamic Diagnostic Manual (PDM) [12].

15.6.1   The British Proposal

Developed by the World Health Organization under the leadership of Professor Michael Rutter, the British proposal [9] represents a refinement of proposals for the improvement in validity of psychiatric diagnoses in childhood and adolescence advanced by him some 25 years earlier [13]. This nosological system is based on Chapter V (F) of the ICD-10 [1], and reorganizes the psychiatric disorders and other related conditions of concern for childhood and adolescence along six axes: 1. Clinical psychiatric syndromes; 2. Specific disorders of psychological development; 3. Intellectual level; 4. Medical conditions; 5. Associated abnormal psychosocial situations; and 6. Global assessment of psychosocial disability.

Among other interesting improvements over the international system, the British proposal includes codes for a normal health state or lack of any diagnostic condition in the child under assessment, as well as codes for superior intellectual functioning (as opposed to different states of mental retardation), and superior or good social functioning. Finally, although it presents a clinical format, and does not include the specific criteria for research, the nosographic descriptions of each disorder is enriched considerably, based on the formidable clinical experience of its proponents.

15.6.2   The Cuban Classification of Childhood Disorders

The third Cuban glossary of psychiatry [10] is an adaptation of Chapter V (F) of ICD-10 [1] to the needs and particularities of the Cuban population and its health system. It organizes the psychiatric disorders and other conditions of interest for patients who present for clinical care along six axes: I. Diagnoses (using the nosological organization of ICD-10, and enriching its descriptions with important description that make it more useful for the local realities); II. Disabilities; III. Adverse environmental and personal factors; IV. Other personal and environmental factors; V. Psychopathogenic mechanisms and needs; and VI. Other meaningful information. Cuban child psychiatrists contributed significantly to review the nosography of child and adolescent clinical syndromes and adjusted in a very effective way those descriptions to adapt them to the realities of everyday clinical practice in child psychiatry. This, in addition to the multiaxial system proposed, provides the clinician with an effective instrument to effectively capture the data that is relevant for effective diagnosis and treatment of the child psychiatry patient.

15.6.3   The Latin American Guide for Psychiatric Diagnosis (GLADP)

Developed by the Section on Diagnosis and Classification of the Latin American Psychiatric Association [11], the GLADP is the product of the participation of an extensive group of mental health professionals from most countries in Latin America. It also represents an annotation of Chapter V (F) of ICD-10 to the needs and realities of the region in matters of mental health. Concerning its diagnostic format, it employs a comprehensive diagnostic model, in line with the World Psychiatric Association's International Guidelines for Diagnostic Assessment [IGDA] ([14] Mezzich, Berganza, von Cranach *et al*, 2003. The GLADP's diagnostic model has three components: the first is a standardized multiaxial one composed of four axes: 1. Clinical disorders; 2. Disabilities; 3. Contextual factors; and 4. Quality of life. The second component is an idiographic diagnostic formulation that allows the clinician to include in natural language a description of what is idiosyncratic to the clinical situation of the patient under assessment. This must be an articulation of the perspectives of the clinician, the patient and his/her family, and includes a contextualized description of the main problems identified by the standardized component, the main positive aspects and strengths of the patient and his/her context, and his/her expectations and those of the family concerning recovery. Finally, the third component is a diagnostic format to compile relevant information for planning and disposition.

This diagnostic format allows the child psychiatrist to easily adapt the diagnostic model to the particular needs of the child or adolescent under their care, in line with what is usually required in the everyday child psychiatric practice.

15.6.4   The French Classification for Child and Adolescent Mental Disorders

Operational since 1983, the French Classification of Child and Adolescent Mental Disorders (FCCAMD) [5] is the classification of reference for all French child psychiatrists, who are very attached to it; they recognize themselves in the clinical and therapeutic methods they find there, and in which they were (and continue to be) trained.

Validated through multicentric studies [15], it is currently used (together with ICD-10) in all the medical-administrative documents in France, and in the existing activity evaluation and project management of the child psychiatry public services (Thevenot *et al,* 1993 and 1999 [16, 17].

The FCCAMD is articulated with the WHO classification of handicaps [18], and comprises a table of conversion with the ICD-10 [1]. A data-processing expert system was built on this classification, testifying to the rigour and the reproducibility of its steps [19].

The FFCAMD is deliberately built according to a hierarchical architecture, seeking in priority to establish, whenever possible, a structural diagnosis as the **main diagnosis**. (see Figure 15.1). This structural diagnosis includes personality characteristics and developmental aspects and is referred to psychodynamic psychopathological categories (neurosis, psychosis, narcissistic and borderline organization, reactional states). A **complementary diagnosis** then has to be established, based on descriptive categories similar to DSM and ICD categories. FCCAMD is thus not pretending to be atheoretical; on the contrary, it clearly assert the theory on which it is based, allowing it to remain closer to the clinical steps in clinical situations, never atheoretical. A second axis classifies contextual and possibly etiological figures, including biological and environmental characteristics; this axis is purely descriptive and completely atheoretical, allowing its use from any etiological perspective.

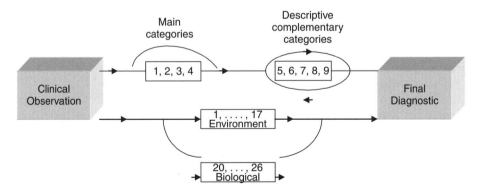

Figure 15.1   Diagnostic process in FCCAMD [5].

15.6.5   The Psychodynamic Diagnostic Manual (PDM)

Clearly supported by the International Psychoanalytic Association, the Psychodynamic Diagnostic Manual (PDM) [12] project proposes to complement DSM-IV [2] by adding the specific contribution of a psychodynamic perspective. For child and adolescent diagnoses, it includes: a) an individual profile of mental functioning (including pattern of relating, comprehending, feelings, coping with stress and anxiety, observing one's own emotions and behaviours, judgements; b) healthy and disordered personality functioning; and c) symptom patterns based on DSM-IV, including differences in each individual's personal or subjective experience of the symptoms.

In the French classification, the overall architecture and the diagnostic process it induces, are based on a psychodynamic theoretical approach, whereas most of its components are not (the complementary diagnoses based on DSM-like descriptive categories, and axis II contextual and possibly etiological factors). In the PDM, it is somewhat the opposite; the PDM remains clearly referred to DSM, to which it adds complementary psychodynamic informed data.

15.7   CONCLUSIONS

Alternative nosological proposals to deal with specificities of diagnosis and classification in child and adolescent psychiatry, then, are numerous. Each of these alternative proposals is, in its own way, trying to overcome the limitations of the current international nosographical system. The British proposal introduces new axes, taking into account psychological and environmental dimensions and giving more attention to intellectual and psychosocial functions; the Cuban classification of childhood disorders and the Latin American guide for psychiatric diagnosis stress the importance of cultural diversity improving the adaptation of the diagnostic model to the particular needs of everyday child psychiatric practice.

These proposals considerably enlarge the domains they take into account in the diagnostic process; they are thus in line with a person-centred psychiatric perspective. The final two proposals (the French classification and the PDM) share this perspective, to which they add an attempt to approach the subjectivity of the person through the psychiatrist's subjective evaluation. To achieve this goal, they are not atheoretical, as are the other three; on the contrary, they clearly assert their psychodynamic theoretical background.

All of these alternative nosographical systems remain referred to an objective nosography based on standardized categories, and consider disorder-centred labelling as merely a part of the person-centred integrative diagnostic process that also requires sufficient attention to other psychological factors (in illness and positive health domains). In that sense, each of them offers a valuable new perspective to classification in child and adolescent psychiatry.

REFERENCES

[1] World Health Organization. *International Statistical Classification of Diseases and Related Health Problems, Tenth Revision [ICD-10]*. Geneva: World Health Organization; 1992.

[2] American Psychiatric Association. *Diagnostic and Statistical Manual of Mental Disorders, Fourth Edition, Text Revision [DSM-IV-TR]*. Washington, DC: American Psychiatric Association; 2000.

[3] Nechmad A, Ratzoni G, Poyurovsky M, *et al*. Obsessive compulsive disorder in adolescent schizophrenia patients. *American Journal of Psychiatry* 2003;160: pp. 1002–1004.

[4] Jeammet PH. Les prémices de la schizophrénie. In: De Clercq M, Peuskens J. (eds.) *Les troubles schizophréniques*. Bruxelles: De Boeck Université; 2000.

[5] Mises R, Quemada N, Botbol M, *et al*. French classification for child and adolescent mental disorders. *Psychopathology* 2002;35: pp. 176–180.

[6] Tordjman S, Ferrari P, Golse B, *et al*. Dysharmonie psychotique et multiplex developmental disorder : histoire d'une convergence. *Psychiatrie de l'enfant* 1997;2: pp. 473–504.

[7] Johnson JG, Cohen P, Skodol AE, *et al*. Personality disorders in adolescence and risk for major mental disorders and suicidality during adulthood. *Archives of General Psychiatry* 1999;56: pp. 805–811.

[8] Diller L. Cola Coca, MacDonald's et Ritaline®. *Enfance et Psy* 2001;14: pp. 137–141.

[9] World Health Organization. *Multiaxial classification of child and adolescent psychiatric disorder*. Geneva: World Health Organization; 1996.

[10] Otero-Ojeda AA, Rabelo-Perez V, Echazabal-Campos A, *et al*. *Tercer glosario cubano de psiquiatría*. Havana, Cuba: Ministerio de Salud Pública; 2001.

[11] Asociación Psiquiátrica de América Latina. *Guía latinoamericana de diagnóstico psiquiátrico*. Editorial de la Universidad de Guadalajara, Mexico; 2004.

[12] Alliance of Psychoanalytic Organizations. *Psychodynamic Diagnostic Manual (PDM)*. Silver Spring MD: Alliance of Psychoanalytic Organizations; 2006.

[13] Rutter M, Lebovici L, Eisenberg L, *et al*. A triaxial classification of mental disorders in childhood. *Journal of Child Psychology and Psychiatry* 1969;10: pp. 41–61.

[14] Mezzich JE, Berganza CE, von Cranach M, *et al*. Essentials of the World Psychiatric Associations International Guidelines for Diagnostic Assessment (IGDA). *The British Journal of Psychiatry*. May 2003;182 (45 Suppl).

[15] Quemada N, Casadebaig F. Caractéristiques cliniques d'une clientèle de secteurs psychiatriques publics. *L'évolution psychiatrique* 1992;57: pp. 201–211.

[16] Thevenot JP, Quemada N. Enquête sur les demandes d'hospitalisation à temps complet en psychiatrie infanto-juvénile en Ile-de-France. Premiers résultats globaux. *L'Information Psychiatrique* 1993;69: pp. 353–358.

[17] Thevenot JP, Quemada N. Les difficultés de l'accès aux soins institutionnels : une enquête épidémiologique en Ile-de-France. *Enfances et Psy* 1999;7: pp. 58–63.

[18] World Health Organization. *International Classification of Impairments, Disabilities, and Handicaps: A Manual of Classification Relating to the Consequences of Disease*. Geneva: World Health Organization; 1980.

[19] Portelli C, Frydmann F, Mises R. JPSY, un système expert d'aide au diagnostic. Inspiré par la classification française des troubles mentaux de l'enfant et de l'adolescent. *L'Information Psychiatrique* 1992;68: pp. 947–954.

CHAPTER 16

Classification in Infant and Child Psychiatry

Sam Tyano

*Professor Emeritus in Psychiatry, Tel Aviv University School of
Medicine, Israel*

Lior Schapir

GEHA Mental Health Center, Tel Aviv University School of Medicine, Israel

16.1 THE NECESSITY OF SPECIAL PSYCHIATRIC CLASSIFICATIONS FOR INFANTS AND CHILDREN

Classification of children's psychiatric disorders evolved with the change in children's status within society. It has progressed from referring to a child as a subject, through perceiving the child as a small adult, to its current form that views the child as a unique being. Diagnosing children is difficult, since they are still in a developmental phase which makes the distinction between normal and abnormal development very difficult. The same phenomenon may be normal at a certain age, while pointing to a disorder at a different age. This begs the question whether the manifestation of a disorder can be exactly the same at different brain maturity stages. Moreover, the same disorder can have different interpretations at different ages, as for example, an eating disorder. When we make an observation at a certain age, what tools do we have to predict the developmental outcome of a symptom or a sign that we find? While one should not base classification on a developmental theory, it is clear that every classification is based on a conceptual understanding. It is not just coincidence that, in the history of psychiatry, the neuroses vanished as rival approaches to psychoanalysis emerged. The recent development seems to be "gene plus environmental influence". Does our classification represent this approach? Many disorders in children have comorbidity. For example, in a recently published study it was found that only 7.6% of the boys and 21.7% of the girls manifested ADHD without any other psychiatric comorbidity [1]. How is this fact expressed in the classification? There are possible implications both for understanding the disorder, and for its treatment.

Psychiatric Diagnosis: Challenges and Prospects Edited by I.M. Salloum and J.E. Mezzich
© 2009 John Wiley & Sons, Ltd

Unlike adult population, in which most of the information is gathered directly from the adult himself/herself, sources of information regarding a child vary. The child itself is of foremost importance in gathering information. Children's reporting may not always be reliable and thus other sources of information are used as well. Parents can provide information a child would not give, leading to diagnoses such as conduct disorders, while a child can report about subjective feelings that the parents may not be aware of, such as depression. The kindergarten teacher or the teacher at school can provide information concerning social disturbances.

In order to gather information, age-adapted scales were constructed, such as the K-SADS [2]. Recent years have seen a significant progression in developmental psychiatry, partly due to improvements in research methodology. Many long-term follow up studies have been published. They discovered that most diagnoses are temporary (with the exception of autism and schizophrenia), and that they may change according to age, risk and protective factors. For example: conduct disorder in children may develop into depression in adolescents. Therefore, we should consider the onset age, as well as risk and protective factors, while keeping in mind that in childhood- development is critical. Assessment of a child is different when it is done to find a diagnosis strictly for academic interest than when it is done in a clinical setting in order to find the right treatment plan. When we assess a child only for the purpose of diagnosing him for an academic study, we use scales and structured questionnaires that make the interview more structured. When we assess a child in order to find the best treatment plan, the interview is quite unstructured, as the parameters being examined, such as inter-personal relationships and inter-subjectivity, are not found in structured questionnaires. The information we gather should be classified in a multi-axial system as in adults. A multi-axial system should refer to: descriptive references, etiological references, pathophysiological references, psychopathological references, behavioral references, dynamic references, structural references, and psychosocial references.

16.2 HISTORY OF CHILD PSYCHIATRY CLASSIFICATION

Table 16.1 Landmarks in the development of psychiatric taxonomies*.

1883	Kraepelin	Proposal for a comprehensive classification system
1948	ICD-6	Psychiatric disorders included
1952	DSM-I	First U.S. official classification system, only a few categories for children
1966	Group for the advancement of psychiatry	Diagnostic system for children
1968	DSM-II	14 disorders include children, from them, only five are exclusively child disorders. Emphasis on theory and Meyer's concept of reaction types
1972	Trajan	Proposed a psychosocial axis
1977	ICD-9	**First Multi-axial system**. Axis I: clinical disorders, Axis II: Intellectual level, Axis III: . . . or Etiology

1980	DSM-III	Fourfold increase in child psychiatric disorders, greater diagnostic precision, multi-axial: Axis-I nine categories of Clinical Disorders, Axis-II Developmental Disorders, Axis-III Physical Illnesses, Axis-IV Psychosocial Stressors, Axis-V Adaptation During Last Year
1987	DSM-III-R	Refinements in criteria, categories. Changing of MR, PDD and LD from Axis-I to Axis-II, thus emphasizing they are developmental disorders, based on a **change in the concept** of these disorders.
1992	ICD-10	Separation of research diagnostic criteria from clinical descriptions
1994	DSM-IV	More emphasis on data based modifications in categories and criteria
2000	DSM-IV-TR	Generally minor revisions in text (not criteria)
2002	DSM-V	Research agenda and white papers
2012	DSM-V	Anticipated publication date

DSM, Diagnostic and statistical Manual of Mental Disorders; ICD, International Classification of Diseases; MR, Mental Retardation; PDD, Pervasive Developmental Disorder; LD, Learning Disorders.
*Adapted from *Lewis's Child and Adolescent Psychiatry: A Comprehensive Textbook*, fourth edition, [3], Copyright © 2007, Lippincott Williams & Wilkins.

16.3   CURRENT MULTI-AXIAL CLASSIFICATIONS FOR INFANT AND CHILDREN'S PSYCHIATRIC DISORDERS – DC: 0-3R, ICD-10, DSM IV–TR, AND OTHER CLASSIFICATION SYSTEMS IN USE

16.3.1   A. Classification of Infant's Psychiatric Disorders

A scientific classification of infants should arise from current understanding of the development of the human psyche. There are many models that try to address the complicated issue of development from infancy to adulthood. Such models include the deterministic constitutional model, the deterministic environmental model, the interactional model, and the transactional model.

The transactional model of development [4] deals with the combined effects of genetics, biology, culture, life events, and psychology. It is widely accepted and forms the basis for infant classification.

According to our model, there are three dimensions of the self: the Biological self, which involves biological factors such as motor skills, genetically-programmed brain characteristics, and cognition, the psychosocial self, involving the emotional intrapsychic and interpersonal development and life events influencing the development of the child, and finally, the cultural self that deals with cultural influences and demands on the developing child.

When assessing an infant, one must identify risk factors resulting in negative developmental outcomes as well as protective factors leading to more favorable outcomes. Both types of factors may be found within the infant, the parents and the environment. Factors found within the infant can be biological, constitutional or experiential. Biological factors may constitute, for example, severe prematurity, congenital diseases, or physical illness, Constitutional factors include vulnerability, resilience or lack thereof, temperament, IQ level, etc., Experiential factors could be adverse relational experiences like insecure or disorganized attachment relationships, abuse, neglect, trauma and loss or the opposite, namely, secure attachments and growth promoting parent-infant relationships. Risk factors that can be found within the parent include: Poor education, low IQ, physical and mental illness, borderline or narcissistic personality disorder, unresolved trauma, losses, past abuse, and disorganized attachment while protective factors comprise maternal education, IQ, healthy personality, well functioning family environment, and a stable marital relationship. Environmental risk factors are poverty, lack of social support and adverse life events vs. protective environmental factors such as social support, high socio economic status, and positive life events. The socio-emotional-cognitive status of the child can be estimated by summing up the relevant protective factors and deleting the risk factors from the sum. The diagnostic challenge in the first three years is linked to the rapid developmental change, the infant's total dependence on the care giving environment, and the difficulty to differentiate normal, temperamental variations from signs of pathology. Furthermore, there are implications to ascribing a diagnosis to an infant. Making a diagnosis means to state that there is a health problem, i.e. a disorder/illness. Such statements can be hazardous especially since nosologies in psychiatry are descriptive rather than etiological. On the other hand, one should keep in mind that the main purpose of making a diagnosis is to plan a therapeutic intervention. There is a need for a classification of very young children. Preschoolers externalizing and internalizing problems are not rare; in a study by Keenan et al. [5] 26.4% of 104 low income five year olds had a DSM diagnosis. Such problems are predictors of negative outcomes years later, and are often quite constant. These children, therefore, have to be treated, thus making it necessary to diagnose them in order to choose a modality of treatment. There are a number of common reasons for referral to infant psychiatry: problems related to withdrawal, feeding-eating disturbances (Failure To Thrive or FTT), sleep disturbances, developmental delays or developmental disturbances, excessive crying, irritability or psychomotor agitation, behavioral problems like abnormal activity level and aggression, relationship disturbances as for example socialization difficulties, inadequate parenting and parental psychopathology. Prior to classifying, one needs to assess the child's mental status, the child's developmental status, the parent's mental status, parenting behavior, marital relationship and the quality of the parent-infant relationship, that is the result of the interplay between the child's and the parent's characteristics.

The Infant-Toddler Mental Status Examination includes:

1. Appearance: size, quality of nourishment, dress and hygiene, apparent maturity compared with chronological age, dysmorphic features, head size, cutaneous lesions.
2. Apparent reaction to situation: (a) Initial reaction to setting and to strangers, and (b) Adaptation: exploration, and reaction to transition.
3. Self-regulation: (a) State regulation, (b) Sensory regulation, (c) Unusual behaviors, (d) Activity level, (e) Attention span, (f) Frustration tolerance, and (g) Aggression.
4. Motor: muscle tone and strength, mobility in different positions, unusual motor pattern, cranial nerves, gross and fine motor coordination.
5. Speech and language: (a) Vocalization and speech production, (b) Receptive language, and (c) Expressive language.
6. Thought processes and content: (a) Specific fears, (b) Dreams and nightmares, (c) Dissociative states, and (d) Hallucinations.
7. Affect and mood: (a) Modes of expression, (b) Range of expressed emotions, (c) Responsiveness. (d) Duration of emotional state, and (e) Intensity of expressed affect.

8. Play: (a) Structure of play, and (b) Content of play.
9. Cognition: play, verbal and symbolic functioning, problem solving.
10. Association: (a) to parents (b) to examiner, and (c) attachment behaviors. In assessing attachment, one can use the Strange Situation Paradigm (research), the Adult Attachment Interview (research) or the Mini-Separation at initial evaluation (clinic). For assessment of temperament, one can use the Observed Temperament, and the Perceived Temperament questionnaires.

The DC: 0-3R (Zero to Three (Organization)) [6] was developed following dissatisfaction with many aspects of the DSM diagnostic system [7] among infant clinicians. The intent was not to replace the DSM but rather to complement it. By its multi-axial structure the DC: 0-3R reflects the transactional approach.

Axis I: Primary diagnosis is equivalent to the "Clinical disorders" of the DSM, and includes posttraumatic stress disorder, deprivation/maltreatment disorder, disorders of affect, and prolonged bereavement/grief reaction. Anxiety disorders in infancy and early childhood include: separation anxiety disorder, specific phobia, social anxiety disorder, generalized anxiety disorder, and anxiety disorder NOS. Depression in infancy and early childhood is divided into: Type I- major depression, and Type II- depressive disorder NOS. In addition there is: mixed disorder of emotional expressiveness, adjustment disorder, regulation disorders of sensory processing (hypersensitive; hyposensitive; sensory stimulation seeking/impulsive), sleep behavior disorder, feeding behavior disorder (6 subtypes), disorders of relating and communicating, multisystem developmental disorder, and other disorders (DSM IV TR or ICD 10 [7–9]). In order to demonstrate the application of the infant classification system in clinical practice, we present results from our field study, which was done in our infant mental health center that is affiliated with Tel-Aviv University [10] (Tables 16.2–16.5).

Axis II: Parent–Infant Relationship disorders uses two tools: the PIR-GAS that relates to the intensity, frequency and duration of the difficulties (81–100: Adapted; 41–80: Features of a disordered relationship; 0–40: Disordered relationship), and the Relationship Problems Checklist that relates to the level of evidence pointing at a

Table 16.2 Distribution of Axis I diagnoses over the first 5 years*

Primary Diagnosis	N	%
No Diagnosis	238	55.2
Eating Behavior Disorder	51	11.8
Sleep Behavior Disorder	43	10
Adjustment reaction Disorder	30	7
Regulatory Disorder	22	5.1
Anxiety Disorder	20	4.6
Attachment disorders	8	1.9
Mixed Disorder of Emotional Expressiveness	6	1.4
Oppositional disorder	6	1.4
Post-traumatic Stress Disorder	5	1.2
Mood Disorder	2	0.5

*Data taken from a field study in the Infant Mental Health Center affiliated with the Tel-Aviv University, Israel [10].

Table 16.3 Distribution of Axis II diagnoses over the first 5 years*

Relationship disorder classification	N	%
No relational diagnosis	207	48.0
Mixed Type	76	17.6
Anxious/Tense Type	52	12.1
Over involved Type	48	11.1
Under involved Type	32	7.4
Angry/Hostile Type	13	3.0
Abusive Type (physical)	3	0.7

*Data taken from a field study in the Infant Mental Health Center affiliated with the Tel-Aviv University, Israel [10].

Table 16.4 Distribution of Axis III diagnoses over the first 5 years*

Medical/Developmental Diagnosis	N	%
No diagnosis	339	78.7
Developmental delays	54	12.5
Failure to Thrive	14	3.2
Medical diagnosis (chronic illness)	12	2.8
Long-term consequences of premature birth	3	0.7

*Data taken from a field study in the Infant Mental Health Center affiliated with the Tel-Aviv University, Israel [10].

Table 16.5 Distribution of Axis IV diagnoses over the first 5 years*

Psycho-social stressors classification	N	%
No Diagnosis	259	60.1
Parental psychiatric problem	94	21.8
Marital conflict	33	7.7
Loss	10	2.3
Divorce	8	1.9
Acute trauma	6	1.4
Birth of sibling	5	1.2
Abuse	2	0.5
Adoption	1	0.2
Other	13	3.0

*Data taken from a field study in the Infant Mental Health Center affiliated with the Tel-Aviv University, Israel [10].

relationship disorder (no evidence; some evidence; needs further investigation; substantial evidence). There are three levels for the various types of relationship disorders: behavioral quality, affective tone, and psychological involvement, which, in turn, can be subdivided into: over-involved, under-involved, anxious/tense, angry/hostile, or abusive (Verbal, physical, sexual).

Axis III: Medical and Developmental Disorders/Conditions. This axis should be used to indicate any physical and/or developmental diagnoses made using other classification systems such as the DSM [7] or ICD [8,9] and other classification systems used by speech/ language pathologists, occupational therapists, physical therapists, special educators, and primary health care providers. Note! If the child meets criteria for a DSM or ICD psychiatric disorder, it should be coded on Axis I.

Axis IV: Psychosocial stressors. The ultimate impact of a stressful event or enduring stress depends on three factors: The severity of the stressor, the infant's developmental level, and the availability and capacity of adults to serve as a protective buffer and to help the child understand and cope with the stressor. There are different types of stressors including: challenges to the child's primary support group, challenges in the social environment, educational/child care challenges, housing challenges, economic challenges, occupational challenges, health care access challenges, issues related to the health of the child, legal/ criminal justice challenges, and other challenges such as natural disaster, terror, epidemic, witness to violence etc.

Axis-V: Functional Emotional Development. Although this axis exists in the official DC 0-3R system, it is rarely used in clinical settings. More research and standardization is probably needed in order to evaluate its usefulness in practice.

During the assessment of a child, one should bear in mind other aspects of the diagnostic process, as well, namely the therapeutic process, including transference and countertransference which start with the first encounter. The working alliance may be facilitated or impinged by the initial contact. The setting is also important and critical information may be obtained using everyday interactions such as play or feeding. In the routine psychiatric evaluation of an infant there is, in fact, a special place for feeding interaction assessment [11]. Mothers of referred infants who were less supportive during feeding provided lower level of appropriate limits, and engaged in less positive and more negative give-and-take interactions with the child. On the other hand, child withdrawal and avoidance behavior, showed different patterns in the play and feeding contexts, and were found to be significantly higher in the referred group, during the feeding session. The location where assessment of an infant is performed may also impact the diagnoses. There is a difference when assessment takes place in the child's natural environment or in other "objective" surroundings (i.e. home vs. clinic vs. daycare etc.). There are many "real-life" issues that complicate the process of assessment, for example, the dilemma of how to diagnose an orphanage-raised infant. The answer to this and other, similar, questions may emerge from results of longitudinal developmental studies.

CLINICAL VIGNETTE

T., a one year and 7 month-old girl, was brought by her adoptive mother for "general guidance", 2 months after her adoption from another country. The mother is a health professional, and a friend recommended her to seek advice because "adopted kids often have problems".

Case History

T. was the fruit of an unwanted pregnancy of an 18 yr-old girl. She was sent to orphanage at the age of one week. At the time of her adoption (1 year 5 months), she looked apathetic. On her way to Israel, she spent most of the flight screaming. Her mother was, naturally, highly distraught.

(CONTINUED)

During the first few weeks post-adoption: T. slept most of the time, made no eye contact, had a flat affect, was startled by minimal sensory stimuli, withdrew when being touched, and preferred to fall asleep by herself with the blanket on her head . . . She refused to eat by herself, and hardly swallowed solid food. The mother felt cheated and bewildered. Her partner was not yet totally committed to her due to an on-going divorce process.

Clinical Status at 19 months: T. had a wild look; her black hair was cut short and she looked small for her age. She made no eye contact, and explored the room without playing. Did not talk, instead produced guttural sounds. She did not seem to be able to understand when addressed directly by her mother. Her affect was completely flat. She tended to slap her head when frustrated or anxious.

Developmental status: Bailey test was done at 21 months. Her performance was suitable for a normative 8 months old girl.

Diagnostic issues: At that time, the differential diagnosis on Axis I included: deprivation/maltreatment disorder, severe early PTSD, autism, or a co-morbidity of the above. Axis III included developmental delay due to deprivation, and mental reardation.

Criteria for Autism/PDD NOS: 1. Impairment in social interactions and recipro-city. 2. Impairment in communication. 3. Restricted/repetitive interests and/or behaviors.

Criteria for Deprivation/Maltreatment Disorder: 1. No evidence for preferring a specific caregiver. This implies either an inability to differentiate among adults, or a preference for unfamiliar adults overfamiliar ones for being comforted by, or a failure to seek comfort when hurt, or a lack of emotional responsiveness to familiar caregivers. 2. Child's mental age of at least 10 months. 3. Does not meet criteria for PDD.

Associated features: Poorly regulated affect; Failure to check back with caregiver; Absence of usually displayed reticence with strangers.

Infant PTSD – Definition: A lasting dysfunction in personal life, that follows from, and is related to an overwhelming experience(s). Note: While the full definition of "traumatic experience" for infants and what it constitutes, is still under debate, it is generally agreed that "threat to own or caregiver's physical integrity" is one of the criteria.

Treatment plan – First stage: Multi-faceted approach, aimed at addressing each possible diagnosis: 1. Dyadic parent-infant treatment to reflect on T.'s behavior, in light of the apparently, adverse past experiences at the orphanage. 2. Paramedical therapies (OT, speech) to address problems in communication and developmental skills. 3. Facilitation of the attachment process by the mother staying at home with the child.

Eight months later: Some attachment behaviors, such as preference for mother and comfort seeking, start appearing. Wider exploratory behavior, but still no play. No interest in peers. She still does not speak. No eye contact. Still slaps herself when easily frustrated.

T. starts kindergarten, and the treatment continues.

1 year and 8 months after beginning the intervention: T. is 3 years and 3 months old and shows further, but still partial, improvement: There is separation anxiety from her mother, but she agrees to stay alone with her father. She makes eye contact; Joint attention and social referencing appear. She looks happier and less vigilant. There is simple imitative play. She is toilet-trained, sleeps and eats well. She still does not talk and still keeps apart from other kids.

Diagnoses revision: She no longer meets criteria for Reactive Attachment Disorder. Severe Language delay and impairment of peer relationships are still predominant, though joint attention, eye contact and social referencing have appeared. The diagnosis of PDD is less fitting. Thus the question arises whether this is a long term sequelae of PTSD, a biological-based developmental delay, or perhaps both.

3 and half years after adoption and intervention: T. is 5yrs old. Her main impairments are: delayed language skills, poor emotional regulation, short attention span and poor peer relationships, namely seeking out children's company, but not knowing how to interact with them.

Main improvements at age 5: There is a clear attachment to her parents, and differentiated relationships with the different therapists. Screaming and self-hitting have ceased. The beginnings of simple symbolic play ("why is the doll sad? The doll has a toothache. . .") are detectable. She participates in all the routines at kindergarten (though she still has difficulties with transitions). She says "I don't want to" (3rd organizer). She shows an interest in her own body and in gender differences. She has a transitional object (Teddy bear).

New revision of diagnosis: Organic Mental Retardation, Long term sequela of deprivation with poor social skills and self-regulation.

16.3.2   B. Classifications of Child Psychiatric Disorders

Diagnosing a child with psychiatric problems is a complex process. Unlike adult assessment procedures which are usually based on self reporting of the patient, child assessment procedures have demonstrated methodological problems such as test-retest attenuation and discrepancies in data from different raters (clinician, parent, teacher, child, class-mate, and so on) [12]. Other important issues in children's classification, that are not as prominent in adults, are the child's developmental stage (i.e. age) and gender differences. Both can influence the clinical significance of symptoms found during the assessment procedure. Similarly, many factors can influence the phenomenology seen in the clinical setting. Some symptoms may be related to different disorders, while other symptoms may indicate a disorder when co-existing. A multi-axial approach helps focusing on specific areas of interest, decreasing the likelihood of overlooking some conditions, and making the selection of treatment modalities more effective in the actual setting of many clinics.

The multi-axial approach however, is not always implemented. Clinicians should make an effort to use it, as it may increase reliability of the diagnoses, and improve communication. Still, the multi-axial system has some difficulties and disadvantages: The number of axes should be as small as possible since a classification including a large number of axes is impractical in normal clinic environments, even when it is possible to list each and every one of the child's problems [13]. When constructing a multi-axes classification system, one should consider issues such as: Which dimensions are important enough to form a separate axis of their own and which can blend with others to form a common axis? What should be done about diagnoses that can be coded on more than one axis? (Ex: enuresis can be derived both from developmental and psychiatric factors).

Another problem is the issue of comorbidity. Some disorders can be a precursor to others; some disorders result from the same risk-factors, while others may just co-exist. How can separate diagnoses for conditions that are mutually inclusive be avoided, but the existence of comorbidity be stressed? ICD-10 provides a different code for conditions with important distinguishing features such as conduct disorder with depression, while the DSM-IV allows for comorbidity, thus coding both conduct disorder, and depression without accounting for their co-existence [7, 8]. Comorbidity is important information for clinicians in order to manage the treatment therefore allowing for comorbidity coding in the classification system is of great consequence, especially in children. Each child follows his or her own developmental path and may develop different disorders at a later developmental stage in accordance to the child's protecting and risk factors. For example, when a child with conduct disorder has a comorbidity of ADHD, he is at eightfold risk for developing an anti-social personality disorder later in life, while a girl with conduct disorder and social isolation is at higher risk for developing depression at a later stage [14]. Thus, in children, comorbidity constitutes a risk factor for the development of other disorders in later life.

An explanation of the impact of development on the diagnosis can be found in the developmental pathways of conduct disorder [15]. Aggressive behavior in infants may be divided into two categories: instrumental aggressiveness and reactive aggressiveness. Infants who have instrumental aggressiveness may also have reactive aggressiveness. In either case, depending on genetic factors, the infants with instrumental aggressiveness are at high risk to develop a psychopathic personality in childhood, which will persist throughout their life into adulthood [16]. Infants who have reactive aggressiveness (not instrumental), or exhibit rule breaking behavior, are often diagnosed as having conduct disorder in childhood [17], especially if they are boys. They tend to have a difficult temperament or neuropsychological difficulties, poor parental limit setting, and experience high parental aggression [18, 19]. Once a child is diagnosed with conduct disorder, his developmental path can diverge into various directions [14]:

One option consists of the child having certain genetic protecting factors (such as MAOA genotypes) which may lead to improvement in adolescence.

A second option is for the child to develop anxiety disorder in adolescence which, in the presence of ADHD comorbidity will increase eightfold the risk for this adolescent to be diagnosed with dissocial personality disorder or to lead to delinquency in adulthood.

A third option is that with the presence of physical abuse and some heritable traits, he is more likely to maintain the diagnosis of conduct disorder in adolescence, while later in adulthood he may be diagnosed as having either some type of personality disorder, or depression.

A fourth option pertains in particular female children who also experience social isolation. These children are at higher risk to develop in adolescence depression that will persist into adulthood.

*Adolescents, who are diagnosed for the first time with conduct disorder, may improve with good school attendance and a functioning family, but may otherwise develop a personality disorder in adulthood.

In other words, having a diagnosis of conduct disorder in childhood can lead to diverse diagnoses later in life (any type of personality disorder, delinquency, anxiety, and depression) depending on the age of onset, risk and protective factors of the child, and on the developmental path. The same principles for developmental pathways as for conduct disorder of childhood apply to various diagnoses of children.

In western countries the most widely used classification systems are the ICD-10, and DSM-IV-TR. Nevertheless, we want to mention the French classification (CFTMEA) [20], which is based on psychoanalytic understanding of the child and adolescent's normal and pathological development. The French child psychiatrists have produced a document specifying the equivalence of diagnoses between the CFTMEA and the ICD-10. In other parts of the world, such as China, there are separate classifications. Currently they are working on harmonizing their classification with the international ones.

According to the psychoanalytic concept, personality disorders cannot be diagnosed in children due to the view that the personality reaches its full intra-psychic consolidation and maturation only in adolescence. Today, as a result of research and clinical experience, it is generally accepted that some personality disorders (such as borderline, narcissistic, and dissocial), can be diagnosed during adolescence [16]. Some personality traits such as psychopathy can be solidly diagnosed even from childhood [21].

16.4 STABILITY

The fastest growing field in child psychiatry is developmental psychiatry. This is mainly due to knowledge emerging from results of long term follow-up studies [21]. These results lead us to the understanding that while the diagnosis is important it does not necessarily constitute the most important factor in development and that the protective and risk factors are as important as the diagnosis itself. These long term studies have shown, for the first time, the stability of the diagnosis. There are three diagnoses in which the same diagnostic criteria can be used in adults as well as in children: Schizophrenia, Depression, and Obsessive Compulsive Disorder (OCD). In OCD, the diagnostic criteria are the same for children as for adults, but the diagnosis is not stable. In other words, a child diagnosed with an OCD, can later in life be without the disorder.

There are different characteristics of the way depression is expressed, at different developmental stages and that mainly in relation to the physiological aspects (sleeping, eating). It is, however, generally accepted that these are almost the only differences attributed to development, and that the rest of the parameters can be evaluated in a manner very similar to their evaluation in adults [22]. They may include depressed mood and affect, guilt feelings, or low self esteem. For decades we did not dare ask children the questions we routinely presented to adults. Only after the existence of depression in children became an accepted fact, children's interviews started following a concept similar to the one followed with adults. It was found that when the "right questions" were asked of children, even at a very young age (i.e. preschoolers), answers characteristic for depression were obtained.

16.5   DIFFERENCES BETWEEN ICD-10 AND DSM-IV-TR

Although efforts have been made to consolidate the main classification systems, a number of important differences between the ICD-10 and the DSM-IV persist. Some of these differences are manifested in the sections dealing with children. The ICD-10 has two different sets of diagnostic criteria; one is a pattern recognition approach for clinical use, and the other a symptom checklist approach used for research. The DSM-IV has only a symptom checklist approach, used for both clinical situations and research. The symptom checklist approach increases reliability, but is cumbersome and not applied rigorously by clinicians. Such an approach can also lead to under-diagnosis in cases when clinicians believe that a diagnosis is present because of the severity of the symptoms, even without sufficient number of symptoms to meet the diagnostic criteria. Comorbidity constitutes another difference between ICD-10 and DSM-IV. The ICD system supports the approach of finding a single diagnosis that fits best the clinical picture, while the DSM and the research diagnostic criteria of the ICD-10 allows selecting all diagnoses whose criteria are met. An additional difference between the classification systems is that in the ICD-10, suggests a different set of multi-axial systems for children and adolescents than it does for adults. The DSM-IV has the same axes for all ages. [23].

A multi-axial approach is the norm in children's classifications. In the ICD-10, the axes refer to [8]:

I.   The clinical psychiatric syndrome;
II. The presence or absence of a specific disorder of psychological development. These include speech and language, reading, spelling and motor development (coded on Axis I in the DSM system);
III. The intellectual level;
IV. Medical conditions;
V.   Associated abnormal psychosocial situations.

The DSM IV-TR does not apply a different set of axes specific for children and adolescents but rather uses the same axes as for adults. The Axes of the DSM are [7]:

I.   Clinical disorders;
II. Mental retardation (in general, personality disorders cannot be diagnosed in childhood with the exception of psychopathic personality);
III. General medical conditions;
IV. Psychosocial and environmental problems;

V. Global assessment of functioning – Here the children's global assessment scale (CGAS [24]); which is an adaptation of the Global Assessment of functioning (GAF) is used.

Axis I: Clinical Psychiatric Syndromes

Table 16.6 Prevalence of several clinical psychiatric disorders in children and adolescents [25]*

Disorder	Prevalence	Comments
Pervasive Developmental Disorders		
Childhood Autism	5–20 per 10,000	
Asperger's Syndrome	3–4 per 1,000	Boys 4 times than Girls
Behavioral and Emotional Disorders with onset usually occurring in Childhood and Adolescence		
ADHD, Hyperkinetic Syndrome	0.5–1% in England	Differences due to difference in criteria
	3–5% in the US	Boys 3–4 times more than girls
Conduct disorders		
Tic Disorders		
Mental and Behavioral Disorders due to psychoactive substance use	For 15–16 y/o teens in the UK	Generally no differences between boys and girls
Alcohol	Near 100% had consumed, >3/4 had been intoxicated	
Cannabinoids	2/5 had used at some time	The illicit drug most commonly used
Heroin, Cocaine, Crack	Less than 2.5%	
Hallucinogens	LSD-1/10 had used, Ecstasy (MDMA)-1/12	
Tobacco	2/3 had smoked, 1/3 in the last month	Girls used more than boys
Volatile Solvents	1/5 had used at some time	
Schizophrenia, Schizotypal and Delusional Disorders		
Schizophrenia	3 per 10,000	
Mood (Affective) Disorders		
Bipolar Disorder	Rare before puberty	Equal frequency in boys and girls
	Preadolescents: 10–15% with depressed mood, 2% meet DSM-III criteria.	Little difference between preadolescent boys and girls.
Depression	Ages 11–16: >3%	Adolescent girls 2 times more than boys
		More common in minority race, low socio-economic status, low school grades

(Continued)

Table 16.6   *(cont.)*

Disorder	Prevalence	Comments
Neurotic, Stress-Related and Somatoform Disorders		
Social Phobia	1%	
Panic Disorder	Less than 1%	
Obsessional conditions	High school students: 3% Subclinical conditions: 19%	
Behavioral Syndromes Associated with Physiological Disturbances and Physical Factors		
Anorexia Nervosa	Adolescent girls: 0.1–0.2%, Age: 6–60, great majority: 14–19	
Night terrors	3–15%, peak age: 4–7	

*Data was taken from Graham P, Turk J and Verhulst F [25].

Axis II: Specific Disorders of Psychological Development

Table 16.7   Prevalence of several psychological developmental disorders in children and adolescents*

Disorder	Prevalence	Comments
Language delay	6–8%	
Developmental expressive language delay	5–6 per 1,000	Boys 2–3 times more than girls, associated to: family size, social class, presence of emotional and behavioral disorder
Receptive dysphasia	1 per 10,000	

*Data was taken from Graham P, Turk J and Verhulst F [25].

Axis III: Intellectual Level
Axis IV: Medical Conditions Often Associated with Mental and Behavioral Disorders
Axis V: Associated Abnormal Psychosocial Situations

It was found that the number of psychosocial adversities is related exponentially to disorder rates [26], and that some diagnoses are related to specific psychosocial situations, such as Conduct disorder and emotional disorders that are associated with a poor immediate psychosocial environment and acute life and school-related chronic stressors, respectively [27].

16.6 DISCUSSION ON THE PRESENT AND THE FUTURE OF PSYCHIATRIC CLASSIFICATION OF INFANTS AND CHILDREN

Classifications have to deal with various challenges, including errors in data collection, developmental variations, comorbidity, and integration of data from various sources [12]. We join those advocating for one generally accepted, agreed upon and validated international classification system, in order to be able to exchange and compare information as well as for research proposes. In this chapter we tried to understand each one of the nosological systems and to determine the developmental pathways from infancy to adulthood. This is important, as it can assist with the detection of first manifestations of a disorder, leading to early interventions that will help avoid its full development. This interpretation of our actual classification is due to the fact that child and adolescent psychiatry is considered as part of general psychiatry and the axis of development is determined by these concepts.

There is another option for conceiving our discipline, namely, to emphasize the age of our patients, and to look at disorders at every age as an integral part of development. We could look at each of the infant, child and adolescent disorders as a manifestation of a gene brain and environmental interaction, and to interpret the meaning and the dynamics of disorders according to the stage of development and to the general health of the patient. If we look at obesity for example, it points to different problems at different ages. In infancy it may point to attachment disorder, in childhood it corresponds to low self esteem, in adolescence it may indicate depression, and in adulthood it may relate to life events. The same rules apply to depression, conduct disorders, dissociative states or hypothyroidism. This approach of interpreting the psychiatric disorder through this single integrated concept of physical and psychiatric disorders may open up a future direction in our discipline, and therefore has its impact on future classifications. In order to consider child and adolescent disorders in such a manner, our discipline should be viewed as related closer to pediatrics than to psychiatry.

REFERENCES

[1] Ghanizadeh A, Mohammadi MR, Moini R. Comorbidity of Psychiatric Disorders and Parental Psychiatric Disorder of ADHD Children. *Journal of Attention Disorders*, 4 March 2008.

[2] Ambrosini PJ. Historical development and present status of the schedule for affective disorders and schizophrenia for school-age children (K-SADS). *Journal of the American Academy of Child and Adolescent Psychiatry* 2000;39(1): pp. 49–58.

[3] Volkmar FR, Schwab-Stone M, First M. *Lewis's Child and Adolescent Psychiatry: a Comprehensive Textbook*. 4th ed. Philadelphia, PA: Lippincott Williams & Wilkins; 2007.

[4] Sameroff AJ, Chandler MJ. Reproductive risk and the continuum of caretaking casualty. In: Horowitz FD. *Review of Child Development Research, Volume 4*. Chigaco: University of Chicago Press; 1975.

[5] Keenan K, Shaw DS, Walsh B, Delliquadri E, Giovannelli J. DSM-III-R disorders in preschool children from low-income families. *Journal of the American Academy of Child and Adolescent Psychiatry* 1997;36(5): pp. 620–627.

[6] Zero to Three (Organization). DC:0–3. Revised ed. Washington: D.C: Zero To Three Press; 2005.

[7] American Psychiatric Association. *Diagnostic and statistical manual of mental disorders: DSM-IV-TR.* 4th ed. Washington, DC: American Psychiatric Association; 2000.

[8] World Health Organization. *The ICD-10 classification of mental and behavioural disorders. Clinical descriptions and diagnostic guidelines.* Geneva: World Health Organization; 1992.

[9] World Health Organization. *The ICD-10 classification of mental and behavioral disorders: Diagnostic criteria for research.* Geneva: World Health Organization; 1993.

[10] Keren M, Feldman R, Tyano S. Diagnoses and interactive patterns of infants referred to a community-based infant mental health clinic. *Journal of the American Academy of Child and Adolescent Psychiatry* 2001;40(1): pp. 27–35.

[11] Feldman R, Keren M, Gross-Rozval O, Tyano S. Mother–Child touch patterns in infant feeding disorders: relation to maternal, child, and environmental factors. *Journal of the American Academy of Child and Adolescent Psychiatry* 2004;43(9): pp. 1089–1097.

[12] Achenbach T. Classification systems and nosology. In: Harrison SI (ed.) Clinical assessment and intervention planning. New York: John Wiley & Sons, Inc.; 1998. p. 10–31.

[13] Rutter M. *Multiaxial Classification of child and adolescent psychiatric disorders.* Cambridge: Cambridge University Press; 1996.

[14] Mason WA, Kosterman R, Hawkins JD, Herrenkohl TI, Lengua LJ, McCauley E. Predicting depression, social phobia, and violence in early adulthood from childhood behavior problems. *Journal of the American Academy of Child and Adolescent Psychiatry* 2004;43(3): pp. 307–315.

[15] Keren M, Tyano S. *The application of core concepts in Developmental Psychopathology to the understanding of continuities and discontinuities of psychopathology from infancy to adulthood.* Submitted. In press.

[16] Blair RJ, Peschardt KS, Budhani S, Mitchell DG, Pine DS. The development of psychopathy. *Journal of the American Academy of Child and Adolescent Psychiatry* 2006;47(3–4): pp. 262–276.

[17] Hofstra MB, van der EJ, Verhulst FC. Child and adolescent problems predict DSM-IV disorders in adulthood: a 14-year follow-up of a Dutch epidemiological sample. *Journal of the American Academy of Child and Adolescent Psychiatry* 2002;41(2): pp. 182–9.

[18] Keller TE, Spieker SJ, Gilchrist L. Patterns of risk and trajectories of preschool problem behaviors: a person-oriented analysis of attachment in context. *Development and Psychopathology* 2005;17(2): pp. 349–84.

[19] Tremblay RE, Nagin DS, Seguin JR, Zoccolillo M, Zelazo PD, Boivin M, *et al.* Physical aggression during early childhood: trajectories and predictors. *Pediatrics* 2004;114(1): pp. e43–e50.

[20] Mises R, Quemada N, Botbol M, Burzsteijn C, Garrabe J, Golse B, *et al.* French classification for child and adolescent mental disorders. *Psychopathology* 2002;35(2–3): pp. 176–180.

[21] Valevski A, Ratzoni G, Sever J, Apter A, Zalsman G, Shiloh R, *et al.* Stability of diagnosis: a 20-year retrospective cohort study of Israeli psychiatric adolescent inpatients. *Journal of Adolescence* 2001;24(5): pp. 625–633.

[22] Keren M, Tyano S. Depression in infancy. *Child and Adolescent Psychiatry Clinics of North America* 2006;15(4): pp. 883–97 viii.

[23] Scott, S. Classification of psychiatric disorders in childhood and adolescence: building castles in the sand? *Advances in Psychiatric Treatment* 2002;(8): pp. 205–213.

[24] Shaffer D, Gould MS, Brasic J, Ambrosini P, Fisher P, Bird H, *et al.* A children's global assessment scale (CGAS). *Archives of General Psychiatry* 1983;40(11): pp. 1228–1231.

[25] Graham P, Turk J, Verhulst F. *Child Psychiatry: a Developmental Approach.* 3rd ed. Oxford: Oxford University Press; 2001.

[26] Rutter M. Psychosocial resilience and protective mechanisms. *American Journal of Orthopsychiatry* 1987;57(3): pp. 316–331.

[27] Steinhausen HC, Erdin A. Abnormal psychosocial situations and ICD-10 diagnoses in children and adolescents attending a psychiatric service. *Journal of Child Psychology and Psychiatry and Allied Disciplines* 1992;33(4): pp. 731–740.

CHAPTER 17

Peri-Natal Mental Disorders

Ian Brockington
Professor Emeritus, University of Birmingham, Birmingham, UK
John Cox
Professor Emeritus, Keele University, Staffordshire, UK
Nicole Garret-Gloanec
Chef de Service de Psychiatric Infanto-Juvenile, Nantes, France
Gisèle Apter-Denon
Responsible Unite Ppumma (Unite de Psychiatric Périnatale d' Urgence Mobile en Maternité), Université Denis Diderot, Paris 7, France

17.1 INTRODUCTION

17.1.1 History

The literature on the psychiatry of childbearing dates back to Hippocrates himself, and includes many illustrious contributions, such as those of Osiander (1797 [1]), Esquirol (1818 [2]) and Marcé (1858 [3]). In the last 50 years, especially the two decades since ICD-10 was finalized, thousands of books, articles and theses have been published. Many more disorders are now recognized. Although most of the research was done in Europe and North America, Cox [4] pioneered studies in Africa and, since then, there has been a flow of papers from the Indian subcontinent, China, South-East Asia, Japan, the Middle East and South America. It is important to provide a nosology appropriate for the world, not the 'West', and especially for those nations that have high birth rates and less access to modern obstetrics. In the context of the International Guidelines for Diagnostic Assessment [5], and the assessment of the patient as a whole person, it is essential that the reproductive process is fully coded, because it will be central to what goes on in the mind and body of the mother presenting for care. Accordingly, this review aims to cover the whole range of disorders found in, or triggered by, pregnancy, parturition and the puerperium.

Psychiatric Diagnosis: Challenges and Prospects   Edited by I.M. Salloum and J.E. Mezzich
© 2009 John Wiley & Sons, Ltd

17.2   WHAT IS SPECIAL ABOUT PERINATAL PSYCHIATRY?

In 1999, at an international workshop in Sweden, the special background of this area of psychiatry was emphasized. Its recommendations, and some others, are listed below:

- A mother must make a complex and profound social and emotional adjustment during pregnancy and after the birth. The birth has a many-sided impact that may threaten her mental health in a variety of ways.
- She must form a relationship with ('bond to') the child.
- Foetal abnormality, development delay or temperamental challenges may be a special form of stress in this phase of motherhood.
- The somatic complications of pregnancy and birth can lead to psychiatric disorders.
- Pregnancy may be unwanted or rejected, and this increases the risk of severe disorders that include child abuse, child neglect and infanticide.
- Mental disorders have a high morbidity for the mother, but also a profound effect on the newborn, her partner or spouse, and the family. Untreated, these effects can be long lasting.
- There are opportunities for prevention, early diagnosis and treatment provided by the additional vigilance, and the systems of help, available in the antenatal and early postpartum periods.
- Perinatal mental disorders clash with the cultural expectation of a smooth 'rite of passage' into motherhood, and confer a stigma that may discourage a mother from seeking help.
- There are special opportunities for research, linking clinical disorders to neuroendocrine and psychosocial triggers.
- There is the need for special services, such as mother-infant day hospitals and inpatient units.

17.3   WHAT IS WRONG WITH PREVIOUS INTERNATIONAL CLASSIFICATIONS

- ICD-8(1967) had a special category for puerperal psychosis.
- ICD-9(1975) made no mention of it.
- ICD-10(1992) permitted the classification of puerperal mental and behavioural disorders only if the onset was within six weeks and could not be classified elsewhere, and only because psychiatrists from 'developing countries' may have 'very real practical problems in gathering sufficient informations'. This complex and confused approach has made it difficult to identify these patients for epidemiological research, public health and policy, and communication between clinicians, researchers and health service managers.
- DSM-IV(1994) acknowledged the specific features of postpartum illness, but had an onset specifier of four weeks, restricted to four diagnoses.
- ICD-10 and DSM-IVmention only a limited number of disorders, omitting some of those that are most important in clinical practice.

17.4   THE NEED FOR AN OBLIGATORY ONSET SPECIFIER

In order to provide epidemiologists and health planners with full access to data, and to fulfil the requirement to cover all key areas of information, it is essential that clinicians *always* code onset when it occurs in pregnancy or in the first postpartum year. This dispenses with the need for ICD-10's category F53. The disorders listed below will find their place under many different headings within the general classification (mentioning their presentation in mothers) but, if rigorously coded, the onset specifier will ensure that they are never lost to researchers and planners. Since different disorders are related to different phases of this time period, the following intervals are suggested:

- Pregnancy. This could be subdivided into trimesters.
- Parturition. Although this event is brief, it is often a time of extreme stress and much psychopathology.
- The early puerperium. This could be subdivided as follows:
    - the first few days are associated with organic disorders and the trauma of infant loss;
    - the first month is when most bipolar and acute polymorphic psychoses begin;
    - the remainder of the first postpartum trimester.
- The rest of the first year of the child's life.

17.4.1   False Pregnancy

Pregnancy can be simulated for social, mercenary or legal purposes. Delusions of pregnancy are common, and can also occur in men; they are seen in a variety of psychoses.

Pseudocyesis is different. These women have no other signs of major mental illness, but firmly believe they are pregnant. They develop somatic signs and symptoms, such as amenorrhoea, morning sickness, breast changes, abdominal swelling, an illusion of foetal movements and moderate uterine enlargement. The belief often lasts the full nine months, ending in a false labour.

17.4.2   Disorders of the Acceptance of Pregnancy

Many pregnancies are unplanned and some are accepted only with difficulty. It is important to distinguish between the following abnormal responses to pregnancy:

- Pregnancy that, because of obesity or imminent menopause, is unnoticed.
- Pregnancy that is deliberately concealed.
- Unwelcome or unthinkable pregnancy met by associative denial.
- Pregnancy that is acknowledged, but emotionally rejected. In the milder degrees, the growing foetus is ignored, and there is no prepartum attachment. In severe cases, the mother may perpetrate foetal abuse.
- Pregnancy that a mother seeks importunately to conclude, occasionally (in the late stages) through self-induced vaginal haemorrhage or other 'obstetric factitious' manoeuvres.

The body changes of pregnancy are sometimes distressing. Dysmorphophobia, with ideas of reference and social avoidance, can ensue.

17.4.3   Mental Illness During Pregnancy

Anxiety

For many mothers, pregnancy is a time of much anxiety. Although its form (panic, or generalized) may have implications for pharmacotherapy, it is helpful also to distinguish between different themes or foci, which indicate psychological treatments. The first trimester may involve an anguished decision whether to continue or to terminate the pregnancy. In mid-pregnancy, women who have previously suffered from prolonged infertility, multiple miscarriages or infant death are prone to anxiety about foetal loss. In the third trimester, anxiety is focused on fear of parturition (tocophobia), foetal abnormality, and/or inability to cope with motherhood.

Depression

Prepartum depression has approximately the same frequency as postpartum depression. It can be recurrent, and there is an association with postpartum depression and puerperal mania. Suicide is less common in pregnant women than it is in the general population, but this may not be true for countries that stigmatize pregnancy out of wedlock.

Addictions

Heavy ethanol abuse has severe effects on the foetus, leading to retarded intrauterine growth, facial dysmorphism and brain damage ('foetal alcohol syndrome'), and neonatal addiction. Abuse of other 'substances' has well-documented effects. For example, narcotic addiction has multiple effects on the foetus, some resulting from the maternal lifestyle; most infants suffer from a withdrawal syndrome, including seizures. Among its other effects, cocaine can cause placental abruption.

Eating Disorders

Most women with anorexia nervosa recover, and resume menstruation. Many have a strong desire for children, and give birth in the normal way. Those who become pregnant while in the throes of the disease may continue to restrict their diet, so that the foetus suffers from malnutrition. Both anorexic and bulimic women tend to relapse in the puerperium, and both disorders sometimes result in deviant mothering.

Psychosis

Pregnancy has no effect on chronic delusional states, but may improve menstrual, bipolar and acute polymorphic psychoses. Nonetheless, acute manic and other psychoses occur during pregnancy, especially in multiparous women with a history of puerperal bipolar disorder.

Two medical complications of pregnancy have psychiatric complications: hyperemesis can cause Wernicke's encephalopathy and Korsakoff psychosis; chorea gravidarum is also associated with organic psychoses.

17.4.4   The Psychopathology of Parturition

Psychopathological complications may be important wherever women give birth without the support of trained professional staff. Delirium can develop without any obvious somatic cause. In obstructed labour, acts of desperation and rage have been described. Unexplained delirium, stupor or coma can occur immediately after delivery or in the first few hours of the puerperium.

These parturient disorders are among the factors involved in neonaticide (the killing of the newborn shortly after the birth). Exhaustion, fainting and delirium after delivery can also endanger the newborn, through neglect.

17.4.5 Infant Loss

The child may be lost for a variety of reasons – termination of pregnancy, miscarriage or ectopic pregnancy, foetal death *in utero*, stillbirth, neonatal death, sudden infant death (SIDS), or relinquishment to adoption. All these events often lead to distress, grief or depression. Abortion like delivery can be followed by bipolar or organic psychoses.

17.4.6 Postpartum Adaptation

For many mothers, childbirth is a supreme moment, and a sense of joy and fulfilment is common. Prolonged euphoric reactions, lasting a week or more, are probably puerperal hypomania, and are often followed by depression.

Newly delivered mothers face a number of challenges, including exhaustion, physical complications, breast feeding, sleep deprivation, social isolation, and the recovery of normal figure and attractiveness. As in pregnancy, some suffer from a state similar to dysmorphophobia. There may be a relative or absolute loss of libido, lasting weeks or months.

The maternity 'blues' is common: this is a sudden, unexpected but brief period of sensitivity and uncharacteristic weeping, occurring a few days after delivery.

17.4.7 Postpartum Mental Illness

Reactions to Traumatic Parturition

After excessively painful or distressing labours, some women suffer from post-traumatic stress disorder. They may avoid further pregnancy (secondary tocophobia) and, if they become pregnant, may experience a return of symptoms, especially in the last trimester.

Another reaction to a severe labour experience is pathological complaining (embitterment disorder). These women complain about perceived mismanagement, and their continuing angry rumination may interfere with infant care.

Anxiety Disorders

Postpartum anxiety disorders have the same frequency as postpartum depression. It is important to identify the focus (as well as the form) of anxiety, because of the possibility of specific psychological therapies. Two themes are particularly important:

- Infant-centred anxiety. Some mothers, especially *primiparae* in isolated 'nuclear' families, are overwhelmed by the responsibility of caring for the newborn. This may progress to phobic avoidance of the infant.
- Pathological anxiety about infant health and survival. These mothers show excessive solicitude, and sensitivity to the slightest indication of illness. In some, the anxiety is focused on the possibility of sudden infant death. Perpetual vigilance can result in excruciating tension, insomnia, exhaustion and distorted mother-infant interactions.

Obsessional Disorders

The puerperium is one of the main precipitants of obsessive-compulsive disorders. In addition to compulsive rituals, a gentle, devoted mother may be disturbed by fantastic thoughts, images, or impulses of child harm ('obsessions of infanticide'); she may avoid her infant, and take extraordinary precautions.

These impulses must be distinguished from pathological anger (see below).

Depression

Depressive disorders are clinically similar to depression at other times, but the social context is distinctive and the adverse impact on the infant considerable; moreover, there are particular foci of management with regard to the mother-infant relationship. Although the prevalence of depression is similar to all women during the reproductive years, whether they are infertile, pregnant, puerperal, menopausal or involved in childrearing, there is often a clustering of new onsets in the immediate postpartum weeks. Some use the term 'postpartum depression' as a rubric for a heterogeneous group of co-morbid postpartum disorders; many mothers with anxiety, obsessional, post-traumatic or other disorders, or with a disturbed mother-infant relationship are depressed, but the settings, causes, and treatments are different. A minority suffer from a mild form of postpartum bipolar disorders.

Whatever its form, severity or associations, maternal depression has serious consequences on family life. It is therefore important to code mild (subsyndromal) disorders, as well as major depression. The suicide rate in the first postpartum year is below the female rate but, in extreme cases, maternal depression can lead to the tragedy of combined suicide and filicide (parental killing of a child over 24 hours old). This rivals child abuse is the commonest cause of filicide.

Mother–Infant Relationship (Attachment) Disorders

The development of the mother-infant relationship is the central psychological process in the puerperium. Sometimes the maternal emotional response is immediate, primed by affiliation to the foetus; but in most mothers attachment develops over the first few weeks, assisted by the baby's burgeoning social responses (eye gaze, smiling, laughing and babbling). Infant characteristics and style, as well as maternal expectations, are major elements that interact in establishing a mutually regulated relationship. In a minority, there is a worrying delay; the mother feels estranged from her infant, and has a distressing lack of emotional response. In a small minority, negative emotions develop, and progress to aversion, hatred and rejection of the baby. These mothers try to persuade relatives to take over, or demand that the infant be fostered or adopted. They may harbour the secret wish that the baby 'disappear' – be stolen, or die. In cases of rejection, there is a risk of child neglect, with impaired interactions and emotional neglect in all, and physical neglect in extreme cases.

Rejection is commonly associated with pathological anger. The infant's demands provoke an aggressive response, which may lead to shouting, cursing, screaming or aggressive impulses. These infants are at risk of various forms of child abuse.

These disorders are usually accompanied by depression (especially in the clinical setting), but can occur with little or no depression. They may respond to antidepressive therapy, but in many cases specific psychological treatment (especially play therapy) is required.

Psychoses

These fall into two main groups – organic psychoses and 'functional' (bipolar or acute polymorphic) psychoses. A third group – reactive or psychogenic psychosis – is most convincingly seen in adoptive mothers and fathers.

Organic psychoses have largely disappeared from Europe and North America, but may still be important in Africa, Asia and Latin America, where the majority of children are born. Historically, the most important causes have been infection and eclampsia. Other causes include vitamin B1 deficiency, chorea, cerebral venous thrombosis (common in India), other vascular disorders, epilepsy, hypopituitarism, ethanol withdrawal, water intoxication and hyperammonaemia.

The form of 'puerperal' psychosis which is still prevalent everywhere, is related to the bipolar (manic depressive) spectrum. But these episodes often have an acute polymorphic ('cycloid') symptomatology, instead of mania, stupor or delusional depression. These 'atypical' psychoses are the historic reason for attempts to define a specific 'puerperal psychosis'; but the clinical syndrome occurs in other contexts, and in men, and the solution is to use the obligatory onset specifier. The onset is acute, usually between 2 and 14 days after delivery. Almost every psychotic symptom may be seen – the whole gamut of delusions, verbal hallucinations, disorders of the will and self, and catatonic features, often with an element of confusion or perplexity. With modern treatment, the duration has fallen to a few weeks. Recurrences occur, especially after subsequent pregnancies. These mothers often have a family history of endogenous mood disorders, and a personal history of other attacks. Episodes are precipitated not only by childbirth, but also by abortion, pregnancy itself (especially the last trimester), post-partum menstruation, menstruation in general, and possibly also weaning. The incidence is somewhat less than 1 in 1000 pregnancies. There is a high heritability – not just for bipolar disorder, but also for the puerperal trigger.

17.5 MAIN RECOMMENDATIONS FOR ICD-11

- It is essential that all clinicians use and code an onset specifier for any mental illness occurring between conception and the end of the first postpartum year.
- Bi-axial diagnosis, using this onset specifier and the syndrome or episode diagnosis, will ensure the identification of all forms and all cases of maternal mental illness. The coding of other associations may also be necessary. In cases of delirium or stupor, a somatic cause (e.g. eclampsia) is usually obvious. Because of its increased risks, unwanted or rejected pregnancy should be one of the codeable contextual factors.
- Disorders of the mother-foetus, and mother-infant relationship must be included in the classification. Unlike some other relationship disorders, with an affect of anger or hatred, maternal attachment disorders are firmly within the clinical domain, and form an important part of the expertise of 'perinatal' psychiatric teams. They are a high-risk group for child abuse and neglect.
- It is important to identify the focus of anxiety disorders in pregnancy and the puerperium, to point the way to specific psychological treatment. This is similar to the identification of agoraphobia, social phobia and specific phobias in general psychiatry.

REFERENCES

[1] Osiander FB. *Neue Denkwürdigkeiten für Ärzte und Geburtshelfer.* Volume 1. Göttingen: Rosenbusch;1797. pp. 52–128.
[2] Esquirol JED. D'aliénation mentale des nouvelles accouchées et des nourrices; 1818. English translation in: *Maladies Mentales*, volume 1, pp. 125–143 (facsimile). London & New York: Hafner; 1845.
[3] Marcé LV. *Traité de la Folie des Femmes Enceintes, des Nouvelles Accouchées et des Nourrices, et Considérations Médico-légales qui se Rattachent à ce Sujet.* Paris: Baillière; 1858.
[4] Cox JL. Psychiatric morbidity and pregnancy: a controlled study of 263 semi-rural Ugandan women. *British Journal of Psychiatry* 1979;134: pp. 401–405.
[5] Mezzich JE. The World Psychiatric Association International Guidelines for Diagnostic Assessment. *World Psychiatry* 2002;1: pp. 36–39.

For a summary of the disorders in this text, please see:
Brockington IF. *Motherhood and Mental Health.* Oxford: Oxford University Press. 1996.

CHAPTER 18

Suicide

Zoltán Rihmer

Professor, Department of Clinical and Theoretical Mental Health,
and Department of Psychiatry and Psychotherapy,
Semmelweis Medical University, Budapest, Hungary

18.1   INTRODUCTION

Suicidal behaviour is one of the most tragic events of human life, causing serious psycho-logical distress among the person's relatives and friends, as well as a great economic burden for society. Globally, around one million deaths from suicide are recorded every year, and the number of suicide attempts is estimated to be10–20 times higher than this [1, 2]. Suicidal behaviour is not a normal response to the levels of stress experienced by many people and, in spite of the fact that almost all suicide victims suffer from a current mental disorder [3, 4, 5], suicide is not a linear consequence of major mental disorders either, as most psychiatric patients do not commit or attempt suicide. Suicide is very complex human behaviour with several 'causes' and many biological, as well as psychosocial and cultural, components. Between 10% and 18% of adults report lifetime suicidal ideation; 3–5% have made a suicide attempt; and up to 0.045% of the population commit suicide every year [1, 6, 7]. Suicidal ideation (including planning suicide), attempted suicide and completed suicide are three different things, but have greatly overlapping signs and symptoms, and the vast majority of suicide attempters and completers come from a population of persons with current suicidal ideation (planning). It should also be noted that more than one third of suicide victims had made at least one prior suicide attempt; this means that about two-thirds of them die at their first attempt [1, 3, 4, 5].

Although the importance of psychosocial and cultural-religious factors in the develop-ment (and prevention) of the suicidal process should never be neglected, suicidal patients, if any, are always provided for mental health care. The focus in this chapter, therefore, is to review suicidal behaviour from a clinical psychiatric viewpoint.

18.2   EPIDEMIOLIOGY OF SUICIDAL BEHAVIOUR

Deaths as a result of suicide account for around 1% of total deaths, and suicide ranks among the ten leading causes of death worldwide. Among people aged 15–34, however, suicide is one of the two leading causes of death. The highest annual suicide rates are reported from Eastern Europe (13–42 suicides per 100 000 persons) followed by Western/Nordic European countries (8–21 suicides per 100 000 persons) and North America and Australia (11–13 suicides per 100 000 persons). Latin America, as well as 'Latin Europe' (Greece, Spain, Italy) and Central Asian countries, report annual suicide rates of less than 10, while suicide is extremely rare in Muslim countries [1, 2, 7].

The reasons for these great differences between national and regional suicide rates have not been fully explained. Geographic, climatic, sociocultural, dietary, religious and economic differences can be taken into account, but differences in psychiatric morbidity, as well as the accuracy of the registration of suicide, the availability of lethal methods and the availability of a social and health care system should also be considered. The importance of religion and related cultural factors in suicide behaviour is underlined by the fact that suicide rates are extremely low in Muslim countries (where suicide is strictly forbidden) and highest in atheist countries (e.g., China and some post-Soviet countries), while Christian, Hindu and Buddhist countries have intermediate suicide rates [1, 7, 8].

Suicide mortality shows a clear gender difference: with the exception of few countries (e.g., China, India), two-thirds to five-fifths of suicide victims around the world are males. This may be a consequence of the fact that, compared to females, males use violent suicide methods (e.g., hanging, shooting, jumping) more frequently, and seek help for their psychological problems (even in the case of acute crisis situation) less commonly. In addition, depression in males is often masked (and suicide frequently triggered) by alcohol and drugs. Homosexual (same-sex oriented) men and women appear to have higher suicide mortality than matched heterosexuals [1, 4, 5, 8, 9].

Suicide rates increase with age in both genders, while the rate of attempted suicide to completed suicide progressively decreases. However, an increase in suicide mortality among young males in several Western societies has been also reported [1, 2, 5, 8].

With regards to ethnicity, African Americans, Hispanic Americans and Asian Americans (both males and females) have much lower rates of completed and attempted suicide compared to white Americans [5, 6, 8].

Suicide rates (like the prevalence of depression), in general, are higher in urban than rural areas; spring/early summer is the season of the highest incidence of suicide and suicide attempts; winter is the season of the lowest. The seasonality of suicide is more pronounced among males, among those using violent methods and in areas with higher geographic latitude. Suicide mortality tends to peak in the late morning and at the beginning of the week; the latter strongly underlines the role of psychosocial factors, at least in triggering suicidal behaviour [8, 10].

In contrast to completed suicides, in the case of suicide attempts, the gender distribution is the opposite: more than two-thirds of suicide attempters are female, and the most commonly used method is overdose or poisoning. While the rate of attempted to completed suicide, in general, is estimated to be about 10–20 to 1, this ratio shows a sharply decreasing tendency with age [1, 5, 8].

18.3   SUICIDE RISK AND PROTECTIVE FACTORS

As the risk factors for attempted and completed suicide show only a few differences, and prior suicide attempt (particularly in patients with major depressive episode) is the most

Table 18.1   Hierarchical classification of clinically explorable suicide risk factors.

1. Psychiatric/medical (primary) suicide risk factors
a. Current (past) Axis I major mental disorders (major depressive episode, substance-use disorders, schizophrenia)
b. Current suicidal ideation, prior suicide attempt
c. Comorbid Axis II (personality) and severe comorbid Axis III (medical) disorders
d. Family history of suicide (first and second degree relatives)

2. Psychosocial (secondary) suicide risk factors
a. Adverse childhood life events (separation, abuse, loss of parents)
b. Permanent adverse life situations (unemployment, isolation)
c. Acute psychosocial stressors (loss events, traumas)

3. Demographic (tertiary) suicide risk factors
a. Male gender
b. Adolescence (boys), old age (both genders)
c. Minority groups (relatives of suicide victims, victims of disasters, bisexuality, same-sex orientation)
d. Vulnerable intervals (spring/early summer, morning hours, premenstrual period)

powerful predictor of completed suicide [3, 4], the risk factors for attempted and completed suicide are not discussed separately in this chapter.

As suicide is a relatively rare event in the community, its precise prediction in individual cases is very difficult. Suicidal behaviour, however, is also significantly associated with a number of suicide risk factors of varying prognostic utility. Taking into account the field of responsibility, as well as the changeable/unchangeable nature of these risk factors, they can be classified hierarchically [3, 4]. The hierarchical classification of clinically explorable suicide risk factors is shown in Table 18.1. Although the statistical relationship between these different demographic (tertiary) risk factors (male gender, old age), as well as psychosocial (secondary) risk factors (unemployment, isolation), and suicidal behaviour is well demonstrated, their predictive utility is very limited in individual cases. Psychiatric-medical (primary) suicide risk factors (major depressive episode, especially in the case of prior suicide attempt) are the most powerful and clinically useful predictors of suicidal behaviour, particularly if psychosocial and demographic risk factors are also present. It is well demonstrated that more than 90% of suicide victims and attempters have at least one current (mainly untreated) Axis I mental disorder, most frequently major depressive episode (56–87%), substance use disorders (26–55%) and schizophrenia (6–13%). Comorbid anxiety and personality disorders, as well as serious medical illnesses, are also commonly present, but they are quite rare as principal (or only) diagnoses [1, 3, 4, 5, 8, 11]. Depression is not only the most common diagnosis among suicide victims but also seems to be the 'final common pathway' in suicide, even among patients with disorders other than depressive, such as schizophrenia and substance use disorders [12]. Clinical studies also show that if patients with major mood disorders commit or attempt suicide, they mostly do so during severe major depressive episodes (78–89%), less frequently in dysphoric mania or mixed affective episodes (11–20%) and very rarely during euphoric mania and euthymia (0–7%), indicating that suicidal behaviour in mood disorder patients is a state- and severity-dependent phenomenon [4, 13, 14]. Between 10% and 15% of severe major depressives die by their own hands [1, 5]. As the majority of patients with depressive disorder never commit

Table 18.2   Clinical indicators of suicidal behaviour in depressed patients.

a. Severe major depressive episode

   hopelessness, guilt
   agitation/depressive mixed state*
   insomnia
   past hypomania or mania (Bipolar II and Bipolar I diagnosis)
   comorbid anxiety, substance use and personality disorder
   inpatient status, short inpatient stay, recent discharge

b. Previous suicide attempt
c. Current suicidal ideating/plan, few reasons for living
d. Family history of suicide (first and second degree relatives)
e. Impulsive-aggressive personality features, cyclothymic temperament

* 'depressive mixed state' means three or more intra-depressive hypomanic symptoms.

suicide and up to half of them never attempt suicide [1, 4], however, special clinical characteristics of depression, such as severe depression, hopelessness, agitation etc [4, 15] (as listed in Table 18.2), as well as some psychosocial factors (see Table 18.1), also play a contributory role in self-destructive behaviour.

In contrast to the numerous suicide risk factors, only a few circumstances are known to have a protective effect against suicide. Good family and social support, having a large number of children, pregnancy and postpartum period, holding strong religious beliefs, having more reasons for living and appropriate medical care seem to have some protective effect [1, 3].

Of course, the absolute precise prediction of suicidal behaviour is impossible. However, the more risk factors that are present in a given patient (Tables 18.1 and 18.2), the higher the risk. A careful and systematic exploration of suicide risk (and protective) factors helps clinicians to identify patients at high suicide risk, with a good chance.

Decreased (dysregulated) central serotonergic system in suicide victims and suicide attempters (particularly in those using a violent method) is one of the most consistent neurobiological findings in psychiatry. Some studies, however, suggest that alterations in other neurotransmitter systems (norepinephrine, dopamine, GABA) might also play a contributory role. Several earlier findings and the most recent findings show that hyperactivity of the hypothalamic-pituitary-adrenal axis (as reflected in the abnormal dexamethasone suppression test), the pathomechanism of which also relates to a disturbed central serotonin mechanism, is a robust predictor of completed suicide, at least in patients with major depressive episode [5].

As decreased central serotonin metabolism is most strongly related to impulsive-aggressive personality features than to any specific psychiatric disorder, these trait-related characteristics highly predispose for suicidal behaviour, particularly in the simultaneous presence of an acute episode of major psychiatric disorder and adverse psychosocial situation, including lack of social support [5, 8, 16]. Based on all of the above, Mann *et al.* [16] proposed the stress-diathesis model of suicidal behaviour in psychiatric patients, in which the risk of suicidal acts is determined not only by the stressor (acute psychiatric illness) but also by a diathesis (impulsive, aggressive, pessimistic personality traits). In spite of the fact that current studies of the biology of suicidal behaviour are very promising, in the everyday clinical praxis (particularly in the case of urgent need of action), clinically explorable risk and protective factors are the most important aids in this complicated and highly responsible task.

18.4   PREVENTION OF SUICIDAL BEHAVIOUR

As suicide is a multicausal (bio-psycho-social) phenomenon, its prevention should also be complex, and the health care system is not the only element that is responsible for it. Given the strong relationship between current major mental disorders and suicidal behaviour, however, health care professionals (primarily psychiatrists and GPs) play a priority role. They should focus primarily (but not exclusively) on the early recognition and adequate acute and long-term treatment of mental disorders [3, 11, 12], which would also be an ideal target even if the fact of suicide were unknown. In spite of the fact that up to two-thirds of suicide victims contact different levels of health care (mostly their GPs) four weeks before their death, and the majority of them suffer from current major depression, the rate of appropriate antidepressant pharmacotherapy among depressed suicide victims is less than 20% [3, 4, 17]. This is quite disturbing, since long-term follow-up studies on severely ill, mainly hospitalized, frequently suicidal, depressive patients consistently show that the successful acute and long-term pharmacotherapy of unipolar depressive and bipolar disorders (antidepressants, mood stabilizers, anxiolytics, antipsychotics) significantly reduces the risk of subsequent suicidal behaviour in the vast majority of patients [4, 7, 18, 19], and the recent widespread use of new-generation antidepressants appears actually to have led to a highly significant decrease in the suicide rates in most countries, particularly in those with traditionally high baseline suicide mortality [7, 12, 20]. There was a marked decline in SSRI prescription for youth depressives in the United States and the Netherlands in 2004 and 2005 (immediately after the FDA's black box warning about the suicidality risk of SSRIs for paediatric depression), after which the suicide rate increased sharply in both countries in this age cohort [21]. If the well-known (but rarely occurring) suicidality potential of some antidepressants does actualize, it must be small enough to be masked by currently favourable trends in national suicide rates. However, doctors must always be vigilant of the rare risk of harm when prescribing antidepressants for patients with depressive disorders where the risk of suicidality is inherently high. Most recent findings suggest that, when antidepressants worsen depression in a few cases, its psychopathological substrate might well reside in an agitated, excited, mentally overstimulated depressive mixed state; recognition of the bipolar nature of depression (including the soft bipolarity) and the concomitant administration of mood stabilizers, anxiloytics and atypical antipsychotics is recommended in such cases to prevent, or at least to minimize, 'antidepressant associated' suicidality [7, 12].

Examining the evidence for the effectiveness of specific suicide-preventive interventions, the authors concluded that physician education in depression recognition and treatment, and restricting access to lethal means are the most important and best documented methods in reducing suicide rates, but promising results have been also published for cognitive therapy, problem-solving therapy and interpersonal psychotherapy [11]. However, because health care workers can help only those who contact them, public education on the symptoms, dangers and treatable nature of mental disorders is also very important. The mass media offers the best possibility for opinion leader suicidologists to

Table 18.3   Suicide prevention strategies.

1. Competence/responsibility of health care
  A. Patient-oriented perspective (targeting high-risk groups)
    a. Elimination of acute suicide danger
    b. Improving the diagnosis and treatment of mood and other mental disorders
    c. Aftercare of persons with high suicide risk
    d. Focus on special subgroups (adolescents, old people)
  B. Public-oriented perspective (targeting general population via media)
    a. Decreasing negative attitudes regarding mental illness and suicide
    b. Responsible media coverage
    c. Education of the public on the symptoms, dangers and treatable nature of mental disorders
2. Competence/responsibility of community leaders
    a. Improve well-being of people (including decreasing unemployment)
    b. Increasing the support for health and social care systems
    c. More restrictive alcohol and drug policies
    d. Decreasing the access to lethal suicide methods (domestic and car-exhaust gas, guns)

achieve a public education that results in decreasing negative attitudes regarding mental illnesses and suicide, and to stimulate journalists to create responsible and professional media coverage of suicide, including avoiding sensational journalism and avoiding the glorification, martyrization or 'mysterification' of suicide [1, 11]. As psychosocial and community factors also play a significant role in suicidal behaviour, it is not only health care workers that are responsible for its prevention [1, 3] (Table 18.3). Improving the well-being of people in general (including decreasing unemployment and providing more support for health and social services), restricting lethal suicide methods (e.g., to reduce domestic and car exhaust gas toxicity and to introduce stricter laws on gun control) and initiating more restrictive alcohol and drug policies – all of which also reduce suicide mortality [1, 3, 11] – already exceed the limits of health care and, rather, are the competence and responsibility of the leaders at any level of society.

REFERENCES

[1] Wasserman D (ed.) *Suicide. An unnecessary death*. London: Martin Dunitz; 2000.
[2] Levi F, La Vecchia C, Lucchini F, Negri E, Saxena S, Maulik PK, Saraceno B. Trends in mortality from suicide, 1965-99. *Acta Psychiatrica Scandinavica* 2003;108: pp. 341–349.
[3] Rihmer Z, Belső N, Kiss K. Strategies for suicide prevention. *Current Opinion in Psychiatry* 2002;15: pp. 83–87.
[4] Rihmer Z. Suicide risk in mood disorders. *Current Opinion in Psychiatry* 2007;20: pp. 17–22.
[5] Carroll-Ghosh T, Victor BS, Bourgeois JA. Suicide. In: Hales RE, Yodofsky SC. (eds.) *The American Psychiatric Publishing Textbok of Clinical Psychiatry*. Washington, DC: American Psychiatric Publishing, Inc; 2003. pp. 1457–1483.
[6] Oquendo MA, Lizardi D, Greenwald S, Weisman MM, Mann JJ. Rates of lifetime suicide attempt and rates of lifetime major depression in different ethnic groups in the United States. *Acta Psychiatrica Scandinavica* 2004;110: pp. 446–451.
[7] Rihmer Z, Akiskal HS. Do antidepressants t(h)reat(en) depressives? Toward a clinically judicious formulation of the antidepressant-suicidality FDA advisory in light of declining national suicide statistics from many countries. *Journal of Affective Disorders* 2006;94: pp. 3–13.

[8] Sudak HD. Suicide. In: Sadock BJ, Sadock VA. (eds.) *Kaplan and Sadock's Comprehensive Textbook of Psychiatry*. 8th ed. Philadelphia: Lippincott Williams and Wilkins; 2005. pp.: 2442–2453.

[9] Rutz W, Walinder J, von Knorring L, Rihmer Z, Pihlgren H. Prevention of depression and suicide by education and medication: Impact on male suicidality. An update from the Gotland study. *International Journal of Psychiatry in Clinical Practice* 1997;1: pp. 39–46.

[10] Partonen T, Haukka J, Pirkola E, Isometsa E, Lönnqvist J. Time patterns and seasonal mismatch in suicide. *Acta Psychiatrica Scandinavica* 2004;109: pp. 110–115.

[11] Mann JJ, Apter A, Bartolote J, Beautrais A, Currier D, Haas A, *et al*. Suicide prevention strategies. A systematic review. *JAMA* 2005;294: pp. 2064–2074.

[12] Akiskal HS. Targeting suicide prevention to modifiable risk factors: Has bipolar II been overlooked? (Editorial). *Acta Psychiatrica Scandinavica* 2007;116: pp. 395–402.

[13] Kessing LV. Severity of depressive episodes according to ICD-10: Prediction of risk of relapse and suicide. *British Journal of Psychiatry* 2004;184: pp. 153–156.

[14] Valtonen HM, Suominen K, Mantere O, Leppamaki S, Arvilommi P, Isometsa E. Suicidal behaviour during different phases of bipolar disorder. *Journal of Affective Disorders* 2007;97: pp. 101–107.

[15] Qin P, Nordentoft M. Suicide risk in relation to psychiatric hospitalization. Evidence based on longitudinal registers. *Archives of General Psychiatry* 2005;62: pp. 427–432.

[16] Mann JJ, Waternaux C, Haas GL, Malone KM. Toward a clinical model of suicidal behavior in psychiatric patients. *American Journal of Psychiatry* 1999;156: pp. 181–189.

[17] Luoma JB, Martin CE, Pearson JL. Contact with mental health and primary care providers before suicide: A review of the evidence. *American Journal of Psychiatry* 2002;159: pp. 909–916.

[18] Angst J, Angst F, Gerber-Werder R, Gamma A. Suicide in 406 mood disorder patients with and without long-term medication: A 40-44-year follow-up. *Archives of Suicide Research* 2005;9: pp. 279–300.

[19] Rihmer Z. Pharmacological prevention of suicide in bipolar patients – A realizable target. *Journal of Affective Disorders* 2007;103: pp. 1–3.

[20] Szántó K, Kalmár S, Hendin H, Rihmer Z, Mann JJ. A suicide prevention program in a region with a very high suicide rate. *Archives of General Psychiatry* 2007;64: pp. 914–920.

[21] Gibbons RD, Brown CH, Hur K, Marcus SM, Bhaumik DK, Erkens JA, Herings RMC, Mann JJ. Early evidence on the effects of regulators' suicidality warnings on SSRI prescriptions and suicide in children and adolescents. *Archives of General Psychiatry* 2007;164: pp. 1356–1363.

COMORBIDITY IN MENTAL AND GENERAL HEALTH

CHAPTER 19

Conceptual and Methodological Considerations in Comorbidity

Ihsan M. Salloum

*Professor of Psychiatry and Director, Division of Alcohol and Substance Abuse:
Treatment and Research, University of Miami Miller School of Medicine, FL, USA;
Section on Classification, Diagnostic Assessment and Nomenclature, World
Psychiatric Association*

Juan E. Mezzich

*Professor of Psychiatry and Director, International Center for Mental Health and
Division of Psychiatric Epidemiology, Mount Sinai School of Medicine, New York
University, NY, USA; Past President of the World Psychiatric Association*

Sandra E. Cordoba

*International Center for Mental Health, Mount Sinai School of Medicine,
New York University, NY, USA*

19.1 INTRODUCTION

Clinical comorbidities have been increasingly recognized as the defining realities of clinical care. The typical case in regular clinical settings is likely to present with multiple difficulties affecting several organ systems requiring different types of interventions. Treatment needs for this population are often unmet within the framework of traditional treatment models of single-disease entity treated in acute care. Primary care models are often challenged by the clinical complexity of these conditions. As a result, the care for these conditions is often fractioned and parcelled among disparate, uncoordinated, service providers.

The challenge of clinical comorbidity has also been addressed by the World Health Organization (WHO) through the establishment of a workgroup of international experts [1].

19.2 THE CONCEPT OF COMORBIDITY

The concept of comorbidity emerged within the context of clinical care, with specific concerns over the impact of additional significant health conditions on the prognosis of an

Psychiatric Diagnosis: Challenges and Prospects   Edited by I.M. Salloum and J.E. Mezzich
© 2009 John Wiley & Sons, Ltd

index disease. The term comorbidity was first introduced in general medicine over 30 years ago, when it was defined as 'any distinct additional clinical entity' and:

> 'such "non-disease" clinical entities as: pregnancy; deliberate dieting in an effort to lose weight; and certain symptomatic reactions, such as nausea, that may occur with various therapeutic manoeuvres [that] has existed or that may occur during the clinical course of a patient who has the index disease under study.' [2],

Thus, this broad definition of comorbidity reflected a primary concern with the prognostic significance of associated health conditions (including disease and non-disease entities) on the effectiveness, choice of treatment, and outcome of the index disease. With an aging world population, the increased prevalence of chronic conditions, and the expanding practice of polypharmacy, the problem of comorbidity is gaining worldwide importance.

Despite the high prevalence and public health significance of clinical comorbidity, a comprehensive approach addressing this complex problem is still lacking. Questions on the interrelationship of coexisting disorders and the resulting effects of multiple ill-health conditions, including a suitable taxonomy, posed more than 30 years ago by Feinstein [2], are still largely unanswered. Within psychiatry, comorbidity presents additional layers of complexity for psychiatric taxonomies [3].

19.3   CLINICAL AND CONCEPTUAL BASES OF THE RELATIONSHIP BETWEEN COMORBID CONDITIONS

Their high prevalence, and the significant impact on health and on health-care systems, have stimulated increasing interest in understanding the true nature of the relationship between co-occurring disorders. Empirical studies, as well as conceptual efforts, have pointed out the multilevel interactions between comorbid disorders.

Comorbid conditions may interact at multiple levels to influence the emergence, manifestations, course and outcome of the conditions involved. Treatment interventions may be ineffective or require significant adaptations in the presence of comorbidity. Significant adverse outcomes, such as suicide, are more likely to occur in the presence of certain comorbidities. Furthermore, the lack of recognition of co-existing morbid conditions, or the minimization of their existence by preconceived notions about attribution, such as treating what is believed to be the primary cause, may delay the implementation of effective treatment of associated comorbidities and result in the prolongation of morbidity and suffering and increased costs.

From a clinical perspective, the relationship between comorbid conditions may involve the following domains: (1) one condition may predispose to the appearance of the second condition, representing a causative or contributing risk factor; (2) one condition may modify the manifestation of the other disorder, causing difficulty in the recognition and accuracy of the diagnosis of the other disorder; (3) one condition may modify the course and treatment responsiveness of the other disorder, thus influencing outcome and the overall prognosis of the disorder. Often, the negative impact on outcome is bi-directional and reciprocal between the comorbid disorders. This may result from consequential behaviour related to the index disorder, such as poor treatment adherence, or to an unknown interaction between the disorders at an underlying causative mechanism.

The lack of etiopathogenic validity and knowledge about the cause and pathophysiology of mental illness poses additional challenges. For example, both the ICD-10 [4] and the DSM-IV

[5] provide a multiaxial system that allows the recording of multiple disorders. This innovative contribution has enhanced the utility of the diagnostic process by focusing attention on all presenting clinical difficulties in need of intervention. The multiaxial system, on the other hand, also highlighted the problem of co-occurring conditions in psychiatry. The lack of etiopathogenic validity for most diagnostic categories of mental disorders raises questions regarding the true versus the spurious or artifactual nature of certain clinical comorbidities.

Several conceptualizations of the relationship between comorbid conditions within the framework of modern classifications of mental disorders have been presented [6]. One perspective that has received some attention is the so-called primary-secondary distinction. This refers to the following potential relationships between comorbid conditions [6].

The first, and most studied, is the chronological sequencing of the disorders without implication of cause and effect relationship. This simply refers to the sequence of onset of the disorders in relation to each other. The second primary-secondary distinction refers to strict causal inference, where a disorder has emerged as a purported direct consequence of a pre-existing one, such as organic mood disorder due to a physical condition or a substance-induced mood disorder. The third distinction refers to the predominance of the clinical feature of one disorder over the other based on the pervasiveness of the syndrome in terms of current acuity and past persistence. Empirical testing of these relationships is still limited.

The chronic disease epidemiology perspective identifies three types of comorbidity: bias comorbidity; coincidental or independent comorbidity; and substantive, dependent, or associative comorbidity [7]. Bias comorbidity is when comorbidity does not reflect a true state of co-existing disorders but results from the presence of bias. For example, Berkson's bias [8] is the finding of a higher rate of comorbidity in people seeking treatment, as those with more than one disorder are more likely to seek help, and thus are overrepresented in treatment settings. Spurious comorbidity is another example of bias comorbidity produced by the imposition of arbitrary diagnostic boundaries in psychiatric classifications.

Coincidental or independent comorbidity is when two independent conditions are expected to co-occur at a rate that equals the product of the prevalence of the separate conditions. The proportion of comorbidity in this case is expected statistically, although comorbidity rates will be higher in sicker populations. It is important to note that, while the disorders may be aetiologically independent from each other, the two co-existing conditions may still have reciprocal negative impact, resulting in an overall worsening of the course and outcome.

Substantive (cluster, dependent, or associative) comorbidity is when the comorbidity rates exceed those that are statistically expected (coincidental), in the absence of bias. Substantive comorbidity may result when the disorders involved share risk factors, or directly or indirectly act as risk factors for one another.

The concept of spectrum disorder is another important related notion that may underlie comorbidity. This genetically-based perspective is often expressed as one predisposing genotype that may manifest itself in a spectrum of several different clinical states or phenotypes. Pleiotropy, or the production of multiple phenotypic effects by a single gene, may be an illustrative example of this mechanism. An alternate view to this perspective is what has been termed 'polygeneity'. Polygenic disorders result from the interaction of multiple common responsible genes. Genetic perspectives may also provide a rich field for understanding comorbidity and the role of epigenetic interactions, including gene-environment interaction in the development of comorbid disorders.

Furthermore, general vulnerability may also exist to develop multimorbidity. A complex interaction between multiple factors, such as genetic and personal vulnerabilities, environmental stressors, and contextual factors may eventuate in higher degree of associated comorbidity. An indication of this general vulnerability is suggested by the findings of a clustering of multiple clinical disorders in a small proportion of the surveyed population. An example of this is the finding of multimorbidity (three or more conditions) concentrated in approximately one sixth of the sample reported by the National Comorbidity Survey [9], a probability sample of the US population ages 15–54 years.

19.4   THE MULTIPLE FACES OF COMORBIDITY IN MENTAL HEALTH

Comorbidity of mental illness includes any combination of different health-related problems that have significant influence on health status and outcome. Mental disorders may co-occur with other mental health disorders, with general health disorders, or with serious social problems. Comorbidity, as it is often the case, may also occur at multiple levels, encompassing all of these domains.

Reporting of comorbidity within mental disorders has become prominent with the advent of the descriptive approach to psychopathology in modern classification systems, such as the DSM-IV and ICD-10, with limited use of exclusionary rules. A major challenge in mental health comorbidity is to separate true versus spurious comorbidity. Comorbidity between mental disorders and physical disorders, including those with communicable diseases, such as chronic viral infections (e.g. HIV, hepatitis viral infections) and non-communicable diseases (e.g cardiovascular and metabolic diseases), are major public health concerns in psychiatry and in the rest of medicine, especially in primary care settings.

The co-occurrence of emotional problems and mental disorders with serious social problems are also highly prevalent. Serious social problems impact key societal building blocks, from core values to community cohesion and to family structure and individual well-being. Poverty, violence and abuse are global issues that erode the fabric of societies and impact on the entire age spectrum, from childhood to old age.

Although many areas may be subsumed under social problems, four broad categories, including violence, abuse, poverty and discrimination, have been the focus of attention.

Violence may be further delineated as domestic violence, delinquency and political violence (such as wars and other armed conflicts), while abuse is specified further as child abuse, spouse abuse and elderly abuse. A review of the number of citations found in Medline Search (1996–2004), cross-referencing social problems with the major categories of mental disorders, indicated that almost 20% of publications from 1996 to 2004 that addressed social problems cross-referenced with some aspect of mental disorders [1].

Political violence had the highest number of citations of mental disorders, followed by delinquency, child abuse, poverty and discrimination. On the other hand, alcoholism, other substance related disorders, depression, schizophrenia and personality disorders were the mental disorders with the highest number of citations cross-referenced with social problems. The three mental disorder categories of non-alcohol substance use disorders, alcoholism and major depression accounted for 80% of all citations cross-referencing domestic violence with mental disorders, with substance abuse and alcoholism accounting for almost half of all citations, and major depression accounting for 30%. Non-alcohol substance use disorders and alcoholism also accounted for 60% of all citations cross-referenced with delinquency, and for over half of those cross-referenced with political violence and war. Two other major psychiatric disorders, major depression and schizophrenia, accounted for 49% of cross-references with political violence and war.

Major depressive disorders, dissociative disorders and personality disorders accounted for over half of cross-references with child abuse. Of note, over 60% of dissociative disorder references were within the child abuse category. Half of the spouse abuse categories were cross-referenced with non-alcohol drug abuse and alcoholism, and 34% with major depressive disorders. Dementia and depressive disorders accounted for 78% of cross-references with elderly abuse.

Major depressive disorders, schizophrenia and anxiety disorders accounted for over half of cross-references with poverty (socioeconomic disadvantage), while drugs or alcohol accounted for one third, and mental retardation and developmental disorders accounted for an additional 10%. Dementia, schizophrenia, major depressive disorder, mental retardation, developmental disorders and attention deficit hyperactivity disorders accounted for approximately three quarters of the cross-referenced citations with discrimination [1].

This broad perspective on comorbidity highlights the importance of considering social and environmental contextual factors. The social problem domains discussed earlier are not exhaustive. For example, depression has been found to be associated with marital discord (e.g. [10]). Elucidation of the role of mental disorders as risk factors or contributors to some social problems, and the role of certain social problems as risk, causative or aggravating factors for some mental disorders would have significant impact on preventative and treatment efforts.

Another facet of comorbidity is when multiple disorders (hyper-comorbidity), either within one domain (i.e. multiple mental disorders) or across multiple domains (mental, general health and social context), are present [11]. There is evidence that a substantial proportion of individuals may be afflicted by more than two comorbid conditions, and that hyper-comorbidity tends to cluster in the same group of individuals [9]. Hyper-comorbidity is a particularly relevant problem in geriatrics [12], an issue of increasing worldwide relevance.

Multi-psychiatric morbidity is associated with increased clinical severity. For example, the number of psychiatric disorders was shown to positively correlate with severity indicators such as history of suicide attempts, work and social impairments, subjective distress, and global severity [13]. Multimorbidity also correlates positively with indicators of increased vulnerability, such as age of onset and family history. It appears that, regardless of whether comorbid disorders are the expression of common underlying cause or the results of independent processes, the presence of multiple disorders is associated with increased clinical severity [13]. Moreover, women with multimorbidity may be differentially affected, experiencing more distress and lower quality of life [14]. Furthermore, multimorbidity within general physical health is highly frequent, and its prevalence increases with age and is associated with an inverse relationship with quality of life in primary care settings [15].

Hyper-comorbidity across multiple domains (mental, physical and social) presents similar or amplified challenges to those presented by simpler forms of comorbidity. For example, some psychiatric and general health disorders comorbidities are highly frequent, with some evidence that they are casually related. General health morbidity appears to predict future development of mental disorders, while the presence of certain mental disorders may increase the rate of general physical disorders. Comorbidity of mental and physical disorders along with social problems is less studied; however, reports of poverty and socioeconomic disadvantage are highly associated. Significant, in this regard, is the high association between substance abuse, other psychiatric morbidity and social problems, as well as SUD, communicable diseases and the social problems mentioned earlier. Tri-aspectual comorbidity may be even more represented among the elderly, with a high frequency of reports on elderly abuse, dementia and depression. Studies of severe mental disorders among the elderly, such as bipolar disorder and schizophrenia, have highlighted the high frequency of multiple health problems in this population [16].

19.5   CONTRIBUTORS TO COMORBIDITY

Causative and contributing factors to comorbidity may include a wide range of domains. Several models have been advanced to explain the increased vulnerability of developing multiple disorders. These include *general susceptibility to illness* [17] versus **morbidity-mediated** models.

Vulnerability factors may involve a constellation of genetic susceptibility, developmental stages, and environmental and contextual domains. Shared antecedent factors, as well as independent risk may be hypothesized across all the spheres preceding the appearance of comorbid conditions. For example, neuroticism, a personality attribute, was found to predict clustering of chronic medical illness, in addition to predicting risk for psychiatric disorders in middle adulthood [18]. Neuroticism may be considered a manifestation of a general susceptibility to illness factor that increases the risk of developing multimorbidity problems.

On the other hand, a **morbidity-mediated model** dictates that the development of one morbid condition may enhance or create vulnerability factors to developing the other condition. The co-existence of two comorbid conditions may also exert a reciprocal negative influence at several levels, from pathophysiological and biological domains, to psychosocial, contextual and environmental realms that would further impact on the manifestation, course and outcome of the disorders involved and ultimately on the individual's prognosis. A **morbidity-mediated model** may provide the opportunity of preventative interventions by which an effective treatment of a specific disorder may prevent the future development of comorbid conditions [19]. A morbidity-mediated model may also provide a conceptual framework where specific, morbidity-mediated risk factors may be separated from pre-existing, generic risk factors.

Studies of the relationship between ill health and major depressive disorder demonstrate the relevance of a morbidity-mediated vulnerability model. Individuals with ill health had a two to four times increased risk of developing major depressive disorders. On the other hand, those with major depressive disorders were four times more likely to develop ill health. The strong association between major depression and physical disorder may be mediated by alterations of the immune system [20]. For example, theories of common immune-mediated vulnerabilities to medical illness and depression are consistent with these associations.

Two models have addressed the influences of early life environment on health in later life. The **latency model** emphasizes the independent effects of discrete events occurring early in life on health status late in life. Events that occur at critical or sensitive periods in brain development would produce disease later in life. Examples that may fit this model include the association between birth weight, placenta size and weight gain in the first year of life and cardiovascular disease in adulthood [19].

The **pathways model** postulates that early life factors are causally linked to disease development in adulthood. This model takes into account the inter-relationships between social and biological risks throughout the life course, as the subsequent social and biological environment may determine the health consequences and outcome of early biological insults. This model emphasizes the full determination of the effects of cumulative social and biological risk factors across the life stages in the inception of disease states in adults. Thus, this model points out the role of early environment on subsequent life trajectories, which in turn influence adult health. The pathways model is an inclusive model of disease development and implicates the cumulative effect of life events along the developmental trajectories. The diatheses of disease development in adulthood result from the overall conditions of life throughout the lifecycle [19]. Several longitudinal studies of disadvantaged populations, such as children and the elderly, have pointed to the importance of socioeconomic status and social position on health outcome.

An early life event, in addition to exerting a 'latent effect', as in the latency model, may also represent the first in a chain of adverse events over the lifecycle, eventuating in a disease state. Furthermore, multiple illnesses may also co-occur when determinants or precursors of the disorders are shared. On the other hand, the presence of any disorder may act as a general facilitator of comorbidity by weakening the general health states, and increase individual vulnerabilities to other ailments and sickness. The role of chronic stress leading to 'allostatic load' has been advanced as a major causative factor in deleterious health effects ranging from decreased immunity to disease causation and increased mortality [21, 22]. A chronic disorder may similarly act as a chronic stress, thus leading to 'allostatic load' and increased morbidity.

Modern epidemiological methods involving multilevel approaches [23], considering both longitudinal unfolding and cross-sectional manifestations may help in the elucidation of the complex web of causative and contributing factors to comorbidity.

19.6   COMORBIDITY AND THE NEED FOR PERSON-CENTRED INTEGRATIVE DIAGNOSIS AND CARE

The clinical complexity presented by comorbidity requires an integrated approach to care. The conventional paradigm of acute, disease-focused care may not be the optimal way to address the complexities of presenting problems associated with comorbidity. A person-centred, holistic, community-oriented and comprehensive approach is key to addressing the complexities of clinical comorbidities. Adequate care for these conditions requires an integrated care model that addresses the various aspects of comorbid conditions, including psychiatric, medical and contextual factors. Important elements of this paradigm are the pointed assessments of both the positive aspects of health and ill health, the involvement of the persons seeking care, their support and the clinician, and the integration of the diagnostic information to support health restoration, recovery, prevention, and health promotion.

19.7   CONCLUSIONS

Clinical comorbidity has become a defining characteristic of presenting health needs, and is becoming a global health problem phenomenon affecting developing and developed countries alike. Clinical comorbidities are becoming the rule in regular clinical care settings, and are associated with increased morbidity, mortality and an overall economic and humanitarian burden. Comorbidity presents with multiple faces, within mental health and across mental health, general health and social problems. Significant social problems appear to be intertwined with psychiatric and medical comorbidity, and may play a key role in the etiopathogenesis and consequence of associated conditions. Management of clinical comorbidity requires a person-centred, community-based integrative approach that addresses the various aspects of comorbid conditions, including psychiatric, medical and contextual factors. Narrow-focused, single-disease, acute care models of care are inadequate to addressing the complexities of clinical comorbidities. There is still an urgent need for research to enhance our understanding of the causative and protective mechanisms involved in the development of and care for comorbid conditions. The growing global public health needs of clinical comorbidities call for the development of appropriate research, treatment, and preventative and educational strategies.

REFERENCES

[1] Mezzich JE, Salloum IM, Bertolote J. Comorbidity: *Clinical complexity and the need for integrated care*. Technical report, unpublished. Geneva: World Health Organization; 2006.

[2] Feinstein AR. The pre-therapeutic classification of co-morbidity in chronic disease *Journal of Chronis Diseases* 1970;23: pp. 455–468.

[3] First MB. Mutually exclusive versus co-occurring diagnostic categories: the challenge of diagnostic comorbidity. *Psychopathology* 2005;38(4): pp. 206–210.

[4] Mezzich JE. On developing a psychiatric multiaxial schema for ICD-10. *British Journal of Psychiatry*. 1988;152(Suppl 1): pp. 38–43.

[5] Association AP. *DSM-IV-TR: Diagnostic and Statistical Manual of Mental Disorders*. 4th ed. Text Revision. Washington, DC: American Psychiatric Association; 2000.

[6] Klerman GL. Approaches to the phenomena of comorbidity. In: Maser JD, Cloninger CR. (eds.) Comorbidity of mood and anxiety disorders. Washington, DC: American Psychiatric Press, Inc.; 1990.

[7] Batstra L, Bos E, Neeleman J. Quantifying psychiatric comorbidity–lessions from chronic disease epidemiology. *Social Psychiatry and Psychiatric Epidemiology* 2002;37(3): pp. 105–111.

[8] Berkson J. Limitations of the application of fourfold table analysis to hospital data. *Biometric Bulletin* 1946;2: pp. 47–53.

[9] Kessler RC, McGonagle KA, Zhao S, Nelson CB, Hughes M, Eshleman S, Wittchen HU, Kendler KS. Lifetime and 12-month prevalence of DSM-III-R psychiatric disorders in the United States. Results from the National Comorbidity Survey. *Archives of General Psychiatry* 1994;51(1): pp. 8–19.

[10] Hollist CS, Miller RB, Falceto OG, Fernandes CL. Marital satisfaction and depression: a replication of the Marital Discord Model in a Latino sample. *Family Process* 2007;46(4): pp. 485–498.

[11] Salloum IM, Thase ME. Impact of substance abuse on the course and treatment of bipolar disorder. *Bipolar Disorders* 2000;2 (3): pp.269–280.

[12] Bartels SJ. Caring for the whole person: integrated health care for older adults with severe mental illness and medical comorbidity. *Journal of the American Geriatrics Society* 2004;52 (12 Suppl).

[13] Angst J, Sellaro R, Ries Merikangas K. Multimorbidity of psychiatric disorders as an indicator of clinical severity. *European Archives of Psychiatry and Clinical Neuroscience* 2002;252(4): pp.147–154.

[14] Gamma A, Angst J. Concurrent psychiatric comorbidity and multimorbidity in a community study: gender differences and quality of life. *European Archives of Psychiatry and Clinical Neuroscience* 2001;251(2).

[15] Fortin M, Lapointe L, Hudon C, Vanasse A, Ntetu A, Maltais D. Multimorbidity and quality of life in primary care: a systematic review. *Health and Quality of Life Outcomes* 2004;2 (1): p. 51.

[16] Depp CA, Jeste DV. Bipolar disorder in older adults: a critical review. *Bipolar Disorders* 2004;6 (5): pp. 343–367.

[17] Hinkle LEJ, Christenson WN, Kane FD, Ostfeld A, Thetford WN, Wolff, HG. An investigation of the relation between life experience, personality characteristics, and general susceptibility to illness. *Psychosomatic Medicine* 1959;20: pp. 278–295.

[18] Neeleman J, Sytema S, Wadsworth M. Propensity to psychiatric and somatic ill-health: evidence from a birth cohort. *Psychological Medicine* 2002;32(5): pp.793–803.

[19] Power C, Hertzman C. Social and biological pathways linking early life and adult disease. *British Medical Bulletin* 1997;53(1): pp. 210–21.

[20] Cohen P, Pine DS, Must A, Kasen S, Brook J. Prospective associations between somatic illness and mental illness from childhood to adulthood. *American Journal of Epidemiology* 1998;147(3): pp. 232–9.

[21] McEwen BS. Mood disorders and allostatic load. *Biological Psychiatry* 2003;54(3): pp. 200–207.

[22] Kopp MS, Rethelyi J. Where psychology meets physiology: chronic stress and premature mortality - the Central-Eastern European health paradox. *Brain Research Bulletin* 2004;62(5): pp. 351–367.

[23] Mezzich JE, Üstün TB. 5.1: Epidemiology. In: Sadock BJS, Virginia A. (eds.) *Kaplan & Sadock's Comprehensive Textbook of Psychiatry*. Philadelphia, PA: Lippincott Williams & Wilkins; 2005. pp. 656–672.

CHAPTER 20

Mental and General Health Comorbidities in Persons Presenting in Primary Care

Michael S. Klinkman

Professor, Departments of Family Medicine and Psychiatry, University of Michigan, MI, USA

Linda Gask

Divisions of Psychiatry and Primary Care, University of Manchester, UK

20.1   INTRODUCTION

The concept of *comorbidity* in the primary health care setting is a difficult one. As the main point of entry to most organized health care systems, individuals often present with a complex mixture of medical, mental health, emotional and social problems, and many of these problems carry labels – and treatment plans – assigned by experts from domains far removed from primary health care. The primary care clinician must identify the most important of these problems and integrate their treatment under severe time and resource constraints. This task is particularly difficult in the mental health domain, where the number of specific disorders multiplies with each revision of DSM and ICD and where 'new' mental and general health comorbidities are 'discovered' each week.

In this chapter, we will describe mental and general health comorbidities as seen from the perspective of primary care clinicians and patients. We will begin by describing the context in which primary care services are delivered in much of the developed world, and the interrelationships between the physical, mental and social problems that make up the everyday work of primary care clinicians. We will then explore the problems seen in applying the psychiatric diagnostic classifications of DSM-IV and ICD-10 to primary care patients before we review our current knowledge about patterns of comorbidity seen in primary care and their clinical importance.

Psychiatric Diagnosis: Challenges and Prospects   Edited by I.M. Salloum and J.E. Mezzich
© 2009 John Wiley & Sons, Ltd

20.2   THE 'CONTEXT' IN WHICH PRIMARY CARE SERVICES ARE DELIVERED

20.2.1   Wide Boundaries and Competing Demands

Primary care has been defined by the Institute of Medicine in the US as the 'provision of integrated, accessible healthcare services by clinicians who are accountable for addressing a large majority of personal health needs, developing a sustained partnership with patients, and practicing in the context of the family and community' [1]. Primary health care is the main point of entry to formal health care for the majority of people who have emotional problems or mental health conditions. However, these problems and conditions occur in the context of acute and chronic medical conditions, medical emergencies, social and personal problems, and significant life events, and they must be identified and managed over time in a series of short, focused clinical encounters in which multiple competing demands are present [2, 3].

20.2.2   Relentless Time Pressure

The average duration of a primary care encounter varies considerably throughout the world, from less than five minutes in some countries in the developing world to 20 minutes or even longer in parts of Northern Europe and North America. After accounting for the duration of encounters and number of problems addressed per encounter, the average number of minutes spent for each presenting problem in Europe and North America is between two and four minutes [4–7]. To manage this enormous time pressure, primary care clinicians must hone their time management skills and develop effective cognitive shortcuts. Unfortunately, these management strategies do not match up well against the protean ways in which mental health problems present to primary care clinicians.

20.2.3   High Prevalence of Undifferentiated and Unfiltered Mental Health Problems

Patients in primary care settings are much less likely to present with clearly identifiable diagnostic syndromes. People present to primary care workers with a wide variety of symptoms, concerns, worries and problems. These are not only *undifferentiated* but also – crucially important at first presentation – *unrehearsed* by prior discussion with doctors versed in the agenda and language of diagnosis.

This situation stands in stark contrast to the way in which patients present to specialist mental health professionals, where they will either be seeking that professional by choice because they consider that the problem is within the clinical domain of that professional (self-acknowledgement and self-referral); or will have already discussed the likely cause of their symptoms and possible diagnosis with a primary care clinician (gatekeeping and referral). The critical point to understand is that primary care clinicians often encounter unfiltered and unrecognized symptoms that may or may not be identifiable as mental health syndromes, while speciality mental health clinicians most often encounter filtered symptoms that are recognized and understood as representative of a mental health problem.

20.2.4   Distress Versus Disorder

The problem of identifying undifferentiated and unfiltered mental health problems in primary care is further compounded by difficulties in separating *distress* from *disorder*. Distress can be present in patients for many reasons other than the presence of a mental health disorder. Many primary care patients have threshold mood disorders without noticeable distress, while others are clearly distressed but do not exhibit other symptoms of mental illness [8, 9]. The adverse consequences of the confusion between these two constructs can be seen in the misidentification of distressed patients as 'depressed' by case-finding instruments such as the CES-D (Center for Epidemiologic Studies Depression Scale) or Hamilton Rating Scale for Depression when they are employed in primary care [10–12]. Misidentification in either direction can have serious consequences for patients.

20.2.5   The Use of Time as a Diagnostic and Therapeutic Tool

Primary care clinicians often cope with the challenges presented by undifferentiated and unfiltered problems, distress, and competing demands by close and repeated observation of their patients over time. For patients whose symptoms do not unambiguously meet criteria for a threshold disorder, clinicians often choose to acknowledge the symptoms and with-hold active treatment while scheduling a follow-up assessment. If symptoms progress over time to the level of a specific disorder, active treatment can be initiated. At present, the degree to which undifferentiated symptoms, distress, or 'subthreshold' or 'mild' disorders progress to threshold level over time is not clear. This is a very important and highly controversial issue (see section 20.4).

20.3   THE COMPLEX RELATIONSHIP BETWEEN PHYSICAL, MENTAL AND SOCIAL PROBLEMS IN PRIMARY CARE PATIENTS

20.3.1   Primary Care 'Diagnosis' as a Three-Dimensional Matrix

We have seen that primary care patients enter the formal health care system with multiple undifferentiated and unfiltered symptoms that may or may not represent mental health disorder. The picture is further complicated in that presenting symptoms may also be related to known or unknown biomedical conditions.

It might be useful to think of primary care as an ongoing three-way interaction among general health problems, mental health problems and social problems. This could be visualized as a three-dimensional space, in which the severity or level of problems in each domain at a point in time can be plotted on an axis (Figure 20.1) as a rough estimate of the overall burden of illness. Over time, the position of the point on each axis will change. These three domains are correlated. For example, changes in the severity of general health problems may create additional social problems or intensify existing mental health problems, and increasing severity of mental health problems may amplify physical symptoms.

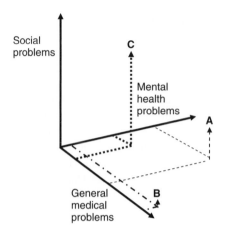

Person A:
- moderate level of general medical problems
- high level of mental health problems
- fairly low level of social problems.

Person B ('classic' biomedical illness):
- high level of general medical problems
- low level of mental health problems
- minimal level of social problems.

Person C:
- low level of general medical problems
- moderate level of mental health problems
- very high level of social problems.

Note: Although person B is often considered to be the most severely ill in medical terms, the overall burden of illness is higher for persons A and C.

Figure 20.1   The three-dimensional matrix of primary care diagnosis.

There is strong evidence supporting the inter-relationships between these domains. Mental health problems are known to occur more frequently in those with common chronic physical illness, such as diabetes, arthritis and heart disease (see section 20.5). Conversely, medical comorbidity plays an important role in how primary care patients experience and cope with their mental health problems [13], and the presence of social problems or the occurrence of significant life events are known to have a major impact on the severity of mental health problems or outcomes of care for chronic physical illness [14, 15].

The message is clear. Mental and general health comorbidities, along with social problems, are the rule rather than the exception in persons presenting to primary care clinicians. They are such a part of the fabric of routine primary care practice that the use of the term 'comorbid', which implies sporadic co-occurrence of independent conditions, is potentially very misleading. Our understanding of primary care might be enhanced by replacing 'comorbidity' with 'multimorbidity' and focusing effort on the integration of diagnosis and treatment across domains [16–18].

20.3.2 Implications for Current and Future Mental Health Classifications

An optimal classification of mental health disorders for primary care would allow primary care workers to accurately record elements of each of the three domains, as well as important elements of the 'context' of care (life events, patient perceptions, goals and preferences) described above. This would provide the information needed to interpret ambiguous symptoms in patients with 'mixed' physical, mental and social suffering.

This expanded primary care classification of mental health disorders could be directly linked to a tailored and expanded therapeutic approach that links different interventions – medication, psychotherapy, social support interventions such as groups, family therapy or community work. This would be very useful in situations where primary care interventions routinely incorporate social interventions, as is the case in Latin America. It could also provide a framework to effectively adapt our current Western-based classifications to fit non-Western cultures: general health and mental health 'disorder' diagnostic domains might require minimal alteration, but the 'context' and 'social problems' domains might be revised to fit the local culture.

20.4 PROBLEMS WITH THE CONCEPT OF PSYCHIATRIC 'CASENESS' IN PRIMARY CARE

Any discussion of comorbidity in primary care must take into account our imperfect understanding of the nature of a 'case' of a specific disorder. Although diagnostic criteria are operationally defined for both DSM-IV and ICD-10 disorders, these criteria have proven quite difficult to validate and apply in everyday primary care practice [19]. Primary care clinicians usually think in terms of mental health **problems** rather than DSM-IV or ICD-10 **diagnoses**. They are far more likely to make a diagnosis of depression if they believe specific treatment is necessary. Formal diagnosis therefore tends to follow management decisions, not precede them, and in mild cases clinicians often record only symptom diagnoses [20–22]. In the US, primary care clinicians are trained to separate patients by level of severity of symptoms, and to carry out full mental health diagnostic assessment only for patients with significant and/or persistent symptoms [23].

There are four major problem areas:

- patients who have transient, fluctuating, or recurrent symptoms;
- ambiguity in the diagnosis of 'subthreshold' conditions in primary care;
- 'overlapping' symptoms that point to more than one mental health or general medical disorder or condition;
- the concept of 'somatization' and 'somatoform' disorder in patients with general medical conditions

20.4.1 Psychiatric 'Caseness' in Individuals with Transient, Recurrent or Chronic Symptoms

The discussion of comorbidity in primary care patients is complicated by the difficulties in establishing a specific diagnosis (or diagnoses) over time. Even when primary care patients meet diagnostic criteria for specific DSM-IV or ICD-10 mental health disorders, their symptoms often fluctuate over time and their 'caseness' may be transient [24, 25]. Of patients with at least one disorder, 20% 'recover' spontaneously within three months [26]. Nosological diagnoses have been demonstrated to last less than four weeks 30% of the time and less than six months 65% of the time [27].

Although primary care clinicians have frequently been criticized for their lack of skill in recognising threshold mental disorders, recognition is itself a complex phenomenon, related in part to the transience of symptoms. Higher rates of detection (and treatment) have been found for patients with more severe symptoms and higher levels of disability [28, 29], and there is some evidence that short-term outcomes for 'detected' and 'undetected' depressed primary care patients are no different [30].

The fluctuating nature of symptoms makes it very difficult to assess the performance of primary care clinicians in recognizing and treating comorbid mental health problems. If a 'comorbid' mental health problem is diagnosed at a point in time and is not present three months later, has it been effectively treated – or did it truly exist in the first place?

20.4.2 Psychiatric 'Caseness' in Subthreshold Disorders

Subthreshold disorders – not meeting full diagnostic criteria for specific diagnoses - are highly prevalent and have been associated with significant disability. The overall prevalence of subthreshold disorders in primary care exceeds that of threshold disorders [31], and individuals with subthreshold disorders report levels of psychological distress, disability in daily activities and perceived health approaching or equal to those with threshold disorder [32, 33]. The high prevalence of subthreshold or mild disorders in primary care has been linked to the development of more severe disorder, and there are many public calls for aggressive treatment of these patients to 'prevent' more serious disorders that are resistant to treatment. However, evidence to support this approach is limited. One long-term longitudinal study of Dutch primary care patients diagnosed as depressed found that the majority had no recurrent episodes over a 10-year follow-up period despite an overall minimal level of treatment [34].

Moreover, subthreshold disorders are also very difficult to reliably diagnose in primary care. In cross-sectional studies, patients with major depression may at the moment of assessment have limited severity and be misidentified as a 'case' of subthreshold or minor depression [8, 35, 36], and subthreshold bipolar disorder may be misidentified as depression or mixed depression-anxiety [37]. In these situations, the correct or 'true' diagnosis may only be clear after repeated assessment over time. Several conceptual frameworks have been proposed over time to accommodate subthreshold conditions [24, 38–41], but their boundaries remain problematic. This creates real problems in any attempt to define or apportion comorbidity between subthreshold disorders and other mental health or general medical conditions in the primary care setting.

20.4.3 Psychiatric 'Caseness' when Common Symptoms Overlap Between Disorders

The third major problem with the concept of comorbidity is that common symptoms may exist at high prevalence across major diagnostic categories (for example, 'fatigue' or 'sleep problems' across anxiety, depression, somatization and substance misuse) in primary care. This coexistence may be cross-sectional in that all these symptoms appear together at the same time, or it may be longitudinal in the sense that one set of symptoms is followed closely in time by another [9]. This problem is compounded by the high prevalence of several of these same symptoms in chronic general medical conditions such as heart disease or diabetes. The cross-sectional studies examining rates of comorbidity have for the most part not addressed this problem, with surveys built 'vertically' to assemble DSM or ICD diagnoses in relation to a specific disorder rather than 'horizontally' to assess the prevalence of common or ambiguous symptoms in the context of other health problems. The limited evidence on the prevalence of individual symptoms over time, or the specificity of symptoms for mood disorder in the presence of chronic medical problems, is inconsistent. [12, 24, 42–45].

20.4.4   The Problem of 'Somatization' in Primary Care

The diagnosis of somatization disorder requires that somatic symptoms be interpreted as a manifestation of underlying psychiatric illness. This presents a tremendous problem in primary care, where undiagnosed symptoms are common, can be followed longitudinally, and are often attributable to the presence of other health problems. The arbitrary diagnostic criteria for duration and number of symptoms do not solve this problem [39]. The creation of a more limited symptom and duration version, somatoform disorder, magnified the problem by lowering the threshold for inclusion while maintaining the hidden attribution of physical symptoms to psychiatric cause. This less restrictive form has been seen as both comorbid with other disorders and independently associated with disability, but in primary care patient samples it is not clear whether it represents a true disorder or simply a count of medical symptoms in patients with multiple health problems [31, 46].

A growing number of researchers are suggesting that the concept of somatization should be replaced, at least in the primary care setting, by the simpler descriptive title 'medically unexplained symptoms' (MUS). In one recent primary care study, a comprehensive psychiatric diagnostic assessment of patients with MUS suggested that depression and/or anxiety characterized MUS patients better than the somatization or somatoform disorder labels [47]. Recent work in Europe casts additional doubt on the validity of these diagnoses in primary care and calls for a new symptom-level classification for MUS to replace somatization and somatiform disorder [48–50].

20.4.5   Summary

This brief discussion of transient symptoms, subthreshold conditions and unexplained somatic symptoms highlights the problems in applying the psychiatric diagnostic classifications of DSM-IV and ICD-10 to primary care patients. There is a clear need for improved symptom-level classification in primary care to better categorize people with physical symptoms and to learn which symptoms represent discrete mental health disorders that require intervention. Until this is in place, it will be very difficult to reliably assess and manage multimorbidity in primary care. With this caveat in mind, we turn to a review of existing evidence on the prevalence of mental health comorbidities in patients presenting to primary care.

20.5   THE MOST COMMON MENTAL HEALTH COMORBIDITIES IN PATIENTS PRESENTING IN PRIMARY CARE

Despite the serious reservations mentioned above regarding the validity of our current constructs of comorbidity, it is important to note the relative frequency of comorbid conditions seen in published work from around the globe, in order to better understand the complexity of mental health problems as they occur in the 'real world' of primary health care.

20.5.1   Comorbidity of 'Threshold' Mental Health Disorders

Much of the evidence regarding mental health comorbidity in primary care was first assembled during the 1990s in the World Health Organization (WHO) Collaborative Study of Psychological Problems in General Health Care [51, 52], conducted in 15 centres in Asia, Africa, Europe and the Americas. This study screened over 25 000 adults between ages of 18 and 65 and carried out detailed diagnostic interviews of a stratified random sample of over 5400 individuals. The results confirmed that 'well-defined' psychological problems (meeting threshold ICD-10 criteria) were frequent in general health-care settings (in about 24% of attenders), and that among the most commonly seen were depression, anxiety, alcohol misuse, somatoform disorders and neurasthenia. The most common co-occurrence of disorders was depression and anxiety [51]. However, subsequent analyses of over 1600 adults with at least three symptoms of anxiety, depression and/or somatization but no formal ICD-10 disorders provided support for the existence of a mixed anxiety-depression category crossing the boundaries of current anxiety and depression disorders [31], setting off the ongoing debate about whether anxiety and depression are comorbid or a single disorder [53, 54].

Subsequent studies by WHO (the World Mental Health Survey, including 17 countries from Europe, America, the Middle East, Africa, Asia and the South Pacific), the US National Institute of Mental Health (the National Comorbidity Survey and NCS Replication) and several European nations have employed a common methodology very similar to that used in the first Collaborative Study. These studies have surveyed representative community samples rather than primary care attenders. Their results have largely confirmed the high level of mental health comorbidity seen in the Collaborative Study [29, 55–58]. For example, the US National Comorbidity Study Replication found a 12-month prevalence of 26.2% for any threshold disorder. Of these, about half met criteria for only one disorder, and a quarter met criteria for three or more disorders. The pattern of comorbidity was complex, with a very high level of comorbidity between anxiety and mood disorders, a surprisingly low level of comorbidity between individual anxiety disorders such as phobia and panic, and high comorbidity between severe internalizing and externalizing disorders [56]. These general patterns appear to hold across different countries, cultures and ethnic groups [55].

Substance misuse is also highly comorbid with anxiety and depression in studies of primary care attenders. A comprehensive New Zealand study revealed that more than one third of people attending their general practitioner had a diagnosable mental disorder during the previous 12 months. The most common disorders identified by standardized diagnostic assessment were anxiety disorders, depression and substance use disorders, and there was high comorbidity of these three groups with the experience of mixed pictures as common as disorders occurring alone [29].

The evidence on mental health comorbidity in subthreshold disorders is both limited and controversial, related in large part to uncertainties about diagnostic boundaries or symptom attribution. One good example can be seen in the difficulty of determining whether patients have subthreshold or atypical bipolar disorder or mixed anxiety-depression [37]. At present, it would seem prudent to approach the diagnosis of subthreshold mental health comorbidity with great caution.

20.6 MENTAL HEALTH AND GENERAL MEDICAL COMORBIDITIES

20.6.1 Chronic Diseases and Mood and Anxiety Disorders: Consistent but Low-Level Association

From the perspective of the primary care clinician, it is important to know whether the presence of chronic medical conditions puts patients at higher risk for comorbid mental health disorders. Several recent publications have calculated odds ratios for the presence of presence of threshold mood and anxiety disorders in patients with self-reported chronic medical problems [59–68]; the results of these cross-sectional studies are presented in Table 20.1.

Table 20.1 Calculated odds ratios for mood and anxiety disorders in patients with selected chronic general medical conditions. All adjusted for age and sex.

	ODDS RATIOS				
CONDITION	Mood disorders	Anxiety disorders	Substance misuse	Comorbid mood/anx	Data source
Heart disease	2.1	2.2	1.4	—	WMHS*
Cardiovascular disease	2.2	2.2	1.6	3.4	Germany^
Back/neck pain	2.3	2.2	1.6	—	WMHS*
Multi-site pain	3.7	3.6	ns	—	WHMS*
Arthritis	1.9	1.9	1.5	—	WMHS*
Musculoskeletal Disease	2.5	2.3	1.3	3.5	Germany^
Diabetes	1.3	1.3	—	1.4	WMHS*
Asthma	1.6	1.5	1.7	—	WMHS*
Chronic lung disease	1.9	2.0	2.0	—	CCHS#
Severe asthma	2.1	2.9–5.5	—	—	Germany^
Non-severe asthma	1.5	2.1	—	—	Germany^
Cancer	2.4	1.7	ns	2.6	Germany^

All studies employed self-report methods for presence of chronic general medical condition, and all used the WHO Composite International Diagnostic Interview (CIDI) to assess for the presence of threshold mental health disorders. All reported values are statistically significant at the p = .05 level.
* data from World Mental Health Survey of 17 countries from Europe, America, the Middle East, Africa, Asia, and the South Pacific.
# data from the Canadian Community Health Survey.
^ data from German National Health Interview and Examination Survey Mental Health Supplement and Epidemiology of Mental Disorders in Medical Rehabilitation Study.

It is important to note that the calculated odds ratios (OR) were modest (most between 2 and 3) and similar across all disorders; the notable exception was diabetes, which had a much lower OR at 1.3 for both mood and anxiety disorders. Ratios were also remarkably stable for mood and anxiety disorders across the 17 countries included in the WMHS, though less so for substance use disorders. Finally, the OR for 'comorbid' mood and anxiety disorder in patients with all classes of chronic disease except diabetes was higher than for individual disorders. The OR for bipolar disorder, where assessed, was slightly higher, ranging from 2.7 to 5.6 (data not shown) [67, 68]. These cross-sectional data do not provide any insights about potential pathophysiologic mechanisms linking the conditions, but some are now proposing that mood disorders are linked to diabetes and cardiovascular disease through shared alterations in metabolic networks [69, 70].

It is clear that the presence of combined mental-physical comorbidity puts patients at higher risk for significant disability. Much has been written about the higher risk of adverse outcomes in patients with depression and cardiovascular disease, depression and diabetes, and multiple other combinations [71–78]. In the WMHS survey, the odds ratios for severe disability in individuals with both mental disorder and each of the chronic medical conditions were significantly greater than the sum of the odds for either type of condition occurring alone [65]. The presence of anxiety disorder or comorbid anxiety-depression in patients with general medical conditions may have a particularly strong negative impact on health-related quality of life [79].

20.6.2   Chronic Medical Conditions and Severe Mental Health Disorders

Individuals with serious mental illness (schizophrenia and affective disorders) also have increased rates of comorbid general medical conditions [80–82]. This has often been attributed to several confounding factors, such as poor diet and obesity, limited exercise, a higher prevalence of smoking, and other social and environmental factors. However, after controlling for smoking and obesity, odds ratios for conditions such as diabetes and heart disease are very similar to those seen with mood and anxiety disorders, and the ORs for chronic lung and liver disease are higher [81]. The interactions here are likely highly complex. There is evidence that antipsychotic medications cause weight gain and elevated blood glucose, and may cause direct liver damage, and the sedation caused by these medications is clearly linked to reduced exercise, apathy, and social withdrawal [83–87]. Primary care clinicians who provide care for patients with serious mental illness should closely monitor for emergence of glucose intolerance or diabetes, and focus significant effort on controlling weight gain and preventing or discontinuing smoking.

20.7   CONCLUSION

Individuals seen in primary care settings often present with a complex mixture of medical, mental health, emotional and social problems. Whether given the label of 'comorbid disorders' or 'multimorbidity', primary care clinicians must identify the most important problems from this mix and manage them in the context of competing demands and long-term relationships with their patients. There is much that we do not yet know about the interrelationships between somatic and mental disorders, but we have learned some important things about how disorders present in primary care. First, it is very common for individuals to have more than one threshold mental disorder. Second, threshold mental health disorders are roughly twice as common in individuals with any of several chronic medical conditions, and are more difficult to treat. Third, serious mental illness puts individuals at high risk of developing chronic medical conditions. These 'facts' can help guide efforts to improve primary care practice. Protocols to screen for the presence of 'comorbid' mental health conditions in patients with a diagnosed threshold disorder or any of several chronic medical conditions can be implemented using few resources, and the simple treatment algorithms created for ICD-10-PC can be refined and linked to screening efforts. As we extend our knowledge about the nature of 'subthreshold' conditions and somatic symptoms and learn which do not need treatment, we may also be able to lighten the burden of formal diagnosis and treatment in primary care.

REFERENCES

[1] Institute of Medicine. *Primary Care: America's Health in a New Era*. Washington, DC: Institute of Medicine Press; 1996.

[2] Klinkman MS. Competing demands in psychosocial care. A model for the identification and treatment of depressive disorders in primary care. *General Hospital Psychiatry* 1997;19(2): pp. 98–111.

[3] Rost K, Nutting P, Smith J, Coyne JC, Cooper-Patrick L, Rubenstein L. The role of competing demands in the treatment provided primary care patients with major depression. *Archives of Family Medicine* 2000;9(2): pp. 150–154.

[4] Beasley JW, Hankey TH, Erickson R, *et al*. How many problems do family physicians manage at each encounter? A WReN Study. *Annals of Family Medicine* 2004;2 (5): pp. 405–410.

[5] Tai-Seale M, McGuire TG, Zhang W. Time allocation in primary care office visits. *Health Services Research* 2007;42(5): pp. 1871–1894.

[6] Flocke S, Frank S, Wenger D. Addressing multiple problems in the family practice office visit. *Journal of Family Practice* 2001;50(3): pp. 211–216.

[7] Gottschalk A, Flocke SA. Time spent in face-to-face patient care and work outside the examination room. *Annals of Family Medicine* 2005;3(6): pp. 488–493.

[8] Coyne JC, Thompson R, Klinkman MS, Nease DE, Jr. Emotional disorders in primary care. *Journal of Consulting and Clinical Psychology* 2002;70(3): pp.798–809.

[9] Katerndahl D. Variations on a theme: the spectrum of anxiety disorders and problems with the DSM classification in primary care settings. In: Gower PL. (ed.) *New Research on the Psychiatry of Fear*. Hauppauge, New York: NovaScience Publishers; 2005. pp. 91–99.

[10] Santor DA, Coyne J. Shortening the CES-D to improve its ability to detect cases of depression. *Psychological Assessment* 1997;9(3): pp.233–243.

[11] Santor DA, Coyne JC. Examining symptom expression as a function of symptom severity: item performance on the Hamilton Rating Scale for Depression. *Psychological Assessment* 2001;13(1): pp. 127–139.

[12] Santor DA, Coyne JC. Evaluating the continuity of symptomatology between depressed and nondepressed individuals. *Journal of Abnormal Psychology* 2001;110(2): pp. 216–225.

[13] Kisely S, Simon G. An international study of the effect of physical ill-health on psychiatric recovery in primary care. *Psychosomatic Medicine* 2005;67(1): pp. 116–122.

[14] Sherbourne CD, Wells KB, Meredith LS, Jackson CA, Camp P. Comorbid anxiety disorder and the functioning and well-being of chronically ill patients of general medical providers. *Archives of General Psychiatry* 1996;53(10): pp. 889–895.

[15] Roy-Byrne P, Stein MB, Russo J, *et al*. Medical illness and response to treatment in primary care panic disorder. *General Hospital Psychiatry* 2005;27(4): pp. 237–43.

[16] Van den Akker M, Buntinx F, Metsemakers JF, Roos S, Knottnerus JA. Multimorbidity in general practice: prevalence, incidence, and determinants of co-occurring chronic and recurrent diseases. *Journal of Clinical Epidemiology* 1998;51(5): pp. 367–375.

[17] Fortin M, Bravo G, Hudon C, Vanasse A, Lapointe L. Prevalence of multimorbidity among adults seen in family practice. *Annals of Family Medicine* 2005;3(3): pp. 223–228.

[18] Batstra L, Bos EH, Neeleman J. Quantifying psychiatric comorbidity - lessions from chronic disease epidemiology. *Social Psychiatry and Psychiatric Epidemiology* 2002;37(3): pp. 105–111.

[19] deGruy FV, 3rd, Pincus H. The DSM-IV-PC: a manual for diagnosing mental disorders in the primary care setting. *Journal of the American Board of Family Practice* 1996;9(4): pp. 274–281.

[20] Dowrick C, Gask L, Perry R, Dixon C, Usherwood T. Do general practitioners' attitudes towards depression predict their clinical behaviour? *Psychological Medicine* 2000;30(2): pp. 413–419.

[21] Susman JL, Crabtree BF, Essink G. Depression in rural family practice. Easy to recognize, difficult to diagnose. *Archives of Family Medicine* 1995;4(5): pp. 427–431.

[22] Rost K, Smith R, Matthews DB, Guise B. The deliberate misdiagnosis of major depression in primary care. *Archives of Family Medicine* 1994;3(4): pp. 333–337.

[23] Klinkman MS, Valenstein M. A general approach to psychiatric problems in the primary care setting. In: Knesper D, Riba M, Schwenk T. (eds.) *Primary Care Psychiatry*. Philadelphia: W. B. Saunders Co.; 1997. pp. 3–8.

[24] Judd LL, Akiskal HS, Maser JD, *et al*. A prospective 12-year study of subsyndromal and syndromal depressive symptoms in unipolar major depressive disorders. *Archives of General Psychiatry* 1998;55(8): pp. 694–700.

[25] Judd LL, Akiskal HS, Zeller PJ, *et al*. Psychosocial disability during the long-term course of unipolar major depressive disorder. *Archives of General Psychiatry* 2000;57(4): pp. 375–80.

[26] Berti Ceroni G, Berti Ceroni F, Bivi R, *et al*. DSM-III mental disorders in general medical sector: a follow-up and incidence study over a two-year period. *Social Psychiatry and Psychiatric Epidemiology* 1992;27(5): pp. 234–241.

[27] Lamberts H, Hofmans-Okkes I. Classification of psychological and social problems in general practice. *Huisarts Wet* 1993;36: pp. 5–13.

[28] Dowrick C, Buchan I. Twelve month outcome of depression in general practice: does detection or disclosure make a difference? *BMJ* 1995;311(7015): pp. 1274–1276.

[29] MagPIe Research Group. The nature and prevalence of psychological problems in New Zealand primary healthcare: a report on Mental Health and General Practice Investigation (MagPIe). New Zealand Medical Journal 2003;116(1171): p. U379.

[30] Coyne JC, Klinkman MS, Gallo SM, Schwenk TL. Short-term outcomes of detected and undetected depressed primary care patients and depressed psychiatric patients. *General Hospital Psychiatry* 1997;19(5): pp. 333–343.

[31] Piccinelli M, Rucci P, Ustun B, Simon G. Typologies of anxiety, depression and somatization symptoms among primary care attenders with no formal mental disorder. *Psychological Medicine* 1999;29(3): pp. 677–688.

[32] Rucci P, Gherardi S, Tansella M, *et al*. Subthreshold psychiatric disorders in primary care: prevalence and associated characteristics. *Journal of Affective Disorders* 2003;76(1-3): pp. 171–181.

[33] Olfson M, Broadhead WE, Weissman MM, *et al*. Subthreshold psychiatric symptoms in a primary care group practice. *Archives of General Psychiatry* 1996;53(10): pp. 880–886.

[34] Van Weel-Baumgarten E, Van den Bosch W, Van den Hoogen H, Zitman FG. Ten year follow-up of depression after diagnosis in general practice. *British Journal of General Practice* 1998;48(435): pp. 1643–1646.

[35] Parker G, Holmes S, Manicavasagar V. Depression in general practice attenders. 'Caseness', natural history and predictors of outcome. *Journal of Affective Disorders* 1986;10(1): pp. 27–35.

[36] Tiemens BG, VonKorff M, Lin EH. Diagnosis of depression by primary care physicians versus a structured diagnostic interview. Understanding discordance. *General Hospital Psychiatry* 1999;21(2): pp. 87–96.

[37] Kessler RC, Akiskal HS, Angst J, *et al*. Validity of the assessment of bipolar spectrum disorders in the WHO CIDI 3.0. *Journal of Affective Disorders* 2006;96(3): pp. 259–269.

[38] Goldberg D. Plato versus Aristotle: categorical and dimensional models for common mental disorders. *Comprehensive Psychiatry* 2000;41(2 Suppl 1): pp. 8–13.

[39] Lamberts H, Magruder K, Kathol RG, Pincus HA, Okkes I. The classification of mental disorders in primary care: a guide through a difficult terrain. *International Journal of Psychiatry in Medicine* 1998;28(2): pp. 159–176.

[40] Pincus HA, Davis WW, McQueen LE. 'Subthreshold' mental disorders. A review and synthesis of studies on minor depression and other 'brand names'. *British Journal of Psychiatry* 1999;174: pp. 288–296.

[41] Druss BG, Wang PS, Sampson NA, et al. Understanding mental health treatment in persons without mental diagnoses: results from the National Comorbidity Survey Replication. *Archives of General Psychiatry* 2007;64(10): pp. 1196–1203.

[42] Suh T, Gallo JJ. Symptom profiles of depression among general medical service users compared with specialty mental health service users. *Psychological Medicine* 1997;27(5): pp. 1051–1063.

[43] Aikens JE, Reinecke MA, Pliskin NH, et al. Assessing depressive symptoms in multiple sclerosis: is it necessary to omit items from the original Beck Depression Inventory? *Journal of Behavioral Medicine* 1999;22(2): pp.127–142.

[44] Simon GE, Von Korff M. Medical co-morbidity and validity of DSM-IV depression criteria. *Psychological Medicine* 2006;36(1): pp. 27–36.

[45] Katerndahl DA. Symptom severity and perceptions in subjects with panic attacks. *Archives of Family Medicine* 2000;9(10): pp. 1028–1035.

[46] Kisely S, Goldberg D, Simon G. A comparison between somatic symptoms with and without clear organic cause: results of an international study. *Psychological Medicine* 1997;27(5): pp. 1011–1019.

[47] Smith RC, Gardiner JC, Lyles JS, et al. Exploration of DSM-IV criteria in primary care patients with medically unexplained symptoms. *Psychosomatic Medicine* 2005;67(1): pp. 123–129.

[48] Fink P, Rosendal M, Olesen F. Classification of somatization and functional somatic symptoms in primary care. *Australian and New Zealand Journal of Psychiatry* 2005;39(9): pp. 772–781.

[49] Fink P, Toft T, Hansen MS, Ornbol E, Olesen F. Symptoms and syndromes of bodily distress: an exploratory study of 978 internal medical, neurological, and primary care patients. *Psychosomatic Medicine* 2007;69(1): pp. 30–39.

[50] Fink P, Rosendal M. Recent developments in the understanding and management of functional somatic symptoms in primary care. *Current Opinion in Psychiatry* 2008;21(2): pp. 182–188.

[51] Sartorius N, Ustun TB, Lecrubier Y, Wittchen HU. Depression comorbid with anxiety: results from the WHO study on psychological disorders in primary health care. *British Journal of Psychiatry. Supplement* 1996(30): pp. 38–43.

[52] Ustun TB, Sartorious N. *Mental Illness in General Medical Care*. Chichester: John Wiley & Sons, Ltd; 1995.

[53] Zimmerman M, Chelminski I. Generalized anxiety disorder in patients with major depression: is DSM-IV's hierarchy correct? *American Journal of Psychiatry* 2003;160(3): pp. 504–512.

[54] Zung WW, Magruder-Habib K, Velez R, Alling W. The comorbidity of anxiety and depression in general medical patients: a longitudinal study. *Journal of Clinical Psychiatry* 1990;51(Suppl): pp. 77–80.

[55] Demyttenaere K, Bruffaerts R, Posada-Villa J, et al. Prevalence, severity, and unmet need for treatment of mental disorders in the World Health Organization World Mental Health Surveys. *JAMA* 2004;291(21): pp. 2581–2590.

[56] Kessler RC, Chiu WT, Demler O, Merikangas KR, Walters EE. Prevalence, severity, and comorbidity of 12-month DSM-IV disorders in the National Comorbidity Survey Replication. *Archives of General Psychiatry* 2005;62(6): pp. 617–27.

[57] Kawakami N, Takeshima T, Ono Y, et al. Twelve-month prevalence, severity, and treatment of common mental disorders in communities in Japan: preliminary finding from the World Mental Health Japan Survey 2002-2003. *Psychiatry and Clinical Neurosciences* 2005;59(4): pp. 441–452.

[58] de Graaf R, Bijl RV, Smit F, Vollebergh WA, Spijker J. Risk factors for 12-month comorbidity of mood, anxiety, and substance use disorders: findings from the Netherlands Mental Health Survey and Incidence Study. *American Journal of Psychiatry* 2002;159(4): pp. 620–629.

[59] Ormel J, Von Korff M, Burger H, *et al.* Mental disorders among persons with heart disease - results from World Mental Health surveys. *General Hospital Psychiatry* 2007;29(4): pp. 325–334.

[60] Harter M, Baumeister H, Reuter K, *et al.* Increased 12-month prevalence rates of mental disorders in patients with chronic somatic diseases. *Psychotherapy and Psychosomatics* 2007;76(6): pp. 354–360.

[61] Demyttenaere K, Bruffaerts R, Lee S, *et al.* Mental disorders among persons with chronic back or neck pain: results from the World Mental Health Surveys. *Pain* 2007;129(3): pp. 332–342.

[62] Gureje O, Von Korff M, Kola L, *et al.* The relation between multiple pains and mental disorders: results from the World Mental Health Surveys. *Pain* 2008;135(1-2): pp. 82–91.

[63] He Y, Zhang M, Lin EH, *et al.* Mental disorders among persons with arthritis: results from the World Mental Health Surveys. *Psychological Medicine* 2008;38(11): pp. 1639–1650.

[64] Scott KM, Bruffaerts R, Tsang A, *et al.* Depression-anxiety relationships with chronic physical conditions: results from the World Mental Health Surveys. *Journal of Affective Disorders* 2007;103(1-3): pp. 113–120.

[65] Scott KM, Von Korff M, Alonso J, *et al.* Mental-physical co-morbidity and its relationship with disability: results from the World Mental Health Surveys. *Psychological Medicine* 2009;39(1):pp. 33–43.

[66] Scott KM, Von Korff M, Ormel J, *et al.* Mental disorders among adults with asthma: results from the World Mental Health Survey. *General Hospital Psychiatry* 2007;29(2): pp.123–133.

[67] Patten SB, Williams JV. Chronic obstructive lung diseases and prevalence of mood, anxiety, and substance-use disorders in a large population sample. *Psychosomatics* 2007;48(6): pp. 496–501.

[68] Goodwin RD, Jacobi F, Thefeld W. Mental disorders and asthma in the community. *Archives of General Psychiatry* 2003;60(11): pp. 1125–1130.

[69] McIntyre RS, Soczynska JK, Konarski JZ, *et al.* Should depressive syndromes be reclassified as 'Metabolic Syndrome Type II'? *Annals of Clinical Psychiatry* 2007;19(4): pp. 257–264.

[70] Golden SH. A review of the evidence for a neuroendocrine link between stress, depression and diabetes mellitus. *Current Diabetes Reviews* 2007;3(4): pp. 252–259.

[71] Evans DL, Charney DS, Lewis L, *et al.* Mood Disorders in the Medically Ill: Scientific Review and Recommendations. *Biological Psychiatry* 2005;58(3): pp. 175–189.

[72] Egede LE, Zheng D, Simpson K. Comorbid depression is associated with increased health care use and expenditures in individuals with diabetes. *Diabetes Care* 2002;25(3): pp. 464–470.

[73] Pirraglia PA, Gupta S. The interaction of depression and diabetes: a review. *Current Diabetes Reviews* 2007;3(4): pp. 249–251.

[74] Stein MB, Cox BJ, Afifi TO, Belik SL, Sareen J. Does co-morbid depressive illness magnify the impact of chronic physical illness? A population-based perspective. *Psychological Medicine* 2006;36(5): pp. 587–596.

[75] Mallik S, Krumholz HM, Lin ZQ, *et al.* Patients with depressive symptoms have lower health status benefits after coronary artery bypass surgery. *Circulation* 2005;111(3): pp. 271–277.

[76] Katon W, Lin EH, Kroenke K. The association of depression and anxiety with medical symptom burden in patients with chronic medical illness. *General Hospital Psychiatry* 2007;29(2): pp. 147–155.

[77] Das-Munshi J, Stewart R, Ismail K, Bebbington PE, Jenkins R, Prince MJ. Diabetes, common mental disorders, and disability: findings from the UK National Psychiatric Morbidity Survey. *Psychosomatic Medicine* 2007;69(6): pp. 543–550.

[78] Surtees PG, Wainwright NW, Luben RN, Wareham NJ, Bingham SA, Khaw KT. Depression and ischemic heart disease mortality: evidence from the EPIC-Norfolk United Kingdom Prospective Cohort Study. *American Journal of Psychiatry* 2008; 165(4): pp. 515–523.

[79] Sareen J, Jacobi F, Cox BJ, Belik SL, Clara I, Stein MB. Disability and poor quality of life associated with comorbid anxiety disorders and physical conditions. *Archives of Internal Medicine* 2006;166(19): pp. 2109–2116.

[80] Carney CP, Jones L, Woolson RF. Medical comorbidity in women and men with schizophrenia: a population-based controlled study. *Journal of General Internal Medicine* 2006;21(11): pp. 1133–1137.

[81] Sokal J, Messias E, Dickerson FB, *et al*. Comorbidity of medical illnesses among adults with serious mental illness who are receiving community psychiatric services. *Journal of Nervous and Mental Disease* 2004;192(6): pp. 421–427.

[82] Dickey B, Azeni H, Weiss R, Sederer L. Schizophrenia, substance use disorders and medical comorbidity. *The Journal of Mental Health Policy and Economics* 2000;3(1): pp. 27–33.

[83] Dickey B, Normand SL, Weiss RD, Drake RE, Azeni H. Medical morbidity, mental illness, and substance use disorders. *Psychiatric Services* 2002;53(7): pp. 861–867.

[84] Newcomer JW. Metabolic risk during antipsychotic treatment. *Clinical Therapeutics* 2004;26(12): pp. 1936–1946.

[85] Newcomer JW, Haupt DW. The metabolic effects of antipsychotic medications. *Canadian Journal of Psychiatry* 2006;51(8): pp. 480–491.

[86] Meyer JM, Koro CE. The effects of antipsychotic therapy on serum lipids: a comprehensive review. *Schizophrenia Research* 2004;70(1): pp. 1–17.

[87] Suvisaari JM, Saarni SI, Perälä J, *et al*. Metabolic syndrome among persons with schizophrenia and other psychotic disorders in a general population survey. *Journal of Clinical Psychiatry* 2007;68(7): pp. 1045–1055.

CHAPTER 21

Comorbidity, Positive Health, and Integration of Services

Juan E. Mezzich

Professor of Psychiatry and Director, International Center for Mental Health and Division of Psychiatric Epidemiology, Mount Sinai School of Medicine, New York University, NY, USA; Past President of the World Psychiatric Association

Ihsan M. Salloum

Professor of Psychiatry and Director, Division of Alcohol and Substance Abuse: Treatment and Research, University of Miami Miller School of Medicine, FL, USA; Section on Classification, Diagnostic Assessment and Nomenclature, World Psychiatric Association

21.1 INTRODUCTION

Addressing clinical complexity has emerged as a key requirement to recognize adequately the richness of the health field, to design fully informative diagnostic models, and to prepare effectively plans for clinical care and health promotion [1]. A major aspect of clinical complexity involves the coexistence of diseases or disorders within and across mental health and general health conditions. Complementing pathology (ill health), it is also important to consider positive health (from adequate functioning to quality of life) for understanding health status, dealing with its problems, and attempting to raise health levels. Advancing in the appraisal and understanding of clinical complexity make a case for integration of care, including mental health, general health and even social services.

The sections that follow address in sequence the importance and forms of comorbidity and of positive health and then the need and prospects for integration of services.

21.2 COMORBIDITY ESSENTIALS

A major form of clinical complexity is **comorbidity**, which is widely recognized as a common feature of regular clinical care. While recognizing the spurious use that has been made sometimes of this term as when two facets of the same condition have been taken as separate disorders, there are many situations where clearly different clinical conditions, such as circulatory problems and depression, are identified as requiring specific attention.

The need to systematically address comorbidity in general medicine was highlighted by Feinstein [2] a professor of medicine and epidemiology at Yale University, who is credited with coining this term. He defined it as "any distinct additional clinical entity that has existed or that may occur during the clinical course of a patient who has the index disease under study". The broadness of "additional clinical entities" under his concept of comorbidity reached physiological conditions requiring clinical attention such as pregnancy.

Comorbidity can be noted among conditions in the same chapter of the International Classification of Diseases (ICD), such as that on mental disorders. It can be noted as well among conditions in different ICD chapters. It can be argued that comorbidity can also apply to the concurrence of disorders and social conditions of clinical significance, such as trauma and child abuse. The intricacy of comorbidity may also be extended to the involvement of multiple sectors such as mental disorders, general medical disorders, and clinically relevant social conditions, a situation that has been referred to as *hypercomorbidity* by the WHO Workgroup on Comorbidity [3].

The US National Comorbidity Survey [4] revealed that 79% of all ill people had comorbid disorders, and that over half of the lifetime disorders identified were concentrated in 14% of the population studied. Comorbidity is particularly common in the elderly, and with world-wide advancing of population age comorbidity is becoming a major global health concern.

21.3 COMORBIDITY AND POSITIVE HEALTH

The wide space between pathology or illness and the totality of health corresponds to large extent to the concept of positive health. In an attempt to map out the complexity of positive health, the following aspects or dimensions can be outlined from an analysis of the international literature, particularly from existing and emerging diagnostic systems [5].

Functioning as a substantial variable here has evolved from the consideration of disabilities and adaptive functioning as opposite poles of the same dimension. It has been regarded as a single integrated variable in DSM-IV Axis V [6] and as a multilevel variable in ICD-10 Axis II [7] in which it is unfolded into personal care, occupational functioning, functioning with family, and broader social functioning.

Another significant aspect of positive health correspond to the notions of *robustness* and *resilience* [8–9]. These are innovative concerns that have not been incorporated yet into standard of official diagnostic systems.

Contextual factors refer to environmental and personal features contextual to clinical problems and which may enhance understanding of such problems and treatment planning. As elements of positive health, they may include a range of personal resources [10] as well as emotional and instrumental social supports. Contextual factors have been considered in the multiaxial schemas of ICD-10 [7] and DSM-IV [6] as well as along with functioning, in WHO's International Classification of Functioning,Disability and Health [11].

A major concept in positive health refers to *Quality of Life*. This variable, commensurate in content with health and life, is often proposed to be evaluated primarily from the view point of the person who consults and is emerging as a compelling feature for health assessment. A number of instruments have been proposed for its evaluation, the internationally-based or culturally-informed tending to range from physical well-being to spiritual fulfillment [12–13]. Quality of life has been recently included in the multiaxial schemas of the WPA International Guidelines for Diagnostic Assessment (IGDA) [14] and the Latin American Guide for Psychiatric Diagnosis (GLADP) [15].

The association of two or more chronic conditions may produce additive or even synergistic negative effects on positive health aspects such as functioning and quality of life. For example, in a study of individuals with bipolar disorder and alcoholism, the impact of these two co-occurring illness on family functioning was highlighted by the fact that only 11% of the participants were still married, while 44% were divorced or separated [16]. The association of these two conditions is likely to place severe burden on family relationship and cause substantial impairment in family and social functioning. The number of psychiatric disorders has been found to be correlated not only with the severity of psychiatric disorders, but also with work and social impairments and subjective distress [17] as well as with lower quality of life among women [18] Impairment in functioning and quality of life have been consistently reported for comorbid depression and physical disorders and also for comorbidity within general health disorders [19].

21.4 THE NEED FOR INTEGRATED CARE

Comorbidity is associated with serious implications for clinical care due to its impact on both diagnosis and treatment. Comorbidity may interfere with the identification of the index disease by creating significant difficulty in symptom attribution leading to delay or incorrect nosological diagnosis. The course of the index disorder may be adversely affected by comorbid conditions leading to increased disability and mortality as well as to higher family and societal burden and suffering. Comorbidity may also lead to limitations in treatment planning, implementation and outcome.

Conventional health care paradigms focusing just on disease and immediate care are often regarded as inadequate. This is particularly true when comorbid conditions are noted. The WHO Comorbidity Workgroup [3] concluded that person-centered care offered the most promising approach when comorbid conditions are involved by facilitating coordination and integration of services. A person-centered approach would also facilitate attention to the positive aspects of health, such as resilience, resources, and quality of life. This is important for clinical treatment, prevention, and rehabilitation.

To be considered also is health promotion, a recently recognized key element of clinical care. This is consistent with the definition of health by WHO [20] not limited to the absence of illness or disease, but involving a state of complete physical, social, and emotional well being. Care planning within this broad framework seems to call for a comprehensive diagnostic model as a cornerstone of patient care where all relevant information about the patient condition is integrated with the goal of supporting health restoration and promotion of well-being. Such formulations as that in the International Guidelines for Diagnostic Assessment (IGDA) [14] may allow for comprehensive assessment of the comorbid disorders at hand, along with co-existing disabilities, contextual factors, and quality of life as experienced by the affected person. It also may include an assessment of strengths, positive factors, and the individual's and family's expectations and attitudes towards healing, recovery, and optimization of health.

There is an urgent need for increased awareness of the challenges to appraise health adequately and to enhance pertinent interventions. Attaining these goals could be facilitated by a multilevel approach to identify and formulate causative and contributing factors to comorbidity. The intricacies of clinical comorbidity require a comprehensive and integrated approach to diagnosis and care. Patient-centered, holistic, contextualized, and comprehensive approaches, as opposed to a narrow, single-disease, acute care models, are critical to addressing the challenges and complexities of clinical comorbidities. Adequate attention to these conditions requires integrated care models that address the various aspects of comorbid conditions, including psychiatric, general medical, and contextual factors, in addition to positive health considerations. Such models must be developed in a truly international fashion, relevant to the interactive world in which we live, with built in flexibility to accommodate local realities and needs.

Understanding clinical comorbidities within the broad framework of both ill and positive health and organizing treatment and health promotion on the basis of person-centered diagnostic and care models may lead to qualitative improvements in clinical service and public health.

REFERENCES

[1] Mezzich JE, Salloum IM. Clinical complexity and person-centered integrative diagnosis. *World Psychiatry* 2008; **7**: 1–2.
[2] Feinstein AR. *Clinical Judgment*. Huntington, New York, Robert E. Krieger, 1967.
[3] Mezzich JE, Salloum IM (Eds). *Report of a WHO Workgroup Meeting on Comorbidity*. Technical Report, Geneva, 2004.
[4] Kessler RC, McGonagle KA, Zhao S, Nelson CB, Hughes M, Eshleman S, Wittchen HU, Kendler KS. Lifetime and 12-month prevalence of DSM-III-R psychiatric disorders in the United States: Results from the National Comorbidity Survey. *Archives of General Psychiatry* 1994; **51**(1): 8–19
[5] Mezzich JE. Positive health: Conceptual place, dimensions, and implications. *Psychopathology* 2005; **38**: 177–179.
[6] American Psychiatric Association. *Diagnostic and Statistical Manual of Mental Disorders, Fourth Edition (DSM-IV)*. Washington, DC, APA, 1994.
[7] Janca A, Kastrup MC, Katschnig H, Lopez-Ibor JJ, Mezzich JE, Sartorius N. *Multiaxial Presentation of ICD-10*. Cambridge, UK, Cambridge University Press, 1997.
[8] Foster JR. Successful coping, adaptation, and resilience in the elderly: An interpretation of epidemiological data. *Psychiatry Quarterly* 1997; **68**: 189–219.
[9] Amering M and Schmolke M. *Recovery in Mental Health: Reshaping scientific and clinical responsibilities*. Wiley-Blackwell, Chichester, UK, 2009.
[10] Schmolke M. *Gesundheitressourcen im Lebens-alltag schizophrener Menschen*. Bonn, Psychiatrie Verlag, 2001.
[11] WHO. *International Classification of Functioning, Disability and Health (ICF)*. Geneva, Author, 2001.
[12] Kuyken W, Orley J. The World Health Organization Quality of Life Assessment. *Soc Sci Med* 1995; **41**: 1403–1409.
[13] Mezzich JE, Ruiperez MA, Perez C, Yoon G, Lin J, Mahmud S. The Spanis version of the Quality of Life Index: Presentation and validation. *J Nerv Ment Dis* 2000; **188**: 301–305.
[14] World Psychiatric Association. Esssentials of the WPA International Guidelines for Diagnostic Assessment (IGDA). *British J Psychiatry* 2003; **182** (suppl 45): 37–66.
[15] Latin American Psychiatric Association (APAL) Section on Diagnosis and Classification. *Latin American Guide for Psychiatric Diagnosis (GLADP)*. Guadalajara, Mexico, Guadalajara University Press, 2004.

[16] Salloum IM, Cornelius JR, Daley DC, Kirisci L, Himmelhoch JM, Thase ME. Efficacy of Valproate Maintenance in Patients with Bipolar Disorder and Alcoholism: A Double-Blind Placebo-Controlled Study. *Arch Gen Psychiatry* 2005; **62** (1) :37–45.

[17] Angst J, Sellaro R, Ries Merikangas K. Multimorbidity of psychiatric disorders as an indicator of clinical severity. *European Archives of Psychiatry & Clinical Neuroscience* 2002; **252**(4):147–54.

[18] Gamma A, Angst J. Concurrent psychiatric comorbidity and multimorbidity in a community study: gender differences and quality of life. *European Archives of Psychiatry & Clinical Neuroscience* 2001; **251**(2)

[19] Fortin M, Lapointe L, Hudon C, Vanasse A, Ntetu A, Maltais D. Multimorbidity and quality of life in primary care: a systematic review. *Health and Quality of Life Outcomes* 2004; **2**(1):51

[20] WHO. *Constitution of the World Health Organization*. Geneva, WHO, 1946.

Diagnostic Models

CHAPTER 22

The Validity of Psychiatric Diagnosis: Etiopathogenic and Clinical Approaches

Kenneth F. Schaffner

University Professor of History and Philosophy of Science,
Professor of Psychiatry,
University of Pittsburgh, PA, USA

22.1 INTRODUCTION

In this paper, I will be discussing several traditional concepts of nosological validity as well as two newer notions: reductive etiopathogenic validity and clinical validity. I also sketch a non-standard prototype-dimensional approach to basic science and psychiatric classification, and relatedly argue that biology (and psychiatry) involves multilevel non-reductive models. In the context of this account, I suggest that 'reality' is multilevel, and includes subjective and intersubjective mental life, and what might be termed 'clinical reality' among its levels. Finally, I briefly readdress the notion of diagnostic validity, and also discuss the relation of the individual to the universal, in the context of the WPA's 'comprehensive diagnostic model,' more recently termed 'person-centred integrative diagnosis' (PID).

These are philosophical issues, but what kind of philosophical perspectives are needed here? I believe that many have an oversimplified view of philosophy that makes it irrelevant at best, or distracting and harmful at worst. In this paper, I hope to offer a more positive, nuanced, and practical view of the role of philosophy, in psychiatry in general and in classification and diagnostic validity in particular. In a short paper, I can only offer readers a framework, and some pointers to the philosophical literature. However, my general philosophical orientation is pragmatic, in the tradition of James, Pierce, and Dewey, [1] but it also has Aristotelian, as well as analytic aspects. And the approach takes the science very seriously.

Psychiatric Diagnosis: Challenges and Prospects   Edited by I.M. Salloum and J.E. Mezzich
© 2009 John Wiley & Sons, Ltd

22.2   CONCEPTS OF VALIDITY, INCLUDING DIAGNOSTIC VALIDITY AND ETIOPATHOGENIC VALIDITY

The validity notion is clearest in deductive logic where it refers to truth preserving inference. In empirical science, the validity concept is involved with the notion of capturing an objective external 'reality'. In psychiatry, the 'validity' issue historically arises out of the psychological testing literature, where a classical source is Cronbach and Meehl's 1955 article 'Construct validity in psychological tests' [2]. There, 'construct validity' assessed whether a test is a good measure of some quality that is not 'operationally defined'.

The traditional concepts of psychiatric validity include a version of construct (or external) validity, for example that diagnosis correlates with expected external validators, such as family history, and neurobiological markers – compare First *et al.* [3]. Additionally, psychiatrists refer to the notion of 'face validity', which is prima facie, first impression validity (and in my view, at best heuristic). Psychiatrists also consider 'descriptive validity', where some define this as whether the features of a category are unique to that category relative to other mental disorders, as well as the very important notion of predictive validity, where a diagnosis predicts future course, complication and treatment response. Other validity concepts have also been discussed in many literatures, including content, internal, interpretive, theoretical, etc. validities.

For our purposes, the notion of 'diagnostic validity' is of special importance. This concept comes from Robins and Guze's classic and extraordinarily influential 1970 article that adapted the construct validity notion to psychiatric diagnosis by using the term 'diagnostic validity' [4]. They proposed a 'method' consisting of five phases: clinical description; laboratory studies; exclusion criteria (to distinguish a diagnosis from other disorders); follow-up studies; and family studies. These were not necessarily a linear sequence, but were expected to be an interactive process. In a series of papers in the 1980s, Kendler refined and amplified on these notions to specify additional criteria, such as antecedent validators (familial aggregation, precipitating factors) and predictive validators (relapse and recovery rates, response to treatment). Importantly, Kendler pointed out that many types of nosological questions, such as conflicts among validators, cannot be answered empirically, but will involve value judgments [5], an issue further developed by Fulford and Sadler (see Fulford's contribution in Chapter 2 of this book). Relatedly, Kendell [6] noting the slow progress of using what Mezzich has termed 'etiopathogenic validity' validators in psychiatry, proposed that advances might be better made by developing studies focused on 'clinical validity', a topic to which I shall return several times in this paper.

Nancy Andreasen, however, in 1995 stressed a 'newer program', complementary to Robins and Guze's, involving genetic and neuroimaging studies, as well as other neurobiological markers [7], and more recently Stephen Hyman suggested a similar approach [8]. Andreasen's and Hyman's proposals hope for strong diagnostic validity based on a neurobiological approach, which can be thought of as a search for 'etiopathogenic validity': looking for validators that point to the cause of a disorder, or that clarify the pathogenetic process involved in a disorder. This approach typically involves a search for neuroanatomical, neurophysiological or molecular genetic factors, and thus tends to be reductive or reductionistic. Thus far, this type of approach is more speculative than empirically validated, though there have been some recent promising advances in schizophrenia genetics, psychiatric oriented neuroimaging, and event-related brain potentials (ERPs). In spite of such preliminary advances, however, Hyman's recent essay indicates that these laboratory findings are not specific enough to likely find their way into either DSM-V or ICD-11 [9].

22.3 CLINICAL VALIDITY

For the in-progress revisions of ICD-11 mental disorders, however, as well as the national DSM-V revision scheduled for 2012, I believe the major work will involve *clinical validity*, a notion initially introduced in Kendell [6] and that I shall re-examine further below. This clinical validity concept carries forward both the Robins and Guze and the Kendler multi-faceted and multilevel approaches, more than it does the reductive Andreasen and Hyman programs, which may achieve success for future ICD-12 and DSM-VI versions.

To assess the proper way that reductive etiopathogenic validity may figure in diagnostic classification, and also to motivate the notion of clinical validity, I want to begin from a provocative but very influential 2003 article by Kendell and Jablensky [10]. Kendell and Jablensky proposed two very strong conditions for validity. First, they wrote:

'We suggest...that a diagnostic category should be described as valid only if one of two conditions has been met. If the defining characteristic of the category is a syndrome, this syndrome must be demonstrated to be an entity, separated from neighboring syndromes and normality by a zone of rarity. ... [i.e., interforms would be very rare]'. [[10], p. 8]

They also proposed another condition, writing:

'Alternatively, if the category's defining characteristics are more fundamental – that is, if the category is defined by a physiological, anatomical, histological, chromosomal, or molecular abnormality – clear, qualitative differences must exist between these defining characteristics and those of other conditions with a similar syndrome.' (10, p. 8)

Though Kendell and Jablensky argue persuasively, I want to take a different approach. In my view, studies of simpler organisms such as regulatory mechanisms in bacteria and behavioural traits in the worm (*C. elegans*) and the fly (*Drosophila*) – more on these organisms later but also see Kendler and Greenspan [11] – suggest that such traits will *not* resolve into discrete forms at the molecular level. I think the evidence demonstrates that there are numerous interforms and *quantitative* traits: *this is dimensionality all the way down*. A good example of this is found in the operon model of gene regulation in bacteria, where there are many interforms – what Lewin, the author of a major textbook on molecular genetics, called 'a panoply of operons' [12]. Expecting discreteness because of fundamentality is, I think, a 'Platonic' prejudice. It can be satisfied in physics, with its fundamental particles, and in chemistry, as in the periodic chart, but it is rare in biology.

22.4 A PROTOTYPE APPROACH

But I believe that variation and dimensionality can still be made tractable, by using an approach that identifies the most robust categories as prototypes, related to other prototypes by similarity. Some, such as Mezzich (see Cantor *et al.* [13]) think that a related fuzzy set, grade of membership, analysis will also assist a prototype approach representation schema;

also see the recent paper from Jablensky's group on a current application of this approach [14] (Hallmayer *et al.*, 2005). I would argue that the prototype approach is supported by the deep structure of biology, and I develop such a prototype approach to biology, including genetics and the neurosciences, in my 1993 book [15]. In this book, I contrast the structure of the physical sciences, such as in mechanics, electromagnetic theory, and quantum mechanics, with an alternative theoretical structure for biology.

In my view, we do not have what Meehl in his 1955 validity article called a simple 'network of [universal] laws' that constitutes a theory, either in biology, psychology, or psychiatry, though we do find such networks frequently in physics, and occasionally in chemistry. (Also compare the comments in Caspi and Moffitt [16] p. 587, on the need for a 'nomological network'.) Rather, in biology, and I would argue eventually in psychiatry, we have families of models or mechanisms with, in any given subdiscipline, a few prototypes. These prototypes are typically interlevel: in biology they *intermingle* ions, molecules, cells, cell-cell circuits, and organs, in the same causal/temporal process – an issue I shall return to in a moment. The prototype models are related to each other by dimensional similarity, and there are many interforms. The prototypes in this view are narrow classes, but do allow for law-like/causal predictions, and explanations, sometimes just for individuals. Extensive variation among the models and mechanisms is a natural consequence of the result of how evolution operates: by replicating entities with many small variations, and assembling odds and ends – thus 'tinkering', as François Jacob has written about evolution.

But a prototype/GoM approach has other independent arguments in its support, in addition to consistency with the way that relationships among biomolecular models seem to behave. Psychologists, beginning with the pioneering work of Rosch in 1975, have argued that prototype representations are closer to the way that humans think naturally than are other more logically strict approaches to concepts. Rosch's work was initially grounded in psychological anthropology. In her investigation, Rosch found, both to her own and others' surprise, that primitive peoples as well as advanced societies do not represent concepts or categories as collections of necessary and sufficient properties. Rather, a category is built around a central member or a prototype, which is a representative member that shares the most attributes with other members of that category and which shares the fewest with members of the contrasting category [17]. Thus, a robin would be a more prototypical bird than either a penguin or a chicken. Rosch wrote:

'Categories are coded in cognition in terms of prototypes of the most characteristic members of the category. That is, many experiments have shown that categories are coded in the mind neither by means of lists of each individual member of the category nor by means of a list of formal criteria necessary and sufficient for category membership, but, rather, in terms of a prototypical category member. The most cognitively economic code for a category is, in fact, a concrete image of an average category member.' [17]

Rosch went on to extend her views to learning in children and to question the sharpness of boundaries between concepts. Her contributions are viewed as major advances in our understanding of memory and knowledge representation, though her account has been construed by some as needing supplementation for complex category representation. The Roschean view of concepts as being built around prototypes shares certain similarities with the philosopher Hilary Putnam's urging we consider meanings as 'stereotypes'.

A prototype approach – again see Cantor *et al.* [13] for an early discussion of this approach in psychiatry by Mezzich's group – can conform well to a polythetic categorical approach in the limiting case. But a prototype approach can also permit a dimensional representation as well. A dimensional approach coupled with a prototype analysis may, in point of fact, be emerging in DSM-V and ICD-11, particularly for the personality disorders. We may see a dimensional approach as a parallel analysis to a standard categorical definition – see First *et al.* [18] and also Helzer and American Psychiatric Association [19] – or we may see some hybrid approaches [20]. Such an approach, whether it be dimensional or hybrid, will have to be carefully developed and rigorously tested for clinical validity and user friendliness. An evidence-based psychiatry is key here. And the prototype-dimensional approach may also be more consistent with etiopathogenic validations to come in the future, perhaps in ICD-12.

22.5 REDUCTIVE VERSUS INTERLEVEL APPROACHES TO NEUROBIOLOGY

I believe a close inspection of the disciplines of molecular genetics and neuroscience, including their research articles and textbooks, will indicate that the prototypes that are used in these sciences are actually and typically interlevel, and *not* unilevel and simply reductionistic: i.e. one does not *only* use molecules in describing the results of studies in these area. These levels include atoms and molecules at the smallest level, but can range up through organisms, social groups, and also include internal (subjective) monologue and intersubjective dialogue, as well as values, at the upper levels.

Recent work on how molecular geneticists explain the difference between social and solitary feeding in the worm, *C. elegans*, shows an interlevel example of a circuit in the worm controlling social feeding from de Bono *et al.* [21] (also see [22, 23] for background on the worm). It may be worth describing this work in some detail to illustrate persuasively how interlevel this kind of 'molecular' explanation in fact is.

The explanation (at a very abstract level) is contained in the title of the de Bono *et al.* 2002 paper, 'Social feeding in *C. elegans* is induced by neurons that detect aversive stimuli' [21]. The specifics of the explanation appeal to a 1998 study published in *Cell* as background, and look at *npr-1* mutants (social feeders), examining what *other* genes might prevent social feeding, thus restoring solitary feeding in *npr-1* mutants. A search among various *npr-1* mutants (again, these would be social feeders) indicated that mutations in the *osm-9* and *ocr-2* genes resulted in significantly more *solitary* feeding in those mutant animals. (Both of these genes code for *components* of a sensory transduction ion channel known as TRPV (transient receptor potential channel that in vertebrates responds to the 'vanilloid' (V) compound capsaicin found in hot peppers). Both the *osm-9* and *ocr-2* genes are required for chemoattraction as well as aversive stimuli avoidance. Additionally, it was found that *odr-4* and *odr-8* gene mutations could disrupt social feeding in *npr-1* mutants. The *odr-4* and *odr-8* genes are required to localize a group of olfactory receptors to olfactory cilia. Interestingly, a mutation in the *osm-3* gene, which is required for the development of 26 ciliated sensory neurons, *restores social* feeding in the *odr-4* and *ocr-2* mutants.

de Bono *et al.* present extensive data supporting these complex findings in the 2002 article. Typically, the reasoning with the data examines the effects of screening for single, double, and even triple mutations that affect the phenotype of interest (feeding behaviours), as well as looking at the results of gene insertion or gene deletion. This reasoning essentially follows Mill's classical methods of difference and concomitant variation (the latter because graded rather than all-or-none results are often obtained), and is prototypical

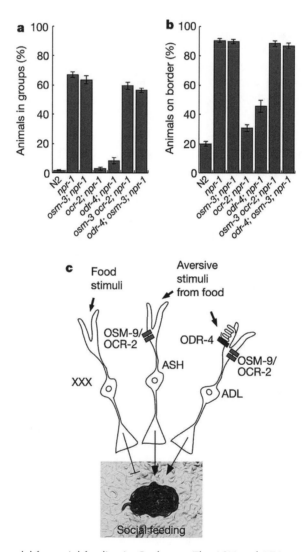

Figure 22.1   A model for social feeding in *C. elegans*. The ASH and ADL nociceptive neurons are proposed to respond to aversive stimuli from food to promote social feeding. This function requires the putative OCR-2/OSM-9 ion channel. The ODR-4 protein may act in ADL to localize seven transmembrane domain chemoreceptors that respond to noxious stimuli. In the absence of ASH and ADL activity, an unidentified neuron (XXX) [involving *osm-3*] represses social feeding, perhaps in response to a different set of food stimuli. The photograph shows social feeding of a group of > 30 npr-1 mutant animals on a lawn of *E. coli*. Reproduced with permission of Nature Publishing Group from de Bono, M., *et al.* (2002), [21].

causal reasoning. Also of interest, are the results of the laser ablation of two neurons that were suggested to be involved in the feeding behaviours. These two neurons, known as ASH and ADL, are implicated in the avoidance of noxious stimuli and toxic chemicals. Identification of the genes noted above (*osm-9, ocr-2, odr-4* and *odr-8*) allowed the investigators to look at where those genes were expressed (by using Green Florescent Protein (GFP) tags). It turned out that ASH and ADL neurons were the expression sites. The investigators could then test the effects of laser beam ablation of those neurons, and showed that ablation of both of them restored a solitary feeding phenotype, but that the presence of either neuron would support social feeding.

The net result of the analysis is summarized in a 'model for social feeding in *C. elegans*' (Figure 5 in de Bono *et al.* [21]; my Figure 22.1).

The work described above suggests that important information, and generalizations, might be obtained at any level of aggregation – in fact, the purely molecular level may not be the best place to identify such information, intervene, and predict. Paying attention to interrelations and possible integrations among different levels of aggregation, often in the 'same process', is an important feature of the biomedical sciences, and also for any science that depends on the basic biomedical sciences [24].

22.6   CLINICAL UTILITY AND CLINICAL VALIDITY

With these considerations as background, let us again return to Kendell and Jablensky's important 2003 paper [10] to consider what type of validity might be feasible in the area of psychiatry. In that seminal paper, Kendell and Jablensky also sharply distinguish diagnostic *validity* from diagnostic *utility*, and write: 'In our view, it is crucial to maintain a clear distinction between validity and utility, and at present these two terms are often used as if they were synonyms.' At this point in their article, they cite Spitzer's classic writings in connection with DSM-III. Kendell and Jablensky then add: 'We propose that a diagnostic rubric may be said to possess utility if it provides nontrivial information about prognosis and likely treatment outcomes, and/or testable propositions about biological and social correlates.' [10, p. 9].

Though the Kendell and Jablensky definition of utility is excellent, *it is also what has traditionally been called 'predictive validity'*, as has recently been noted by First *et al.* [3]. And to a philosophical pragmatist such as myself, such *utility* is constitutive of what we think of as *reality*, and thus such utility is an indicator of an appropriate form of validity (as predictive validity) in the realm of clinical reality.

How might we best try to think further about this very complicated notion of 'reality'? From my perspective, a philosophical pragmatist does not think we can directly access an independent reality. Rather, we can only 'triangulate' – maybe better 'converge' – on it through multiple useful indicators and interventions in the world. There is no simple 'gold standard' waiting 'out there'. The great American pragmatist, Charles Saunders Pierce, suggested we would only get to true reality at the end of time, or when we had a completed science. Some of these triangulating indicators and interventions that help us towards a pragmatic reality do involve sophisticated technologies and long chains of inference, e.g. gene action and fMRI results. But information from *all* levels, including high levels such as interpersonal experience – which may be 'more real' for many purposes for a pragmatist than molecular pathways – will continue to be key for psychiatry. Again, we can think of this multilevel reality as what the psychiatrist encounters in the clinic, or as 'clinical reality' requiring studies that are 'clinically valid' to insure the best possible patient care.

Clinical validity can be furthered by several types of empirical studies suggested in 1989 by Kendell. Some of these studies are difficult to carry out, and can be expensive, but in the absence of short-term advances in etiopathogenic validity, they deserve to be carefully considered by the workgroups and task forces involved with DSM-V and ICD-11. Kendell [6] outlined four types of studies, which I list below, along with a few parenthetical comments on their problems as well as current status:

- prospective follow-up studies based on serial interviews (expensive);
- therapeutic trials involving a broad spectrum of diagnostic categories (ethically problematic);
- family studies involving a broad spectrum of diagnostic categories (actually underway by a number of researchers);
- twin studies involving alternative definitions of syndromes (some work by McGuffin and colleagues, maybe others).

Finally, there is a related issue concerning the validity of our psychiatric disorders and classification schemas, which has been discussed both in the philosophical and the psychiatric literature. This is whether, as we go forward with our more sophisticated understanding of molecular genetics and neuroscience, what we take to be reality – especially involving the standard set of mental disorders such as schizophrenia and depression – might radically change. The multilevel 'reality' that we commit to as a result of this on-going (scientific) process is, I think, always provisional. Thus it could be subject to major modifications via scientific revolutions of a Kuhnian sort, as described by Kuhn in his extraordinary book, *The Structure of Scientific Revolutions* [25]. It is thus *possible* that our current classification categories will radically change and be replaced as a result of advancing genetics and neuroscience, a thesis that I have speculated on along with Harris (see [26]).

However, my best guess at present is that current ICD-10 and DSM-IV-TR categories will *slowly* evolve etiopathogenically, and at the margins, rather than suffer a catastrophic collapse and replacement with some as yet unforeseeable psychiatric classification system. But we should also keep in mind yet another possibility – that our 'Ptolemaic' ICD-10/ DSM-IV classification system may continue as mainly *clinically valid*, while an etipathogenic, but horrendously complex and virtually *clinically useless* 'Copernican' system, slowly emerges. (Though some have said the 'Copernican' system is simpler, that view disregards the fact that at the time of Copernicus there were no dynamics to replace the Aristotelian physics then still entrenched in science.)

I have described this changing view of reality as 'conditionalized realism' in my 1993 book, and I will not go into this technical notion in the present paper. In the book, I also show how two different senses of universal can be distinguished, a distinction that allows for universal-like causal predictions for individuals (the idea here is that 'same conditions yield the same effects' can work for particulars). This analysis is a response to worries that we do not have any 'laws' in biology, such as we do in physics. Pragmatism tolerates considerable flexibility, but it also prizes stable classifications and strong predictability.

In summary, I think that 'reality,' and attempts to validate our constructs in this reality, will take the form of provisional multilevel prototypes that interrelate dimensionally. I believe we will encounter these both in the clinical validity area, as well as ultimately, i.e., but perhaps not for many years to come, in the etiopathogenic area, since we do not have well-confirmed etiopathogenic reductionist prototypes, even in such well plumbed areas as schizophrenia, as yet – see for example Harrison and Weinberger [27].

22.7   A 'PERSON-CENTRED INTEGRATIVE DIAGNOSIS'

What does this account of pragmatic validity and realism suggest for the diagnosis of *individual patients*, within the nosological philosophy just sketched? I think it argues that we need to pay attention to multiple levels and their interactions simultaneously, and that this includes objective and subjective elements, as well as values held both by patient and the treating psychiatrist. The analysis sketched above also urges a scientific approach to individualized prediction and decision-making.

I believe that this account thus constitutes an excellent fit with the 'comprehensive diagnostic model' – more recently designated as 'Person-Centred Integrative Diagnosis' – of the WPA's International Guidelines for Diagnostic Assessment (IGDA) (see [28] and World Psychiatric Association. Essentials of the World Psychiatric Association's international guidelines for diagnostic assesment (IGDA). Br J Psychiatry 2003;182 (Suppl. 45): s37–s66. http://bjp.rcpsych.org/cgi/reprint/182/45/s62 as well as [29]). A Person-Centred Integrative Diagnosis mandates we pay attention to the place of an individual's problems in the context of a standard nosology, thus allowing us to integrate the general and the particular circumstances affecting a disorder, and also emphasizes that we attend to the particulars, including the values and a positive notion of comprehensive health for that patient. Though this is a multilevel bio-psycho-social approach, it is *not* utopian, but represents true realism. Such integration is practical and doable, as the Ms. Y example from IGDA, 2001 indicates – see pp. 53 – 55 at http://bjp.rcpsych.org/cgi/reprint/182/45/s62 for this detailed case example, as well as the clinical report forms in which the Person-Centred Integrative Diagnosis is implemented. This approach has been adopted by the Latin American Psychiatric Association through its Latin American Guide for Psychiatric Diagnosis (Guia Latinoamericana de Diagnostico Psiquiatrico, GLADP) [30].

22.8   CONCLUSIONS

Let me sum up my conclusions. These are that diagnostic validity is best pursued as clinical or predictive validity, supplemented with attempts to develop etiopathogenic validators, as we can. In addition, etiopathogenic validators will best be understood in a framework of biological prototypes related dimensionally. Further, a prototype-dimensional approach may also assist disorder reconceptualization, perhaps as hybrid models, as well as clinical validation, and ultimately comport best with emerging etiopathogenic biological validators. I also emphasized that the prototypes we find in biology are interlevel, and suggest that psychiatrically relevant prototypes will similarly be interlevel, and likely will slowly become more molecular as research continues, but never purely molecular. I argued that reality is not a simple 'gold standard' to which we can appeal, and that validation is by a complex triangulation that changes the vision of multilevel prototypic 'reality' over time. Finally, I suggested that the prototype dimensional inter-level analysis developed here permits individualized predictions and explanations, and can serve well as a framework for the multilevel and individualized Person-Centred Integrative Diagnosis of the WPA.

ACKNOWLEDGMENTS

Special thanks to Drs. Gottesman, Jablensky, Kendler, Mezzich and Salloum for discussions and for sharing their work with me. I also want to express gratitude to the United States' NSF and NIH, and to the Greenwall Foundation, for support for my work on both etiopathogenic and clinical dimensions of genetics, neuroscience, and psychiatry. Not all those mentioned in the previous sentences, however, will necessarily agree with my conclusions.

REFERENCES

[1] Konvitz MR, Kennedy G. *The American pragmatists; selected writings.* New York: Meridian Books; 1960. p. 413.

[2] Cronbach LJ, Meehl PE. Construct validity in psychological tests. *Psychological Bulletin* 1955;52: pp. 281–302.

[3] First MB, *et al.* Clinical utility as a criterion for revising psychiatric diagnoses. *American Journal of Psychiatry* 2004;161 (6): pp. 946–954.

[4] Robins E, Guze SB. Establishment of diagnostic validity in psychiatric illness: its application to schizophrenia. *American Journal of Psychiatry* 1970;126(7): pp. 983–987.

[5] Kendler KS. Toward a scientific psychiatric nosology. Strengths and limitations. *Archives of General Psychiatry* 1990;47(10): pp. 969–73.

[6] Kendell RE. Clinical validity. *Psychological Medicine* 1989;19 (1): pp. 45–55.

[7] Andreasen NC. The validation of psychiatric diagnosis: new models and approaches. *American Journal of Psychiatry* 1995;152(2): pp. 161–162.

[8] Hyman SE. Neuroscience, genetics, and the future of psychiatric diagnosis. *Psychopathology* 2002;35(2-3): pp. 139–144.

[9] Hyman SE. Can neuroscience be integrated into the DSM-V? *Nature Reviews Neuroscience* 2007;8(9): pp. 725–732.

[10] Kendell R, Jablensky A. Distinguishing between the validity and utility of psychiatric diagnoses. *American Journal of Psychiatry* 2003;160(1): pp. 4–12.

[11] Kendler KS, Greenspan RJ. The nature of genetic influences on behavior: lessons from 'simpler' organisms. *American Journal of Psychiatry* 2006;163(10): pp. 1683–1694.

[12] Lewin B. *Genes V.* Oxford, New York: Oxford University Press; 1994. pp. xxiv; 1272.

[13] Cantor N, *et al.* Psychiatric diagnosis as prototype categorization. *Journal of Abnormal Psychology* 1980;89(2): pp. 181–193.

[14] J. Hallmayer, L. Kalaydjieva, J. Badcock, M. Dragovic, S. Howell, P. Michie, D. Rock, D. Vile, R. Williams, E. Corder, K. Hollingsworth, A. Jablensky (2005) Genetic Evidence for a Distinct subtype of Schizophrenia characterized by Pervasive cognitive Deficit. *The American Journal of Human Genetics*, Volume 77, Issue 3, pp. 468–476.

[15] Schaffner KF. Discovery and Explanation in Biology and Medicine. In: Hull DL. (ed.) *Science and Its Conceptual Foundations.* Chicago: University of Chicago Press; 1993.

[16] Caspi A, Moffitt TE. Gene-environment interactions in psychiatry: joining forces with neuroscience. *Nature Reviews Neuroscience* 2006;7(7): pp. 583–590.

[17] Rosch E, Mervis CB. Family resemblances: Studies in the internal structure of categories. *Cognitive Psychology* 1975;7: pp. 573–605.

[18] First MB, Bell CC, Cuthbert B, Krystal J, Malison R, Offord D, Reiss D, Shea T, Widiger T, Wisner K. Personality Disorders and Relational Disorders: A Research Agenda for Addressing Crucial Gaps in DSM. In: Kupfer DJ, First MB, Regier DA. (eds) *APA Research Agenda for DSM-V.* Washington, DC: American Psychiatric Association; 2002. pp. 123–99.

[19] Helzer JE, American Psychiatric Association. *Dimensional approaches in diagnostic classification : refining the research agenda for DSM-V.* (1st ed.) Arlington, VA: American Psychiatric Association; 2008. pp. xxvii; 136.

[20] Pilkonis PA. *Personal communication*, 2004.

[21] de Bono M, *et al*. Social feeding in *Caenorhabditis elegans* is induced by neurons that detect aversive stimuli. *Nature* 2002; 419(6910): pp. 899–903.

[22] Schaffner KF. Genes, Behavior, and Developmental Emergentism: One Process, Indivisible? *Philosophy of Science* 1998;65(June): pp. 209–252.

[23] Schaffner KF. Model Organisms and Behavioral Genetics: A Rejoinder. *Philosophy of Science* 1998;65: pp. 276–288.

[24] Schaffner KF. Reduction: the Cheshire cat problem and a return to roots. *Synthese* 2006;151(3): pp. 377–402.

[25] Kuhn TS. *The structure of scientific revolutions*. 2nd ed.Chicago: University of Chicago Press; 1970. pp. xii; 210.

[26] Harris HW, Schaffner KF. Molecular genetics, reductionism, and disease concepts in psychiatry. *Journal of Medicine and Philosophy* 1992;17(2): pp. 127–153.

[27] Harrison PJ, Weinberger DR. Schizophrenia genes, gene expression, and neuropathology: on the matter of their convergence. *Molecular Psychiatry* 2005;10(1): pp. 40–68.

[28] Mezzich JE. Comprehensive diagnosis: a conceptual basis for future diagnostic systems. *Psychopathology* 2002;35(2-3): pp. 162–165.

[29] Mezzich JE. Psychiatry for the Person: articulating medicine's science and humanism. *World Psychiatry* 2007;6 (2): pp. 65–67.

[30] GLADP, Asociacion Psiquiatrica de America Latina (APAL). *Guia Latinoamerica de Diagnostico Psiquiatrico (GLADP)*. Guadalajara, Mexico: Seccion de Diagnostico y Clasificacion de la APAL; 2004.

CHAPTER 23

The Overall Development of ICD-11

T. Bedirhan Üstün
Robert Jakob
Office of Classifications, Terminologies, and Standards,
World Health Organization,
Geneva, Switzerland

23.1 INTRODUCTION

The International Classification of Diseases (ICD) is a member of the World Health Organization Family of International Classifications (WHO-FIC), which provides the basic building blocks for health information systems across the world for information exchange and comparison. The ICD provides a global standard to classify and organize diseases and related health problems [1]. In the study of illness, causes of death and health expenditures, a standard classification of diseases and related health problems is essential and has to be up to date with current scientific knowledge. The ICD has been the global standard and international public tool to fulfil this requirement since its first appearance as an international common list for causes of death in 1851 [2].

Diseases are numerous, and have multiple features. Capturing all of this complex information within a classification is a challenging task. A classification has to be scientific and architecturally sound to serve the many purposes, ranging from diagnosis and management of a single patient to decisions at population level for public health purposes.

23.1.1 Unit of Classification in ICD

A classification covers a universe of numerous entities. These entities must share a similar feature as the 'unit of classification'. To maintain coherence and be internally consistent, the unit of classification must share similar characteristics, such as: 'animals', 'plants', 'vegetables', 'fruits'... etc. The unit of classification for the ICD is naturally understood to be 'diseases'. However: (1) the disease construct has not been operationally defined; and (2) in the ICD it also includes, under the loose heading of health conditions: 'disorders', 'injuries

Psychiatric Diagnosis: Challenges and Prospects   Edited by I.M. Salloum and J.E. Mezzich
© 2009 John Wiley & Sons, Ltd

and other external causes' and 'signs and symptoms', and these entities are sometimes used for 'reason for encounter' (e.g. why people seek care) purposes. Therefore, the intent and purpose of the use of the classification category has to be clear.

23.1.2   Uses of ICD

The use of a classification may have different purposes for different users. For example, Linnaean botanical classification, which is a perfect scientific classification, may not even be relevant for a botanical shop that basically categorizes plants as indoor and outdoor plants. Similarly, for the ICD, the categorization may be driven by other purposes. In general, doctors or health care workers need detailed information for clinical diagnosis and differential diagnosis, whereas decision makers may use higher level aggregation across populations for summary purposes. Likewise, different levels of detail (i.e. granularity) in grouping are needed for patient safety, resource allocation, reimbursement (e.g. case-mix systems) or prevention programmes (e.g. screening). Ideally, th ICD has to serve to link each level of detail across different uses (i.e. zooming in and out between different levels of granularity).

23.1.3   ICD: Cause of Death, Main Reason or Clinical Diagnosis

The ICD is applied on the diagnosis formulated in the health records, such as hospital records or death certificates. The ICD provides categories and rules of application that allow correct identification of cases for different purposes. Most clinical activities evolve around diagnosis. Diagnosis is the formulation of what is wrong with the patient. The ICD allows a framework for diagnostic formulation. Certain chapters of the ICD, such as those on mental disorders, tumours and neurological disorders, have additional information that serves to define the categories, either in more detail or in operational rules. This type of information increases the diagnostic accuracy.

23.1.4   Financial and Political Aspects

The categories of the ICD that are used by physicians as diagnosis, also serve reimbursement purposes by insurance companies or other payers. Health care authorities use payment groups based on the ICD. Similarly, drug indications or interventions may be formulated based on ICD categories. Most importantly, the ICD provides a common base for international health statistics and comparisons. In line with the WHO's International Nomenclature Regulations, approved in 1969, all governments in the world have agreed to a treaty to report health statistics in line with the ICD.

23.1.5   ICD and Health Information Systems

The ICD is used in formulating different aspects of health information, such as: mortality, morbidity, quality, safety, reimbursement or resource allocation. It, therefore, plays a key role in health information systems. The outcome of health services could be monitored and evaluated using the ICD in terms of diseases and health conditions. In addition to the ICD, there are other building blocks in health information systems that cover other domains, such as the International Classification of Functioning Disability and Health (ICF), health interventions, and other elements in the WHO Family of International Classifications. (WHO-FIC) [3].

23.2   REVISION OF THE ICD

The ICD is scheduled to be revised in 10-yearly revisions '. . . to revise as necessary. . .' [4] and updated annually, in line with the constitution and recommendations of the governing bodies of the WHO [5, 6]. That preserves the scientific currency and public health utility of the classification and allows consistency to be maintained between the members of the WHO Family of International Classifications.

In the most recent (10th) revision of the International Classification of Diseases (ICD-10), the mental disorders chapter has been considerably expanded, and several different descriptions are available for the diagnostic categories: the 'clinical description and diagnostic guidelines' (CDDG) [7]; a set of 'diagnostic criteria for research' (DCR) [8]; 'diagnostic and management guidelines for mental disorders in primary care' (PC) [9]; a 'pocket guide' [10]; and a multiaxial version [11] and a lexicon [12]. These interrelated components all share a common foundation of ICD grouping and definitions, yet differentiate to serve the needs of different users.

In the ICD-10, explicit diagnostic criteria and rule-based classification have replaced 'the art of diagnosis' with a reliable and replicable descriptive scheme that has considerable predictive validity in terms of effective interventions. Its development has relied on international consultation and has been linked to the development of assessment instruments. The mental disorders chapter of the ICD-10 has undergone extensive testing in two phases to evaluate the CDDG [13] as well as the DCR [14] and agreement between different assessors, as measured by the kappa statistic, was over 0.70 for most categories, indicating very good agreement. Low agreement categories were later revised so as to improve the reliable use of the classification.

All chapters of the ICD will be revised in the process towards the ICD-11. In each area of health care, the classification will be systematically reviewed along three interconnected main lines: for scientific evidence, clinical usefulness and public health usefulness. This work will be carried out by a core team of WHO investigators along with a group of international collaborators and advisors. An Internet-based knowledge management and sharing portal will allow a worldwide audience to participate in the revision.

23.3   OBJECTIVES OF THE ICD REVISION PROCESS

The ICD-11 will be a user-friendly, scientifically credible classification that is useful in public health, supports clinical decisions and management, and should be integrated in routine practice in different settings including primary care, clinical care and research, while preserving the statistical continuity. Accordingly, the ICD-11 may be presented in different but compatible versions to be used interchangeably at different levels and in the various specialities of the health sector. Statisticians and coders might prefer a view that will look like the current version of ICD-10. A clinician's view might follow body systems, for instance. For example, more than 100 categories directly mention kidney disease. These are spread over 13 chapters of ICD-10. In the ICD-11, access through body systems might show those all together to the clinician; still, the code will remain the same in any kind of projection.

23.3.1   Use of the Classification in Multiple Levels

It is clear that the ICD is used in various settings with different levels of granularity, ranging from a set of 100 codes to tens of thousands. A classification (and a coding scheme) that can zoom in and out across various levels, will satisfy such demands. An ICD-11 primary care version should focus on the most frequent conditions in primary care that are generally broad categories (e.g. depressive disorder). A clinical version would include all clinical conditions with diagnostic guidelines (e.g. unipolar, bipolar depressive disorder mild, moderate, severe . . .). The research version would include detailed, standardized criteria for the diseases and disorders. A computer application will tailor a master version to generate several special versions, as for primary care, clinical care, and research. Accordingly, such versions have compatible categories that can be used interchangeably in different levels of health care.

23.3.2   Taxonomic Rules and Definitions for an Applied Ontology

The ICD should be clear about what it classifies: its units of classification (groups of diseases, individual diseases, disorders, findings, symptoms . . .) and definitions of these units; its organization in terms of its structure; and relationships among its units. These categorizations should be fit for the purpose that they are used in such areas as clinical, public health and research.

Key taxonomic principles need to include ontological definitions, and pragmatic conventions as a result of common consensus, in order to represent the health knowledge in a fashion to be useful in health information systems. Clear definitions of categories and diseases in the ICD guide coders to better find the appropriate code, allow translations to be consistent with the original meaning and allow establishing linkages to electronic health records using standardized clinical terminologies.

To allow these aims to be achieved, an information model has been put up, to guide the revision work to identify each rubric in the ICD as a set of dysfunction(s) in any of the body systems defined by:

1. *symptomatology – manifestations*: known pattern of signs, symptoms and related findings;
2. *etiology*: an underlying explanatory mechanism;
3. *course and outcome*: a distinct pattern of development over time;
4. *treatment response*: a known pattern of response to interventions;
5. *linkage to intrinsic (genetic) factors*: genotypes, phenotypes and endophenotypes;
6. *linkage to interacting environmental factors*.

Each category of the ICD will be defined along this model, linking each ICD category with other defined terminologies and ontologies.

Each ICD rubric will be identified, whether it is a disease or another entity, as disorder, injury, sign, or symptom. Each such entity has to be defined and identified with appropriate properties, and their relationships, as shown in Figure 23.1.

Each entity in ICD is defined by attributes

Name of disease, disorder, or syndrome

1. Textual definition
2. Synonyms
3. Index terms -

Definitional characteristics

1. **Type** [pick one]
   Disease, disorder, syndrome, injury, sign, symptom, exposure to external causes, health problem, reason for encounter;

2. **Pathophysiology**

3. **Anatomical site** (at the most specific level relevant to the condition)

4. **Manifestation Attributes**
   1. **Symptoms**
   2. **Signs**
   3. **Diagnostic results**
   4. **Functional impact**

5. **Etiology**
   1. **Causal agents**
   2. **Mechanism**
   3. **Genomic characteristics**

6. **Temporal Relations**
   1. Chronicity (including acute)
   2. Episodicity

7. **Severity and/or Extent**

8. **Treatment/Prevention**

9. **Hierarchical relationships**
   (parents and children in ICD structure)

Maintenance attributes

A. **Subset, adaptation, and special view flag**
   E.g. Primary Care, Clinical Care, Research, Special indices (e.g. Public Health Indices or Resource Groupings)

B. **Unique identifier**

C. **Mapping relationships**
   (Linkages to other systems like SNOMED etc.)

D. **Sanctioning rules**

Figure 23.1   Draft information model. Each entity in the ICD will be defined with known ontological properties.

The ICD, in summary, will be a compilation of all relevant diagnostic knowledge. It will thus represent clinical signs, symptoms and laboratory findings in operational definitions in line with the above information model. This can be understood as similar to the clinical diagnostic guidelines or diagnostic criteria. Apart from the earlier formulations for mental and behavioural disorders in Chapter V of ICD, these definitions will be presented digitally (i.e. in computerized algorithms) so that the data in electronic health records could be linked to the ICD for various applications. In short, one of the major aims of the ICD revisions is to have the ICD ready for digital health information systems.

It is essential that the ICD diagnosis could be linked to clinical terminologies so that the electronic health records could process the information in a meaningful way. For example, Figure 23.2 illustrates how F32 Depressive Disorder will be captured as SNOMED CT terms, each coded and defined, such as low mood; loss of interest; low energy; appetite problems (low appetite, binging . . .); sleep problems (insomnia, early awakening . . .); sexual problems (libido loss); guilt; thoughts of death and suicidal ideation or acts. All these terms are coded in SNOMED CT so that the computers could process the data in electronic health

Definition: Depressive Disorder F32.0	
A. **Low mood**	{41006004}
Loss of interest	{417523004}
Low energy	{248274002}
B. Appetite	(*decrease, increase*) {64379006, 72405004}
Body weight	(*decrease, increase*) {89362005, 8943002}
Sleep	(*decrease, increase*) {59050008, 77692006}
Psychomotor	(*decrease, increase*) {398991009, 47295007}
Libido loss	{8357008}
Low self esteem	{286647002, 162220005}
Guilt, self blame	{7571003}
Thoughts of death . . .	
Suicide Ideation	{102911000, 6471006}

Figure 23.2 Linkages between diagnostic criteria of ICD-10 category F32.0 and SNOMED.

records. Using the operational definitions in the ICD or DSM linked to terminologies will allow this functionality.

This same process will be done for all domains of the ICD, together with international experts in the related fields. WHO's previous work on speciality adaptations (such as classification of tumours and ICD-O, mental health etc) and joint work with CIOMS on the International Nomenclature of Diseases (IND) will enable populating the information model. Other work already existing in knowledge bases will be incorporated in a similar fashion (i.e. in rare diseases from Orphanet).

23.3.3   ICD Development Process Phases

Towards an ICD-11, three major phases are planned:

1. **ICD-10-Plus**: this phase aims to compile all suggestions and user needs. A web-based platform called ICD-10-Plus brings together three main sources:

   I. A combination of all additional codes from national modifications of the ICD (e.g. USA, Canada, Australia, Germany, Thailand, Korea . . .), primary care versions, and speciality adaptations (oncology, mental health, neurology, headache, sleep disorders, dentistry and stomatology, paediatrics . . .).
   II. Suggestions from different users and user groups: any interested person or group could make a structured proposal for a possible change in the ICD system.
   III. Definitions of disease entities, as of the International Nomenclature of Diseases and other reliable sources, should be reviewed in line with the information model above.

2. **ICD-11 alpha draft: will be compiled by the WHO assigned editors and Topic Advisory Groups (TAGs)** for an initial review by the core users as the WHO FIC network. It will contain reviewed conceptual structure and definitions at the level of detail that corresponds to blocks and three character categories of the ICD-10.
3. **ICD-11 beta draft**: will be the field trial version for testing for its feasibility, reliability, utility and other predefined objectives. It will be simultaneously presented in six WHO official languages, and tools for translations to other languages will be provided. The beta draft will have a structure similar to an ICD-10 fourth edition, with possible field test options to test the conversion from the 10th to the 11th version. This convergence will allow users to switch from the ICD-10 to the ICD-11 in a seamless fashion, and preserve statistical continuity.

23.3.4   Web-Based Distributed Development

Former ICD revisions were conducted through conferences and editorial groups communicating through conventional means (see the introduction to Volume 1 of the ICD-10). Given technological advancements, the ICD-11 drafting environment is planned as a wiki-like structured joint-authoring tool based on a semantic wiki application that incorporates a structured information model and identified terminology system. This tool is called HiKi. Selected groups of experts will be given the mandate of drafting portions of the ICD-11. Each working group will place their draft into the WHO web portal. Each rubric will be taxonomically reviewed and clarified by WHO experts, as needed. Expert groups for disease domains in collaboration with user groups for use cases will scientifically review rubrics, thus ensuring the quality of the submitted drafts, as for completeness, adequacy, clinical utility, or relevance for information systems.

The revision process is open to many experts from all over the world. In order to facilitate better **communication** and **collaboration**, the revision process will be open for comment to public. The revision portal will be the *single point of access* for the update and revision process with different user interfaces, levels of access and editing rights. The revision website will also include different components, such as a calendar of activities, discussion forums, collaborative document creation process, document libraries, linkage to publications, other practical tools etc.

23.3.5   Multilingual Versions of ICD-11 Drafts

It is a specific goal to make the ICD multilingual in six WHO official languages, with further guidelines and tools to make it available in other languages, as it is important for the public good internationally. Currently, the ICD-10 exists in 40 different languages and it is expected that the ICD-11 will also be available in as many as 40. Given previous experience in multilingual production, WHO will use English as the master working version during the revision process, with near-simultaneous production in six official languages. This means that the master English version will be generated as a representation of language independent constructs, and it will be represented with the best possible terms in other languages.

23.4 METHODS

The main methods for the revision process are to make systematic reviews and distillation of knowledge in the following areas: scientific stream; clinical stream; and public health stream. The results will be tested against a set of use cases for ICD-11.

23.4.1 Scientific Stream

The scientific stream will explore the scientific basis of diseases. To achieve this specific aim, systematic reviews of literature will be carried out by selected expert groups. Specific questions in this area may include:

- Do the new discoveries in etiologic agents require classification or coding changes?
- Do the new discoveries of drugs or other treatment require specific coding changes (e.g. drug resistance, the human papilloma virus (HPV)-vaccination against cervical cancer)?
- Does the availability of genetic information on human genome and disease specific genes (e.g. genes for Alzheimer's disease, gene patterns for breast cancer, genetic association of lymphoma) have implications in the design and use of the classification?

23.4.2 Clinical Stream

The clinical stream will aim to make the ICD-11 useful in the daily practice of various clinicians in different settings, such as primary care, hospital settings, rehabilitation and long-term care. The involvement of clinicians from the very beginning, and the web-based applications, are the relevant parts of the design of the revision process, in order to attain this goal. The clinical utility will be tested in questions such as: does the classification represent the actual clinical cases? Does it enable clinicians to make better diagnostic formulations, differential diagnosis? Is it helpful in generating patient reports? Is it helpful in identifying treatment need and monitoring outcomes? Other aspects of utility will also arise in the revision process. The proposed changes and options will be tested involving various clinical practitioners in a prospective systematic field-testing trial organized as a global practice network. Ease of use, relevance, utility, reliability and achievability will be the core quality criteria for the ICD-11, among other properties relevant to such global indicators.

23.4.3 Public Health Stream

This stream will serve to explore the public health usefulness of the ICD and make necessary updates and revisions, to better serve the needs of users in the public health field. The topics of exploration are:

- **Mortality**: implementation in countries, codes used, who makes the coding, which tools they use, accuracy of coding, suggestions for improving standardization, reliability. The information will be gathered through an online questionnaire and will also be displayed as full text to allow for verification by the community. A pilot test has been conducted on a set of countries and the system will be online soon.

- **Morbidity**: the same topics as for mortality, and in addition: analysis of the differences and communalities of existing clinical modifications in use and their background (Australian, Canadian, French, German, Thai and others). First analyses have shown common foci of interest. Ways for harmonization of these modifications will be explored, and whether other countries would be willing to adopt these changes. In a first step, the change categories will be compiled in one place. That allows for browsing, and will provide an impression of what the different countries have done to accommodate their needs for morbidity (ICD-XM).
- **Case-mix systems**: Exploring the context of uses of the ICD-10 in reimbursement systems will allow the needs of case mix systems better to be met.
- **Electronic health records**: A high level of detail is necessary for information storage in electronic health records. Information must not be wasted at the very beginning of the information chain. The extent to which ICD-11 can accommodate these needs will be explored, together with areas where formally developed linkages between the categories' definitions and standard terminologies have to fill in the gaps. Best practice guidelines for linkages and for their verification have to be established. The ontological tools mentioned below may prove useful for this exercise.

The clinical, public health and scientific streams will be woven together in an architecture that allows scaling for use in primary care, clinical care, research and other settings. The architecture will be built on categories, and will also allow the ICD to be presented in the way it is published now. The categories will be placed into a technical structure, thus ensuring that they are used in the same way in various representations of the classification (see Figure 23.3).

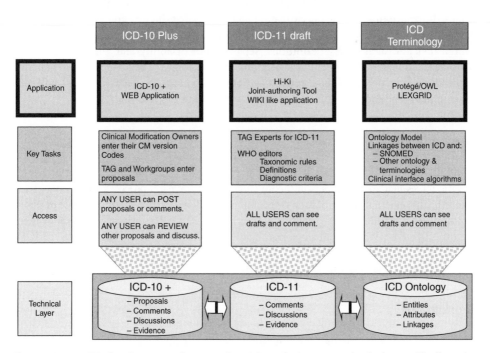

Figure 23.3 ICD development phases and revision platform; a web platform will allow the development of the ICD-11 and field tests.

Open access to this system will allow for online data sharing and unrestricted discussion among participants from any relevant discipline throughout the world, as the revision process evolves. The activity will thus produce a *permanent internet-based workspace* that will document the evidence-based systematic reviews and meta-analysis of available data, and will be a discussion forum open to international multidisciplinary participants.

This platform will facilitate communication within expert workgroups and make the expert workgroup processes transparent to the field.

23.4.4   Organizational Structure

WHO headquarters will coordinate the overall ICD revision in consultation with the WHO member states and multiple professional organizations, to ensure that the final revision is broadly responsive to the many different aspects of health care. The work will be mainly carried out by the Revision Steering Group, topic advisory groups and workgroups, as shown in Figure 23.4 and described below.

The Revision Steering Group (RSG)

The Revision Steering Group (RSG) will serve as the planning and steering authority in the update and revision process. This includes overseeing the broad revision domains, general progress of the revision process, and giving advice for the coordination of workgroups. The RSG will identify uses of the classification and ensure that the revision process addresses the needs of users. It will identify basic taxonomic and ontological principles across the overall revision, such as key definitions, separation of disability and joint use with ICF, attributes, and linkages to other classifications and ontologies. The RSG will also generate suggestions to resolve problems related to field test options, as necessary, and will also develop plans and tools for transition from the ICD-10 to the ICD-11.

Topic advisory groups (TAGs)

Topic advisory groups (TAGs) will serve as the planning and coordinating advisory bodies for specific issues that are key topics in the revision process revision process, such as oncology, mental health, external causes of injury, communicable diseases, non-communicable diseases, rare diseases and others to be established (see Figure 23.4). The primary mission of these groups is to advise WHO in all steps leading to the revision of topical sections of the ICD-10 in line with the overall revision process. The TAGs will consist of experts within each major domain of the classification's chapters.

Workgroups

Workgroups will serve as the key functioning units for the review of evidence and the generation of merged draft ICD-11 proposals for a specific topic in the classification. For example, the TAG in the mental health area will be responsible for the whole of Chapter V

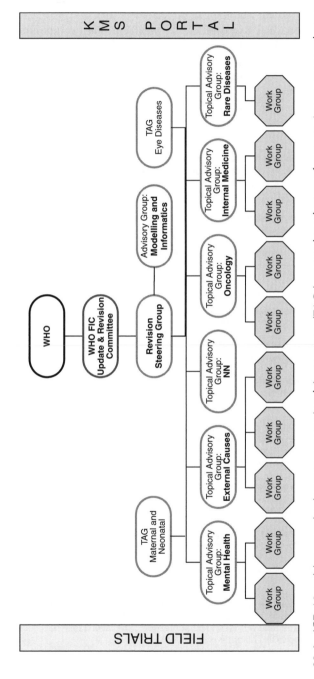

Figure 23.4 ICD-10 revision organization structure: topic advisory groups (TAGs) cover a broad range of content. As necessary, subgroups can be formed, to work on specific items (e.g. accidents). The process will be coordinated by the Revision Steering Group (RSG) and by the Update and Revision Committee (URC) under the overall supervision of WHO. All groups will have access to facilities to carry out field trials. All steps of the revision will occur on the KMS portal.

(Mental and behavioural disorders) of ICD-10 and its linkages, whereas it may generate from five to ten working groups to carry out the systematic reviews on special sections of the chapter, such as schizophrenias and psychosis; mood and anxiety disorders; or topics such as children and youth, common brain disorders and others. Each workgroup is expected to include between five and twelve members. The workgroups are asked to consider core issues that they will seek to address for each diagnostic entity in their content domain, and to develop a preliminary position on each issue based on their pre-existing knowledge of this domain. The initial set of core diagnostic issues to be considered by each workgroup is listed in Figure 23.5. These points may be further expanded by each workgroup to meet the key classification issues on the topic of interest.

I. **Definition of the diagnostic entity as a medical disease or disorder.** Given the key taxonomic guidelines and definitions each group should draw a line around the disorder of interest, identifying its critical properties. How does the workgroup fundamentally view the disorders/diseases in this chapter and identify key criteria and level of evidence?.

II. **Clustering of signs, symptoms, and operational characteristics.** Identify the features that are necessary and sufficient to define the disease/disorder.

III. **Link to underlying pathophysiology and genetic markers.** Identify the intra-individual markers that are associated with the disease/disorder, considering their biological plausibility, their measurement properties (e.g., reliability, specificity, predictive power), and their role in treatment response.

IV. **Clinical utility of the classification entity.** Consider the usefulness of the classification entity in predicting treatment response, course, and outcome.

V. **Reliability of the use of the classification entity.** Consider the stability of the classification entity over time and its consistency of detection across assessors and measurement instruments.

VI. **Validity of the classification entity.** Consider the associations of theoretically relevant variables with measures of the disorder and the support they provide for the validity of the diagnostic construct.

VII. **Separation of disease and disability elements.** Identify the features that signal the presence of the disease/disorder, defining the disease/disorder without reference to the distress, impairment, or other consequences that it produces. Suggestions to link to WHO ICF and operationalize specifically the criteria on disability and distress related rubrics.

VIII. **Cultural elements that need to be attended.** Consider variability in the presentation of the disease/disorder across cultures. Identify ways to achieve cross-cultural comparability and utility of diagnostic criteria rather than listing separate culture-bound syndromes or formulations.

IX. **Threshold considerations.** Identify the number and nature of diagnostic criteria that should be required to qualify for the classification entity. Consider the nature of the boundary separating the disease/disorder from normality, including evidence for the categorical/continuous distinction. Consider the classification entity boundaries with other classes, including challenges of differential diagnosis.

X. **Other nosological issues relevant to this entity** Identify any other aspects of the classification entity that the workgroup believes to be in need of evaluation, including potentially controversial aspects of the disorder that will need to be addressed. This list of additional issues may change as the evidence related to this disorder is reviewed.

Figure 23.5 The 10 core diagnostic issues for the ICD: this set of axioms and related questions makes sure that all working groups consider the same set of comprehensive aspects relevant to the revision of the ICD-10, and that all they do it the same way.

The workgroups **survey the available evidence** for each diagnostic entity to address the core diagnostic issues described in Figure 23.5. Evidence will be reviewed through systematic review of the published literature along a set of guidelines comparable to those used in health technology assessment.

The workgroups will **formulate suggestions** for updating and revising the ICD-10 diagnostic categories, operational criteria and coding structure, based on their evidence-based reviews. The recommendations will be reported to the coordinating TAG and the global community through the KMS portal.

Public **comments**, comments from the scientific society and other ICD stakeholders will be continually collected and reviewed by WHO staff, who will screen them for content and relevance before forwarding them to the appropriate workgroups.

The provisional revised diagnostic criteria recommended by the workgroups will be tested in one or more iterations of field trials, as described below.

The workgroups will prepare a **final report** with the key evidence as the authoritative source of the recommendation.

The resulting proposals will be published in one or more of several possible forums, including the ICD-11 text itself, the ICD website, books published by WHO on the ICD update and revision process, or a companion workbook accompanying the newly-published ICD-11.

Membership of any of the groups has to take into account several aspects, such as experience and knowledge, geographic representation, age (availability for next revision/ participation in the ninth revision) and possible conflicts of interest.

23.4.5   Field Trials

A global network of practitioners will be created in collaboration with the WHO-FIC Network and different Non-Governmental Organizations (NGO), in relation to WHO. This Global Health Practice Network (GHPN) will include health professionals throughout the world participating in quarterly web-based surveys. It has its own Internet platform. The surveys will provide different types of information about patient characteristics to inform the ICD update and revision process. Both clinicians' ratings of individual patients, and patient self-report questionnaires collected by the participating clinicians, will be used as part of such ongoing surveys. The GHPN platform will enable real-time collaboration to obtain direct patient assessments on crucial diagnostic questions among current patients within practices throughout the world. In addition to providing a venue for fast, large-scale data collection to inform the review of evidence and development of diagnostic criteria, the GHPN platform will also serve as the main tool in field trials. That will allow us to test the provisional revised criteria and evaluate their reliability, validity and clinical utility in a range of clinical settings around the world. The GPHN platform is currently being pilot tested.

23.5   CONCLUSION: FUTURE STEPS

The active phase of the ICD update and revision process began in 2007. Annual updates of the ICD-10 continue, with major updates and cumulated updates published every three years. Two major drafts of the ICD-11 will be developed. An alpha version will be developed by 2010, and a beta version by 2012 for systematic field trials. The field trials will focus on the feasibility, reliability, clinical utility and validity of the classification. A penultimate version for public viewing and response from all interested parties will be produced following the field trials, and the final ICD-11 version is intended to be submitted to the World Health Assembly for approval by 2014.

The manual for the classification will be developed along the formulation of the pre-final version. Index and transition tables will be the product of the ontological and terminological tools used in the revision process. The implementation of the ICD-11 can start in 2015.

Given the interest of multiple stakeholders and available resources, the overall revision process is able to give to the global health community and multiple stakeholders the opportunity for participation. Web-based tools will render the revision process transparent to all users and will make use of the large synthetic capacity of evidence through the participation of all interested parties.

REFERENCES

[1] Chronicle WHO Vol.II, No 6, 1948, WHO press.
[2] WHO (2004), International Classification of diseases, 10th revision, 2nd edition, WHO press.
[3] Jakob R, Ustun T, (2007), The Family of International Classifications, Bundesgesundheitsblatt.
[4] World Health Assembly. WHO Constitution 1948.
[5] World Health Assembly (1990), ICD Resolution (WHA 43.24).
[6] World Health Assembly (1967), WHO Nomenclature Regulations (WHA20.18).
[7] World Health Organization. *The ICD-10 classification of mental and behavioural disorders: clinical descriptions and diagnostic guidelines*. Geneva: World Health Organization; 1992.
[8] World Health Organization. *The ICD-10 classification of mental and behavioural disorders: diagnostic criteria for research*. Geneva: World Health Organization; 1993.
[9] World Health Organization. *Diagnostic and management guidelines for mental disorders in primary care: ICD-10 primary care version*. Bern: Hogrefe and Huber; 1996.
[10] Cooper JE. *Pocket guide to the ICD-10 classification of mental and behavioural disorders, with glossary and diagnostic criteria for research*. Edinburgh: Churchill Livingstone; 1994.
[11] World Health Organization. *Multiaxial presentation of the ICD-10 for use in adult psychiatry*. Cambridge: Cambridge University Press; 1997.
[12] World Health Organization. *Lexicon of psychiatric and mental health terms*. Geneva: World Health Organization; 1989.
[13] Sartorius N, Kaelber CT, Cooper JE, Roper MT, Rae DS, Gulbinat W, Ustun TB, Regier DA. Progress toward achieving a common language in psychiatry. Results from the field trial of the clinical guidelines accompanying the WHO classification of mental and behavioral disorders in ICD-10. *Archives of General Psychiatry* 1993;50: pp. 115–124.
[14] Sartorius N, Ustun TB, Korten A, Cooper JE, van Drimmelen J. Progress Toward Achieving a Common Language in Psychiatry, II: Results From the International Field Trials of the ICD-10 Diagnostic Criteria for Research for Mental and Behavioral Disorders. *American Journal of Psychiatry* 1995;152: pp. 1427–1437.

CHAPTER 24

The Revision of ICD Classification of Mental and Behavioural Disorders

Shekhar Saxena

*Programme Manager, Department of Mental Health and Substance Abuse,
World Health Organization, Geneva, Switzerland*

Benedetto Saraceno

*Director, Department of Mental Health and Substance Abuse,
World Health Organization, Geneva, Switzerland*

Note: The opinions expressed in this paper are of the authors only and do not represent the official views of the World Health Organization.

24.1 INTRODUCTION

A classification of diseases can be defined as a system of categories to which morbid entities are assigned according to established criteria. The ICD is the longest-standing and historically most important of WHO's classifications. Its core purpose is to permit the systematic recording, analysis, interpretation and comparison of mortality and morbidity data collected in different countries or areas and at different times. WHO is the only organization with the ability to secure global cooperation and international agreement on these issues and is therefore in a unique position to initiate and promote global health standards. WHO's classification systems are the basis for tracking epidemics and disease burden, identifying the appropriate targets of health care resources, and encouraging accountability among member countries for public health at the population level. WHO's classification systems are also among the core building blocks for the electronic health information systems that are of increasing importance in many countries.

Classifications also serve other important functions, like making communication possible between health professionals, and between them and other sectors of the society (policy-makers, judicial systems, insurance companies, users of health services, the medical and pharmaceutical industry and, last but not least, society at large). Finally,

Psychiatric Diagnosis: Challenges and Prospects Edited by I.M. Salloum and J.E. Mezzich
© 2009 John Wiley & Sons, Ltd

classifications facilitate comparative studies (epidemiological and clinical) and the training of health professionals across countries and cultures.

The International Classification of Diseases and Related Health Problems, Tenth Edition (ICD-10) is the latest edition of this official international classification [1]. The last systematic survey to assess the ICD-10 implementation status was conducted in 2002 [2]. A country was considered as having fully implemented ICD-10 if it was currently used for mortality and morbidity reporting to WHO. Globally, 138 (64%) countries reported implementation for mortality but only 99 (46%) for both mortality and morbidity. The highest levels of implementation were reported from the regions of the Americas and Europe, while the African and Eastern Mediterranean regions were reporting much lower rates.

Mental and behavioural disorders are covered in the Chapter 5 of ICD-10. The work undertaken to develop Chapter 5 of ICD-10 was gigantic, involving consultations with an international group of experts, and a series of field trials to assess the utility of the categories and criteria. Fifty countries were involved in field trials, involving more than 150 centres, 1 000 clinicians and 35 000 patients.

Chapter 5 of the 'Reference Classification' provides brief glossary definitions and is conceived for clinician and statistical users. Derived and adapted versions that have been produced subsequently are:

- Clinical Descriptions and Diagnostic Guidelines, which is for use in clinical work and contains narrative descriptions;
- Diagnostic Criteria for Research, which provides inclusion and exclusion criteria and diagnostic algorithms (onset, duration, clustering, episodes);
- Primary Health Care Version, which is a selection of 27 psychiatric conditions with diagnostic and management guidance;
- Multiaxial Presentation for Use in Adult Psychiatry, which presents three axes: clinical diagnosis, disabilities, contextual factors (psychosocial and environmental);
- Multiaxial Classification of Child and Adolescent Mental Disorders, which presents six axes: clinical syndromes, disorders of psychological development, intellectual level, medical conditions, associated abnormal psychosocial situations and psychosocial disability.

24.2   REVISION OF ICD-10 MENTAL AND BEHAVIOURAL DISORDERS

WHO has decided to revise the International Classification of Diseases and Related Health Problems, Tenth Edition (ICD-10). The revision of the ICD-10 is an important normative function of WHO, and is scheduled to be completed by 2011. WHO's Classification and Terminology Team has developed a common strategy and work platform for all chapters of the ICD. The Department of Mental Health and Substance Abuse is taking a lead in the revision of Mental and Behavioural Disorders, working closely with the Classification and Terminology Team. The revision will be done in close collaboration and consultation with all stakeholders, including health care researchers, public health experts, non-governmental organizations, and consumer and family groups. The scope of these collaborations and consultations will be international and multiprofessional/multidisciplinary, with adequate consideration of regional and gender balance.

WHO has constituted a high-level WHO International Advisory Group for the Revision of ICD-10 Mental and Behavioural Disorders. The Advisory Group has the primary task of advising WHO in all steps leading to the revision of mental and behavioural disorders in ICD-10 in line with the overall revision process. The Advisory Group consists of a small number of experts from all regions of WHO, and also representatives of international associations of mental health professionals. The Advisory Group meets twice every year; summary reports of its meetings are available on the WHO website [3].

Even though the revision of classification of ICD-10 mental and behavioural disorders is in an early phase, a number of issues have emerged that require close attention. A brief description of these follows.

24.2.1   Universality of Categories

Universality of specific categories of mental illness is an inherent assumption in ICD-10. This assumption is not proven and, in spite of the call for more attention to culture in psychiatric diagnosis by some authors (e.g. [4, 5, 6]), the 'image of a global ecumene tends to view culture as a distraction from the project of developing a body of universal knowledge' [6]. Attention to cultural framework cannot be an option but should become a key element in developing future classification and diagnostic criteria. The increasing trend of basing psychiatry exclusively on the biological underpinnings of mental disorders fits quite well with the 'global ecumene' and still considers such variables as culture and socio-economic status a 'soft' variable:

'... the study of variation is a cornerstone of science, and the diversity of symptoms, outcome and prevalence of mental illness offers a tremendous opportunity to test the way human cultures and environments shape the formation, distribution and manifestation of disorders. So far this opportunity has been neglected.' [5]

While attention has been given to differences and possible harmonization between the ICD-10 Chapter 5 and the American DSM, not very much attention has been paid to examining the discrepancies from Western nosological systems and other systems, for example, the Chinese Classification of Mental Disorders. China, in fact, has a national system of classification of mental disorders first published in 1979 and then revised in 1981 and 1984. In spite of this version (called CCMD-2) sharing a broadly comparable architecture with ICD-10, there are several differences and discrepancies between it and the international classifications.

'The complicated language of psychiatry based on philosophical concepts of nineteenth century Europe makes it very difficult for the non-European to contribute effectively. The rich philosophical heritage of other world cultures like Indian, Islamic or Chinese is not reflected in the terminology used in psychiatry today'. [7]

24.2.2   The scope of a diagnostic manual

An issue related to the scope of a diagnostic manual is whether it should include information that pertains to the disorders but is not directly essential to making a diagnosis.

A distinction needs to be made between the purpose of a diagnosis and classification system, and that of a textbook (e.g., see [8]). The information that is included for each diagnosis in the ICD-10 Classification of Mental and Behavioural Disorders: Clinical Descriptions and Diagnostic Guidelines [9] includes an introduction, a clinical description, diagnostic guidelines, and a short section on differential diagnosis. DSM IV-TR [10] often includes a long introduction and information on associated features and disorders (including associated descriptive features and mental disorders, associated laboratory findings, associated physical examination, and general medical conditions), specific features related to culture, age, gender, prevalence, course, familial patterns, differential diagnosis and, finally, the diagnostic criteria for the disorder.

Some have argued that, when there is strong evidence for the use of particular treatments for particular disorders, the mention of these should be included in the diagnostic classification, though both psychopharmacologic and psychotherapeutic treatments tend to be effective across a variety of disorders and evidence for their specificity is poor [11, 12]. A key question here is whether a diagnostic classification should attempt to be a therapeutic manual or textbook, and, if so, what should be the limits of the information provided.

24.2.3   Public health aspects of diagnosis and classification system

There is a need to enhance attention given to the public health implications of diagnosis and classification during the revision process. One of the critical issues is the vast treatment gap. Out of the 450 million people suffering from neuropsychiatric disorders, more than half are practically excluded from any kind of treatment [13]. Among the half who are receiving some kind of treatment, the vast majority are receiving inappropriate treatment and poor quality of care, and in many instances are exposed to systematic violations of human and civil rights, including massive disrespect of their dignity. One could legitimately ask: what is the added value of changes in diagnosis and classification in those countries where this double gap is large? A case can be made that, even in countries where mental health care is based on very basic skills, services and drugs, proper diagnosis is worthwhile because it increases the likelihood of proper, even if basic, treatment. Furthermore, regulatory practices for drug availability also depend on available diagnostic systems in both rich and poor countries.

Diagnosis and classification are largely considered statistical reporting, clinical, research and educational tools, with almost no consideration given to public health implications. A number of important public health aspects related to mental disorders prevention and care are related to diagnosis and classification systems. Some of the most salient of these issues are as follows.

Public Health Implications of Definition of Mental Disorders

The definition of mental disorders has direct consequences for public health action. It affects the estimates of prevalence of disorders, the evaluation of the outcome of health interventions, the legal protection of people against abuse by psychiatry and by society, and a number of other public health issues. ICD-10 Clinical Descriptions and Diagnostic Guidelines [9] refers to the term 'disorder as the existence of a clinically recognisable set of symptoms or behaviour associated in most cases with distress and with interference with personal functions. Revision process will need to ascertain whether this concept of mental disorders has been useful and whether it is sufficiently operational.

Forensic and Legal Issues

Diagnoses and classification categories are used in the practice of forensic psychiatry. The ICD revision process needs to review the evidence around the use of psychiatric diagnostic terms in law, the capacity of legal profession and their clients to understand diagnostic information and decisions, and the provisions concerning chronicity and long-term impairment in diagnostic manuals.

Economic Consequences

The financing of mental health services is closely related to diagnostic categories. The financing of government mental health services, as well as by social or private insurance, is likely to be impacted by changes in categories and criteria of mental and behavioural disorders. Attention also needs to be paid to issues like pensions and welfare benefit entitlements, reimbursement and parity of care in relation to diagnostic categories. One important issue is whether severity of impairment and distress should be included in relevant diagnostic definitions and criteria.

Statistics and Information Systems

The impact of new classifications on how countries collect and report statistics is an important consideration. A large amount of effort goes into the training of diagnostic data coders and medical librarians. Changes in diagnostic names and codes makes this task even more complex. There are also public health implications of a new diagnostic system on the reporting of mental health conditions (e.g. suicide, mental retardation, substance use disorders).

Education and Training of Professionals

The introduction of new diagnosis and classification systems into real life settings needs mental health care professionals to be trained in its use. Revisions must take these needs into account, including the (re)training of primary care staff.

Primary Care

Since most people with mental disorders are treated in primary care, it is important that any diagnostic system is useful in these settings. Whether a primary care version should be an adaptation after the full version has been developed, or whether both versions need to be developed simultaneously, is not only a conceptual issue but also an issue of practical significance.

Prevention of Mental Disorder

Should a diagnostic manual be concerned only with clinical syndromes, or should it include information on risk and protective factors and sub-clinical states? With an increasing number of interventions available for prevention of mental and behavioural disorders [14, 15], this question is more relevant now than earlier.

24.2.4 Harmonization with DSM

The American Psychiatric Association has begun work on the creation of DSM-V. Because the overall timeframes for the development of ICD-11 and DSM-V are similar, there may be a unique potential to harmonize the two revision processes and work towards the maximum possible uniformity or harmonization between ICD-11 and DSM-V. However, it should be recognized that there may be important and legitimate differences between the two systems, based on their different purposes and constituencies. Other differences that may be relevant include ownership, range of participation, and financial interests. ICD is owned by an international organization with a recognized charter to work on behalf of the public good in global health and health care. It is made available by WHO to its intended users at no cost. DSM is a commercial product owned by a national association representing a single professional guild, which derives a significant portion of its revenues from the sale of DSM and its related products.

While recognizing that these factors may influence the development of the two classifications such that they are not completely reconcilable, careful consideration needs be given to the mechanisms needed to harmonize the two revision exercises, the barriers to harmonization that can be anticipated, and what can be done to avert or minimize those barriers.

24.3 CONCLUSIONS

The Revision of ICD is a unique opportunity to assess the strengths and weaknesses of current diagnostic concepts and criteria in the area of mental and behavioural disorders. Sufficient attention needs to be given to the new evidence on nosology and diagnosis, how the current classification systems are used (and not used) and what can be done to enhance the use. The process of classification revision can also be used to bring the public health implications of diagnosis and classification to the foreground.

REFERENCES

[1] World Health Organization. *International Classification of Disease and Related Health Problems*. 10th Revision. Volume 1. Geneva: WHO; 1992.
[2] World Health Organization. *Global summary of the ICD-10 implementation status in 2002* Geneva: WHO; 2002. WHO/GPE/CAS/C/02.17.
[3] World Health Organization. *Summary Reports of Meetings of the International Advisory Group for the Revision of ICD-10 Mental and Behavioral Disorders*. 2008. www.who.int/mental_health/evidence/en/ (accessed on 31 January 2008)
[4] Patel V, Winston M. Universality of Mental Illness Revisited: Assumptions, Artefacts and New Directions. *British Journal of Psychiatry* 1994;165: pp. 437–440.

[5] Kleinman A, Cohen A. Psychiatry's global challenge. *Scientific American* 1997; March: pp. 74–77.

[6] Kirmayer L. Culture, Context and Experience in Psychiatric Diagnosis. *Psychopathology* 2005;38: pp. 192–196.

[7] Wig NN. Requirement for classification of mental disorders in the world today. In: Stefanis CN. (ed.) *Psychiatry: A world perspective, Volume* I. Amsterdam: Elsevier Science Publishers BV; 1990.

[8] Sadler JZ. *Values and psychiatric diagnosis.* New York: Oxford University Press; 2004.

[9] Health Organization World . *The ICD-10 Classification of Mental and Behavioural Disorders: Clinical descriptions and diagnostic guidelines.* Geneva: WHO; 1992.

[10] Psychiatric Association American. *Diagnostic and statistical manual of mental disorders.* 4th ed. Text Revision. Washington, DC: American Psychiatric Association; 2000.

[11] Charney DS, Barlow DH, Botteron K, Cohen JD, Goldman D, Gur RE, *et al.* Neuroscience research agenda to guide development of a pathophysiologically based classification system. In: Kupfer DE, First MB, Regier DA. (eds.) *A research agenda for DSM-V.* Washington, DC: American Psychiatric Association; 2002. pp. 31–83.

[12] Lambert MJ, Ogles BM. The efficacy and effectiveness of psychotherapy. In: Lambert MJ(ed.) *Bergin and Garfield's Handbook of Psychotherapy and Behavior Change.* New York: John Wiley & Sons, Inc.; 2004. pp. 139–193.

[13] Kohn R, Saxena S, Levav I, Saraceno B. Treatment gap in mental health care. *Bulletin of the World Health Organization* 2004;82: pp. 858–866.

[14] Health Organization World . *Prevention of Mental Disorders Effective interventions and policy options: Summary Report.* Geneva: WHO; 2004.

[15] Saxena S, Jané-Llopis E, Hosman C. Prevention of mental and behavioural disorders: implications for policy and practice. *World Psychiatry* 2006;5 (1 February 2006); pp. 5–14.

CHAPTER 25

Experience with the Diagnostic and Statistical Manual of Mental Disorders and Preparations for the Future

Michael B. First

Professor of Clinical Psychiatry, Columbia University, NY, USA;
Research Psychiatrist, New York State Psychiatric Institute,
New York, NY, USA

25.1 INTRODUCTION

Although DSM-IV was produced by the American Psychiatric Association in 1994 primarily for use in the United States, it is also used in many other countries. It is overwhelmingly favoured by researchers internationally [1] and is also the preferred system for clinical purposes in a number of non-US countries (e.g., New Zealand [2]). DSM-IV follows the diagnostic paradigms first established by DSM-III in 1980. Acknowledging the field's lack of knowledge and understanding of the underlying etiology of mental disorders, DSM-III eschewed basing the structure of the classification and definition of disorders on hypothesized but unproven etiological theories in favour of a descriptive approach in which disorders were defined in terms of their presenting symptomatology. DSM-III also defined each disorder using operationalized diagnostic criteria, which were designed to enhance communication and improve diagnostic reliability. In order to facilitate research into the underlying etiology and pathophysiology of disorders, DSM-III attempted to identify homogenous subgroups of patients by establishing a number of diagnostic subtypes (e.g., melancholic depression) as well as splitting broad diagnostic groupings into narrower categories that shared specific diagnostic features, resulting in a large expansion of the number of categories (as compared to DSM-II) and increasing rates

Psychiatric Diagnosis: Challenges and Prospects Edited by I.M. Salloum and J.E. Mezzich
© 2009 John Wiley & Sons, Ltd

of diagnostic comorbidity. Furthermore, each disorder definition was also accompanied by descriptive text intended to enhance the diagnostic assessment process, clarify differential diagnostic issues, and provide information that would make it useful for educational purposes (such as associated features, prevalence, course, predisposing factors). These innovations were largely responsible for the overwhelming acceptance of the DSM by mental health professionals, students, administrators, and patients and their families – each edition of the DSM has sold well in excess of one million copies, making it one of the top selling medical books of all time.

After DSM-IV was published in 1994, it was decided that the pace of the diagnostic revision process should be slowed down, at least partly in response to criticism that disruptions caused by updating the diagnostic criteria at seven-year intervals was not justified [3]. Anticipating publication of DSM-V around 2010, the American Psychiatric Association took advantage of this delay by partnering with the National Institute of Mental Health (NIMH) and the World Health Organization (WHO) to undertake a two-phase research planning process with the goal of enriching the research base in advance of the formal beginning of the DSM-V and ICD-11 revision processes. (Because of a number of factors, the DSM timelines have slipped, so that is it expected that DSM-V will be published in 2012).

A large part of the impetus for this endeavour was the general frustration expressed by both researchers [4] and clinicians [5] with the descriptive approach taken by DSM-IV and ICD-10. Disorders in the DSM and ICD are defined in terms of syndromes, i.e., symptoms that have been observed to co-vary together in individuals. In adopting this approach, DSM-III presumed that, as in general medicine, the phenomenon of symptom covariation could be explained by a common underlying etiology and pathophysiology. Although based largely on expert consensus, there was a general understanding that the DSM-III criteria would be continually revised in subsequent editions of the DSM with the goal of improving diagnostic validity based on new research findings, ultimately culminating in the identification of the underlying disease processes.

Unfortunately, in the more than 25 years that have elapsed since the publication of DSM-III, the goal of determining the underlying pathophysiology of the DSM mental disorders has remained elusive. Despite the discovery of many promising candidates over the years, not one single laboratory marker has been shown to be diagnostically useful for making any DSM diagnosis [6]. Epidemiological and clinical studies have demonstrated extremely high rates of comorbidities among the disorders, undermining hypotheses that the DSM-defined syndromes have distinct etiologies. Validating DSM categories based on treatment response or genetics, as suggested in Robins and Guze's classic 1970 paper [7] has also been problematic. Treatments from widely different drug classes are effective for the same diagnosis (e.g., lithium, anticonvulsants, and antipsychotics for treatment of acute mania) and the same drug can be effective for treating disorders across the diagnostic spectrum (e.g., SSRI's are effective for depression, panic, generalized anxiety disorder, posttraumatic stress disorder, social anxiety disorder, body dysmorphic disorder, obsessive-compulsive disorder, pathological gambling, trichotillomania, borderline personality disorder, etc.). Twin studies have also contradicted many of DSM's assumptions that separate syndromes have a distinct underlying genetic basis (e.g., evidence suggests that major depressive disorder and generalized anxiety disorder have the identical genetic risk factors [8]).

25.2 DSM-V RESEARCH PLANNING PHASE I: DEVELOPMENT OF A RESEARCH AGENDA

The main impediment to basing the DSM classification on underlying etiology is, of course, the enormous gaps in our understanding of the pathophysiology of mental disorders. Therefore, in order to help move the field forward towards the ultimate goal of having a primarily etiological classification, a series of 'white papers' was commissioned under the joint sponsorship of the American Psychiatric Association (APA), the National Institute of Mental Health (NIMH), the National Institute for Alcoholism and Alcohol Abuse (NIAAA), and the National Institute for Drug Abuse (NIDA). Research planning work-groups responsible for the development of these white papers were constituted with two goals: (1) to stimulate research that will enrich the empirical data base prior to the start of the DSM-V revision process; and (2) to devise a research and analytic agenda that would facilitate the integration of findings from animal studies, genetics, neuroscience, epide-miology, clinical research, cross-cultural research, and clinical services research, which will eventually lead to the development of an etiologically-based, scientifically-sound classification system. Rather than having the white paper workgroups focus on the tradi-tional diagnostic categories, the workgroups were instructed to focus instead on cross-cutting issues. These included:

1. a basic nomenclature workgroup, focusing on a variety of issues that had to do with the way disorders are classified in the DSM;
2. a neuroscience and genetics workgroup whose focus was to develop a basic and clinical neuroscience and genetics research agenda to guide the development of a future pathophysiologically-based classification;
3. a developmental science workgroup which outlined a research agenda to inform the developmental aspects and evolution of psychiatric disorders;
4. a workgroup focusing on two major gaps in the DSM-IV, namely inadequacies in the classification of personality disorders and relational disorders;
5. a mental disorders and disability workgroup, which focused on disentangling the concepts of symptom severity and disability;
6. a culture and psychiatric diagnosis workgroup which considered cross-cultural issues in diagnosis and classification.

Given the breakthrough nature of the suggested research and the relatively short time-frame leading up to the anticipated publication of DSM-V and ICD-11, it was understood from the outset that most of the proposed research agenda was unlikely to bear fruit until DSM-VI or later.

A closer examination of the Basic Nomenclature and Neuroscience and Genetics white papers illustrates the cross-cutting focus of these white papers. Issues addressed in the Basic Nomenclature white paper [9] include:

1. whether a new mental disorder definition can be developed that might be useful as a criterion for considering proposals for new disorders in DSM-V;
2. setting up a hierarchy of validators to handle potential conflicts among external valida-tors (e.g., using family history as a validator supports a broad definition of schizophrenia that would include schizotypal personality disorder, whereas using diagnostic stability as a validator would support a narrow definition that requires a chronic course);

3. addressing the misleading appearance that the knowledge base supporting each disorder is equivalent (e.g., schizophrenia appears to have as strong an empirical basis as does histrionic personality disorder) by possibly rating the quality and quantity of supportive information.

The Neuroscience and Genetics white paper [6], noting that current DSM definitions are virtually devoid of biology despite evidence that most mental disorders are biologically-based, discussed why progress has been so limited and offered strategic insights that may lead to a more etiologically-based diagnostic system. Reviewing genetic studies, brain imaging, post-mortem and animal studies, the paper argues that limitations in technology and techniques have been the main impediment to further progress.

The six white papers were published by the American Psychiatric Association in a 2002 monograph entitled *A Research Agenda for DSM-V* [10]. Three additional white papers, one focusing on gender issues, one focusing on diagnostic issues in the geriatric population, and one focusing on mental disorders in infants and young children, were commissioned subsequently and appear in a second volume of the research agenda. [11].

25.3   DSM-V RESEARCH PLANNING PHASE II: RESEARCH PLANNING CONFERENCES

The second phase of the DSM-V Research Planning Process consists of 12 research planning conferences (plus a methods conference) from 2004–2008, under the title 'The Future of Psychiatric Diagnosis: Refining the Research Agenda'. These conferences were organized in collaboration with the World Health Organization and are co-funded by APA, NIMH, NIAAA, and NIDA. Unlike the white papers in the first phase, which focused on general cross-cutting issues, these conferences for the most part focus on specific diagnostic topics. The primary goal of these conferences is to stimulate the empirical research necessary to allow informed decision-making regarding crucial diagnostic deficiencies identified in DSM-IV and ICD-10. A secondary goal of these conferences is to promote international collaboration in order to increase the likelihood of having a unified DSM-V and ICD-11. The entire conference series was structured so that there are equal US and international participation in terms of chairs, attendees and sites: each conference has two co-chairs, one from the US and the other outside the US; each includes an equal number of US and international participants; and half the conferences took place outside of the US. The 12 diagnostic-topic focused conferences covered: Dimensional Approaches to Personality Disorders (December 2004, Arlington, VA); Substance-Related Disorders (February 2005, Rockville, MD); Stress-Induced and Fear Circuitry Disorders (June 2005, Arlington, VA); Dementia (September 2005, Geneva, Switzerland), Deconstructing Psychosis (February 2006, Arlington, VA); Obsessive-Compulsive Spectrum Disorders (June 2006, Arlington, VA); Dimensional Approaches to Diagnosis (July 2006, Bethesda, MD); Somatic Presentations (September 2006, Bejing, China); Externalizing Disorders of Childhood (February 2007, México City); Comorbidity of Anxiety and Depression (June 2007, London, UK); Public Health Implications (September 2007, Geneva, Switzerland); and Autistic Spectrum Disorders (February 2008, Sacramento, California).

In order to illustrate the types of issues discussed at these conferences, two of the conferences that tap into issues that will feature prominently in the DSM-V preparations are briefly described here. (Summaries of all 12 conferences are posted on the DSM-V web site (www.dsm5.org) and monographs describing the presentations at each of the conferences are being published by the American Psychiatric Association [12–17]). DSM-IV and ICD-10 are both categorical classifications; that is, an individual either has or does not have a particular diagnosis. Categorical systems or typologies are the predominant approach used in medical classifications for several reasons. Classifying the world into categories is a fundamental characteristic of human mentation embodied in the nouns of everyday speech (e.g., animals, plants, planets, chemical elements). Furthermore, clinical practice is characterized by a number of yes/no decisions, i.e., whether or not to treat, whether or not to hospitalize, etc; a categorical approach to diagnosis facilitates such decision-making. Moreover, it has traditionally been assumed that most medical diseases are discrete entities. Although psychiatrists in the past have assumed that mental disorders are likewise discrete entities, with the exception of only a few conditions (e.g., Down syndrome, fragile X syndrome, Alzheimer's disease, Creutzfeldt-Jakob disease), research evidence strongly suggests that psychiatric disorders do not have discrete boundaries between them or between them and normality [18–20]. For this reason, there has been great interest in exploring whether dimensional approaches can be introduced into DSM-V and the Personality Disorders research conference illustrates the establishment of a research agenda specifically with the goal of moving the DSM-V personality disorders in a dimensional direction. Questions have also been raised about the organizational structure of DSM-IV and alternative ways to group the disorders together have been proposed (e.g., [21]). The Obsessive-Compulsive Spectrum Disorders conference explored research issues regarding what kind of evidence would be needed to justify creating an Obsessive-Compulsive Spectrum grouping in DSM-V.

25.4 DIMENSIONAL APPROACH TO PERSONALITY DISORDERS CONFERENCE

This conference, a follow-up to the personality disorders white paper that recommended a dimensional approach to classification of personality disorders [22], was co-chaired by Thomas Widiger, PhD and Erik Simonsen, MD. There are a number of serious problems with the personality disorder diagnoses in DSM-IV, many if not most of which can be attributed to the use of a categorical approach for these essentially dimensional constructs. For example, severely ill patients typically meet criteria for three, four, or even more personality disorders. However, rather than actually having several co-occurring independent personality disorders, these patients more likely have a single, albeit very severe personality disorder, the comorbidity being an artifact of the large number of personality disorder items present across the various categories. In contrast, the kinds of patients typically treated as outpatients often fail to meet the criteria for any of the specific DSM-IV personality disorders, necessitating the use of the Personality Disorder NOS diagnosis. Finally, because of their reliance on a fixed (and arbitrary) item count cut-off, personality disorders appear to come and go over time as the number of items present naturally wax and wane around the diagnostic threshold. In contrast, dimensional approaches to personality disorder view the components of personality as being on a continuum, and avoid the use of arbitrary thresholds. One impediment to adopting a dimensional approach to personality has been the multitude of alternative approaches that have been proposed by researchers over the past 20 years; it is far from clear which approach should be adopted. Recognizing that each model has its strengths and weaknesses, the conference participants proposed a strategy to combine the various dimensional models into a single integrated model, given that most models converge on four dimensions (i.e., extraversion versus introversion, antagonism versus dependence, impulsivity versus constraint, and emotional dysregulation versus emotional stability). During the conference, papers were presented on various aspects of these personality dimensions, such as childhood antecedents (i.e., the same four dimensions can be identified in children), neurobiological markers (i.e., for which there is limited evidence; the only well-documented relationship is between serotonin and impulsivity), and cross-cultural applicability (i.e., variation of personality traits between cultures is only one-third of the magnitude of variation among individuals within the same culture). The monograph summarizing the conference presentation was published in 2006 [12].

25.5   OBSESSIVE-COMPULSIVE DISORDERS SPECTRUM CONFERENCE

Obsessive-Compulsive Disorder (OCD) is classified among the Anxiety Disorders in DSM-IV. This placement reflects the DSM-IV convention that bases disorder groupings primarily on common presenting symptomatology; i.e., patients with OCD typically present with anxiety resulting from their obsessions and compulsions. Besides this superficial similarity, however, OCD appears to have little in common with the other anxiety disorders in terms of treatment response (e.g., OCD responds only to medications that affect the serotonin system whereas other anxiety disorders respond to a broader range of medications), family history, neurocircuitry, and comorbidity patterns, suggesting that OCD belongs in its own diagnostic grouping. This conference, co-chaired by Eric Hollander MD and Joseph Zohar MD, examined which other disorders in the DSM might be considered for inclusion in an Obsessive-Compulsive Spectrum grouping, based on phenomenology, comorbidity, course of illness, treatment response, genetics, neuroimaging and other validators [23]. Proposed candidates for inclusion in the OC spectrum include: obsessive-compulsive personality disorder (OCPD), hoarding, tic disorders, Syndenham's and other PANDAS, trichotillomania, body dysmorphic disorder, hypochondriasis, autism, eating disorders, pathological gambling and other behaviour addictions, and substance dependence. Overall, the participants of the conference concluded that the strongest evidence for inclusion in an OC spectrum exists for tics, body dysmorphic disorder, and hypochrondriasis, with less support for hoarding, trichotillomania, PANDAS, and OCPD.

25.6   LIKELY DIRECTIONS FOR DSM-V

Despite the field's hope that DSM-V will be etiologically-based, based on the material presented at these research conferences it is unlikely that genetics, neuroimaging findings, or biological markers will be incorporated into the diagnostic criteria for disorders in

DSM-V. Evidence from the conferences does strongly support the incorporation of dimensional approaches along with categorical approaches in DSM-V; the challenge will be to formulate dimensions that will be useful to both researchers and clinicians [24]. Furthermore, it is likely that there will be major changes in the diagnostic groupings in DSM-V; besides the possibility of creating an Obsessive-Compulsive Spectrum grouping, other suggested regroupings include the establishment of a distress disorders grouping that would include both Major Depressive Disorder and Generalized Anxiety Disorder (from the GAD and Depression conference) and the dismantling of the Somatoform Disorders section (from the Somatic Presentations conference). Other likely directions include taking a more developmental approach to psychopathology, with diagnostic definitions being modified to reflect differing presentations across the life span. Finally, there will be an increased effort to be sensitive to cultural and gender considerations in the definitions of psychiatric disorders.

REFERENCES

[1] Mezzich J. International surveys on the use of ICD-10 and related diagnostic systems. *Psychopathology* 2002;35(2-3): pp. 72–75.
[2] Mellsop G, Dutu G, Robinson G. New Zealand psychiatrists' views on global features of ICD-10 and DSM-IV. *Australian and New Zealand Journal of Psychiatry* 2007;41(2): pp. 157–165.
[3] Zimmerman M. Why are we rushing to publish DSM-IV? *Archives of General Psychiatry* 1988;45(12): pp. 1135–1138.
[4] Parker G. Beyond major depression. *Psychological Medicine* 2005;35: pp. 467–474.
[5] McHugh P. Striving for Coherence: Psychiatry's Efforts Over Classification. *JAMA* 2005;293: pp. 2526–2528.
[6] Charney D, Barlow D, Botteron K, Cohen J, Goldman D, Gur R, *et al*. Neuroscience research agenda to guide development of a pathophysiologically based classification system. In: Kupfer D, First M, Regier D. (eds.) *A research agenda for DSM-V*. Washington, DC: American Psychiatric Association; 2002. pp. 31–84.
[7] Robins E, Guze S. Establishment of diagnostic validity in psychiatric illness: its application to schizophrenia. *American Journal of Psychiatry* 1970;126(7): pp. 983–987.
[8] Kendler KS. Major depression and generalized anxiety disorder: same genes, (partly) different environments—revisited. *British Journal of Psychiatry* 1996;168(suppl. 30): pp. 68–75.
[9] Rounsaville B, Alarcon R, Andrews G, Jackson J, Kendell R, Kendler KS. Basic Nomenclature Issues for DSM-V. In: Kupfer D, First M, Regier D. (eds.) *Research Agenda for DSM-V*. Washington, D.C.: American Psychiatric Association; 2002. pp. 1–30.
[10] Kupfer D, First M, Regier D. (eds.) *A Research Agenda for DSM-V*. Washington, D.C.: American Psychiatric Publishing, Inc.; 2002.
[11] Narrow W, First M, Sirovatka P, Regier D. *Age and Gender Considerations in Psychiatric Diagnosis: A Research Agenda for DSM-V*. Arlington, VA: American Psychiatric Association; 2007.
[12] Widiger T, Simonsen E, Sirovatka P, Regier D. *Dimensional Models of Personality Disorders: Refining the Research Agenda for DSM-V*. Arlington, VA: American Psychiatric Association; 2007.
[13] Saunders J, Schuckit M, Sirovatka P, Regier D. (eds.) *Diagnostic Issues in Substance Use Disorders. Refining the Research Agenda for DSM-V*. Arlington, VA: American Psychiatric Association; 2007.
[14] Sunderland T, Jeste D, Baiyewu O, Sirovatka P, Regier D. (eds.) *Diagnostic Issues in Dementia. Advancing the Research Agenda for DSM-V*. Arlington, VA: American Psychiatric Association; 2007.

[15] Helzer J, Kraemer H, Krueger R, Wittchen H, Sirovatka P, Regier D. *Dimensional approaches in diagnostic classification: refining the research agenda for DSM-V*. Arlington, VA: American Psychiatric Publishing; 2008.

[16] Andrews G, Charney D, Sirovatka P, Regier D. *Stress-Induced and fear circuitry disorders: refining the research agenda for DSM-V*. Arlington, VA: American Psychiatric Publishing; 2009.

[17] Dimsdale J, Xin Y, Kleinman A. *Somatic presentations of mental disorders: refining the research agenda for DSM-V*. Arlington, VA: American Psychiatric Publishing; 2009.

[18] Van Os J, Gilvarry C, Bale E, Van Horn E, Tattan T, White I, *et al*. A comparison of the utility of dimensional and categorical representations of psychosis. *Psychological Medicine* 1999;29: pp. 595–606.

[19] Krueger R, Piasecki T. Toward a dimensional and psychometrically-informed approach to conceptualizing psychopathology. *Behaviour Research and Therapy* 2002;40(5): pp. 485–499.

[20] Goldberg D. A dimensional model for common mental disorders. *British Journal of Psychiatry* 1996;168(suppl. 30): pp. 44–49.

[21] Phillips K, Price L, Greenberg B, Rasmussen S. Should the DSM diagnostic groupings be changed? In: Phillips K, First M, Pincus H. (eds.) *Advancing DSM: Dilemmas in psychiatric diagnosis*. Washington, D.C.: American Psychiatric Association; 2003. pp. 57–84.

[22] First M, Bell C, Cuthbert B, Krystal J, Malison R, Offord D, *et al*. Personality Disorders and Relational Disorders: A Research Agenda for Addressing Crucial Gaps in DSM. In: Kupfer D, First M, Regier D. (eds.) *A Research Agenda for DSM-V*. Washington, D.C.: American Psychiatric Publishing, Inc.; 2002. pp. 123–200.

[23] Hollander E, Kim S, Zohar J. OCSDs in the forthcoming DSM-V. *CNS Spectrums* 2007;12(5): pp. 320–323.

[24] First M. Clinical Utility: A Prerequisite for the Adoption of a Dimensional Approach in DSM. *Journal of Abnormal Psychology* 2005;114(4): pp. 560–564.

CHAPTER 26

Experience and Implications of the Latin American Guide for Psychiatric Diagnosis

Ángel Otero-Ojeda

*Professor, Havana University School of Medicine, Cuba;
Section on Diagnosis and Classification, Latin American
Psychiatric Association;
Executive Committee on the Latin America Guide for
Psychiatric Diagnosis; Cuban Glossary of Psychiatry*

Carlos E. Berganza

*Professor of Child Psychiatry, San Carlos University School of Medicine, Guatemala;
Past President, Executive Committee on the Latin American Guide for
Psychiatric Diagnosis*

26.1 INTRODUCTION: HISTORICAL BACKGROUND AND DEVELOPMENT

History is not a randomly distributed anarchic storage of facts, but a sequence of dialectically related events, in which the earlier ones, by their very development, create the need for those occurring afterwards, and the latter ones implicitly or explicitly containing the essence of the former. Concerning psychiatric classification, the passage of time, the very development of the International Classification of Diseases (ICD), of humanity in general and the different communities that are integral part of it, as well as of science and technology, have made it necessary for regional glossaries to emerge, to harmonically integrate the universal and the particular of the diagnostic and classification process.

In fact, there are two kinds of phenomena relevant to psychiatric diagnosis and nosology: those of a universal nature, which take place anywhere (although their forms of expression, intensity, and other non essential characteristics may vary in different settings); and those

Psychiatric Diagnosis: Challenges and Prospects   Edited by I.M. Salloum and J.E. Mezzich
© 2009 John Wiley & Sons, Ltd

of a local nature, which only take place in certain environments. A dialectical relationship exists between both types of phenomena, such that one cannot be understood without taking the other into account. The ICD is not excluded from this rule. In psychiatry, a single diagnostic and statistical manual that is based only on the clinical practice and research of highly developed countries can be considered neither universal nor the most appropriate tool for all local realities around the world.

On the other hand, the mere substitution of the ICD by a group of regional or national classifications would not be the solution, since the harmonization of local and general factors is mandatory for an effective two-way communication across different realities, and regional adaptations of the ICD to the local characteristics of people seems to be the best way to achieve it [1].

Concerning international psychiatric diagnosis and taxonomy, the above-mentioned need for integration began to be apparent when the World Health Organization (WHO), confronted with the task of developing ICD-8 [2], identified as one of its main challenges the removal of the multiplicity of classifications being used across the world, such as the one being used in the US at the time, which tended to hinder fluid international communication. In line with this, the international body asked all countries that were signatories of the ICD to adopt the newly born ICD-8, adding to it their respective local glossaries, in order to facilitate mutual understanding.

As all this was happening, conditions in Latin America were already ripe for regional manuals to surface. All through Latin American countries, melted in the crucible of centuries of shared history and a background of similar socioeconomic adversities, conditions had been created for the emergence of a Latin American culture and for glossaries specific for this region to appear (see Tables 26.1 and 26.2).

Table 26.1 Bases for the formation of a culture.

---

1. Encounter, fights for domination and colonization (crushing of the cultural values and ethnic dignity of the autochthonous peoples and syncretism between the cultures of conquerors and subjugated).

2. Hybridization among different cultures:

 (a) Africans brought as slaves;
 (b) colonialists;
 (c) Asians brought as manpower.

3. Emergence of a national identity:

 (a) fights for emancipation;
 (b) materialization of a sense of nationality and a mestizo (ethnically mixed) culture
 (c) immigration:
     (i) internal (basically from the countryside to the cities);
     (ii) regional (from one country to another within the region);
     (iii) international (towards and from countries of the first world);
     (iv) mutual influence of the cultural interchange among these groups;
 (d) scientific and cultural hybridization:
     (i) professionals trained in foreign countries (basically USA, Europe or third world countries)
     (ii) professionals working in foreign countries with a close interaction with those others working in their countries of birth.

Table 26.2 Prerequisites for the emergence of local annotations.

1. A human group whose members:

   (a) have common cultural and historical roots;
   (b) share peculiarities *sui generis* in their idiosyncrasies, world conception, values, socioeconomic status and form of expression of distress and illness;
   (c) respond to a common label accepted by most as defining them as a group;
   (d) exhibit a common sense of belonging and loyalty, cognitively and affectively;
   (e) share (with exceptions) a geographic zone of the world or an ideology.

2. A scientific development mature enough to reflect those identifying characteristics of the group.

3. The emergence of leaders recognized by the community, capable of generating and leading the project.

On the basis of a double hybridization, of their mother culture on one hand and the place of their academic training on the other, prominent professionals from the region had developed an autochthonous scientific thinking and advanced substantial contributions to universal nosology. Of the many illustrations of this, we can mention the contributions of A. Seguín in Peru on stress related disorders; Javier Mariátegui in Peru and C.A. Cabral in Argentina on magic thinking and the Andean world; Bustamante in Cuba on transcultural psychiatry; Acosta Nodal in Cuba on idiographic diagnosis; and, more recently, Alarcón [3] from Peru on mixed ethnicity; Horacio Fábrega (USA and Panama) on comprehensive psychiatric diagnosis; Sergio Villaseñor (México) on ethnopsychiatry; and Juan E. Mezzich (Peru) on psychiatric nosology and classification.

There was also wide experience in the region in the use and design of diagnostic and classification instruments, as well as in tasks of coordination and collaboration with international organizations in matters of psychiatric nosology and taxonomy.

At the dawn of the 19th century, already, it was a Mexican, Jesús E. Monjarás, who made the first application of the Bertillon code. In Cuba, Ortelio Martínez constructed a glossary on the ICD, chapter V, in 1946. Curiel and associates established a collaborating centre for the ICD in 1954, while Leme Lopes [4], Horwitz and Marconi [5] and Fábrega advanced pioneering contributions to the multiaxial and objective diagnosis of the specialty [6]; and Efrén Ramírez (Puerto Rico) designed and applied an octagonal model for the diagnosis of and recording of information about mental patients [7].

Within this context, a Latin American country took up the challenge: on 28 August 1971, at the Hospital Psiquiátrico de la Habana [Havana Psychiatric Hospital], its then director, Dr. Eduardo B. Ordaz, took the first step in the creation of what would eventually become the first national glossary in the Spanish language, the First Cuban Glossary of Psychiatry, by naming an executive committee, presided by Professor Carlos Acosta-Nodal, for its construction.

After this manual (GC-1; [8]), a second one followed (GC-2; [9]) and a third (GC-3; [10]), with a multiaxial format, published in 2000; until the publication of the Latin American Guide for Psychiatric Diagnosis (GLADP), these were the only regional glossaries of the ICD produced systematically in the world of the Romance languages.

26.2   CONSTRUCTION OF THE GLADP

In the late 1990s, the Latin American Psychiatric Association's section on Diagnosis and Classification named a provisional, *ad hoc* committee in charge of preparing the conditions to initiate the development of a regional nosological manual. This committee was integrated by professors Carlos Berganza (Guatemala), Miguel Jorge (Brazil), Juan Mezzich (Peru -USA) and Ángel Otero (Cuba).

The formal elaboration of the GLADP started in October 1998, when an extensive group of experts in psychiatric diagnosis was convened to a formal meeting during the 20th Latin American Congress of Psychiatry in Havana, Cuba [11]. During this meeting, attended by over 60 participants, the executive and advisory committees were elected and the respective commissions were structured, with the task of developing different sections of the diagnostic manual. The coordinator of each section was selected, based on his or her specific expertise within the field, and most members of each commission were designated, making sure that most if not all countries in Latin America were effectively represented.

The process of GLADP construction was informed by the very same principles that had led to the successful completion of the Cuban Glossaries of Psychiatry, namely:

1. compatibility with ICD, as regional glossaries ought to be versions of the ICD, not parallel diagnostic systems;
2. bottom-up construction, promoting the active participation of final users of the manual;
3. a deliberate effort to harmonize different points of view concerning psychiatric diagnosis and classification;
4. systematic participation of as many psychiatrists, psychologists and other concerned mental health professionals as it was possible to include.

Finally, the general rules of the ICD-10 annotation process were spelled out, to harmonize the work of each commission.

Several major consecutive meetings followed the Havana meeting, to allow progress to be made in the construction of the manual, among them: Margarita Island, Venezuela, November 1999; Panama City, Panama, March 2000; Chicago, Illinois, USA, May 2000; Guadalajara, Jalisco, México, August 2000; and, finally, Guatemala City, Guatemala July 2002, where the completed manual was presented in its totality to the leadership of APAL in its electronic version. It took two more years, and the support of the University of Guadalajara, for the manual to be finally presented in its printed version [12]. The first printing totalled 1000 manuals. This is considered the official publication of the manual, and took place in San Carlos de Sonora, México, during a meeting of the Northern section of the Mexican Psychiatric Association in 2004. In 2006, a second printing of 2000 manuals was undertaken, to be distributed through the different academic regional meetings.

In addition to the printing of the manual, the GLADP was uploaded on the web pages of the Mexican Psychiatric Association, APAL and the World Psychiatric Association, and there are plans to upload it on the web pages of the Havana Psychiatric Hospital in the near future. All this has the purpose of facilitating access to the GLADP for potential users across Latin America and the rest of the world. The printed manuals have been widely distributed (at no cost) in México and, to a lesser extent, through several symposia carried out in most countries in Latin America during national and regional psychiatric meetings.

To date, more than 8000 copies of the manual have been downloaded from the websites hosting it; this would imply that there are more copies of the GLADP circulating in Latin America than copies of the ICD-10.

26.3   THE GLADP PROJECT

From the very beginning, the GLADP was conceived not as a simple diagnostic manual, but as a much more ambitious project bringing together the efforts of Latin American mental health professionals in an enterprise with a more general objective of protecting and reinforcing the cultural and scientific treasure of our peoples and humanity, under the premise that, 'wealth is not abundance; wealth is diversity'.

As specific objectives, we have tried to advance the scientific thinking and research in the region as ways to promote the universal recognition of our values, as well as to enrich world nosology, complementing it with our contributions and with the dialectical interaction between its general and particular aspects.

26.3.1   General Principles of the Project

We strongly believe that regional glossaries of psychiatry should not be conceived as a mere listing of local adjustments to the international classification, or the addition of the so-called 'culture-bound syndromes' and local forms of expressing distress. On the contrary, regional glossaries must represent the true basis for the participation of all concerned in the creation of a true bottom-up diagnostic system, enriched by the experience, scientific thinking and particular cosmological view of professionals across the globe. We are convinced that only that way can we promote enough flexibility within the system to allow for capturing the rich variability of the conditions and problems of the human beings that present for care in the four corners of the globe.

26.3.2   Architecture and Main Components of the GLADP

The GLADP is organized around four main parts: Part I, historical and cultural framework; Part II, comprehensive diagnostic process and formulation; Part III, psychiatric nosology (including major classes of ICD-10 and Latin American cultural syndromes); and Part IV, appendices. Five documents, in addition to a bibliography and an alphabetical index were included as appendices: (1) an illustrative clinical case; (2) conditions taken from other chapters of ICD-10, frequently associated with mental and behavioural disorders; (3) a lexicological dictionary; (4) concepts and proposals for future diagnostic systems; and (5) a listing of all participants.

26.3.3   Comprehensive Diagnostic Assessment and Formulation

In line with the major recent advances in psychiatric nosology, the Latin American Guide for Psychiatric Diagnosis incorporates a comprehensive diagnostic system that includes three components. The first component is a standardized one, composed of four axes and several sub-axes (wherever necessary). The four axes proposed by the GLADP are the following:

Axis I. Clinical Disorders and Related Problems. These include mental and general medical disorders formulated in either one or two separate sub-axes according to need, specified and codified according to ICD-10 [13].

Axis II. Disabilities. These are assessed in four areas (personal care, occupational/academic functioning, family functioning, and social functioning in general) according to a combination of frequency and intensity of the limitations in each of those areas, as specified by the *Multiaxial Presentation of ICD-10 for Use in Adult Psychiatry* [14].

Axis III. Contextual Factors. An axis mainly to describe psychosocial or environmental problems pertinent to the presentation, course or treatment of the clinical disorders listed in Axis I. They can be denoted with the Z codes of ICD-10, Chapter XXI [13].

Axis IV. Quality of Life. This is an axis not contemplated in the *Multiaxial Presentation of ICD-10 for Use in Adult Psychiatry* (from which the first three axes are derived) and has emerged in recent years as an important area to describe the status of health of a person, and as an index of the treatment outcome.

The second component of the GLADP comprehensive diagnostic formulation is a rather innovative idiographic formulation, which is a statement of discursive nature with natural language, summarizing what is idiosyncratic for the particular patient under consideration, and critical for disposition and management. The idiographic component must reflect the integrated perspective of the clinician, the patient and his/her family; and must also reflect the way in which major disagreements among the individuals participating in the diagnostic process are approached, negotiated and resolved. Finally, the third component is a format for the convenient and practical formulation and codification of all diagnoses.

26.3.4   Implementation and Dissemination

The project implementation and dissemination tasks have implied an ample plan of teaching activities. Workshops on its use have been carried out in most member countries of APAL and in all APAL congresses that have taken place since the publication of the manual. Over five hundred mental health professionals from the region have been trained on the use of the GLADP, and a number of them have created work groups in their own countries to disseminate and teach the use of this Latin American diagnostic manual. This has included the development of research projects with or about the manual. Special mention in this regard should go to México, where, with the support of the Mexican Psychiatric Association, workshops, lectures and symposia have been presented in all zones of the country; and to Cuba, where, with the support of the Ministry of Public Health, an educational programme is being carried out (already about 75% completed) on the application of the Cuban Glossaries and the GLADP in the everyday clinical practice, education and research. Significant efforts at the teaching and implementation of the manual have also taken place in Peru and Ecuador. Outside the

Latin American region, symposia and other educational activities have been presented in countries on all five continents, among them the Francophone Caribbean, USA, UK, Turkey and Australia.

In addition to the comprehensive report on its educational activities on the GLADP, presented by the APAL Section on Diagnosis and Classification through its newsletter [15], a number of reports on the GLADP have been published by prestigious journals and textbooks. These include *Psychiatric Clinics of North America* [11]; *Acta Psychiatrica Scandinavica* [16]; *Psychopathology* [17]; Sadock and Sadock's *Comprehensive textbook of psychiatry* [18]; *Investigación en Salud* [19, 20]; and *Interpsiquis* [21]. Finally, an impressive number of online publications make reference to the GLADP for a variety of reasons, concerning its innovative diagnostic format.

26.3.5   Research

The first systematic research projects have focused on the validity, reliability and feasibility of the diagnostic instrument. Results from initial reports tend to be encouraging. Otero, in Cuba, surveyed about 200 psychiatrists in 6 of the country's 13 provinces and found that, of those surveyed, 98.21% expressed a positive judgment on the diagnostic formulation of GLADP; and 97.3% expressed a positive judgment on its architecture and diagnostic categories. Alonso and Otero [22] reported in Dr. Alonso's graduation thesis a diagnostic agreement superior to 95% among clinicians, using the diagnostic criteria of the GLADP (which are also those of ICD-10); and 97% of diagnoses assigned following the criteria of experts also fulfilled the diagnostic requirements of GLADP.

In Peru, Saavedra *et al* [23] have studied the validity, reliability and feasibility of the idiographic component of the comprehensive diagnostic model of GLADP. Some of their results are: concerning Section I (Clinical Problems and their Contextualization), 39.8% of interviewers indicated that it had 'a lot of' or 'excellent' utility, and 81.6% 'some' to 'excellent' utility; for Section II (Positive Factors of the Patient), in 34.8% of cases, the interviewer considered that it had 'a lot of' to 'excellent' utility, and 42.2% 'more or less'. Concerning difficulties experienced by interviewers when applying the GLADP during the assessment of patients, only about 13% of interviewers reported excessive difficulties with the idiographic component of the diagnostic model.

26.3.6   GLADP Casebook

This is being prepared as a complement to the educational activities of GLADP. It should consolidate the experience of applying the diagnostic manual through the multiplicity of opportunities for the assessment of individuals who present for mental health diagnosis and care in the region.

26.4   CONCLUSIONS

Throughout the process of development, implementation and dissemination of GLADP, the APAL Section on Diagnosis and Classification has worked in close collaboration with the corresponding section of the World Psychiatric Association, and members of the GLADP executive committee also participated in the development of the WPA's International Guidelines for Comprehensive Assessment [24]. At the present time, APAL, through its global Section on Diagnosis and Classification, as well as through each section of its member societies, is collaborating with the WPA Global Network of National Classification and Diagnosis Groups, enhancing the possibilities for an effective participation of mental health professionals in Latin America in the development of the WHO'S upcoming ICD-11, and the WPA's Person-Centred Integrative Diagnostic Model. The entities in charge of developing ICD-11 have also requested that the professionals responsible for the design of the Cuban Glossaries of Psychiatry, and those of the GLADP, join other national psychiatric societies, such as the Chinese and the American, to help review the corresponding chapters of ICD-10 [13, 25] towards the development of the new revision.

REFERENCES

[1] Otero-Ojeda AA. Unity and diversity in international diagnosis. In: *Proceedings of the World Psychiatric Association International Congress*. Istanbul, Turkey; 12–16 July 2006.

[2] World Health Organization. *Manual of the International Statistical Classification of Diseases, Injuries and Causes of Death*. 8th revision (ICD-8). Geneva: World Health Organization; 1967.

[3] León CA. Cuadros psiquiátricos de la región [Psychiatric disorders in the region]. In: Vidal G, Alarcón R. (eds.) *Psiquiatría*. Buenos Aires: Editorial Médica Panamericana; 1986. pp. 630–635.

[4] Leme-Lopes J. *As dimensôes do diagnóstico psiquiátrico*. Rio de Janeiro, Brazil: Agir; 1954.

[5] Horwitz J., Marconi, J. El problema de las definiciones en el campo de la salud mental. Definiciones aplicables en estudios epidemiológicos [The problem of definitions in the field of mental health. Definitions applied in epidemiological studies]. *Boletín de la Oficina Sanitaria Panamericana* 1966;60: p. 300.

[6] Mezzich JE, Kleinman A, Fábrega H, *et al. Culture and psychiatric diagnosis: A DSM-IV perspective*. Washington, D. C.: American Psychiatric Press; 1996.

[7] Ramírez E. *Manual Operacional para la Evaluación Octagonal* [Operational Manual for the Octagonal Assessment]. San Juan, Puerto Rico: Secretaría Auxiliar de Salud para la Salud Mental; 1989.

[8] Acosta-Nodal C. *Glosario Cubano de la Clasificación Internacional de Enfermedades Psiquiátricas* [Cuban Glossary of the International Classification of Psychiatric Diseases]. 1st ed. Havana, Cuba: Hospital Psiquiátrico de la Habana; 1975.

[9] Acosta-Nodal C. *Glosario Cubano de la Clasificación Internacional de Enfermedades Psiquiátricas* [Cuban Glossary of the International Classification of Psychiatric Diseases]. 2nd ed. Havana, Cuba: Editorial Científico-Técnica; 1986.

[10] Otero-Ojeda A.. *Tercer Glosario Cubano de Psiquiatría* [Third Cuban Glossary of Psychiatry]. Havana, Cuba: Hospital Psiquiátrico de la Habana.; 2000.

[11] Berganza CE, Mezzich JE, Otero-Ojeda AA, *et al*. The Latin American Guide for Psychiatric Diagnosis: An Overview. *Psychiatric Clinics of North America* 2001;24: pp. 433–436.

[12] Asociación Psiquiátrica de América Latina. *Guía Latinoamericana de Diagnóstico Psiquiátrico*. Guadalajara, Jalisco, Mexico: Editorial de la Universidad de Guadalajara; 2004.

[13] World Health Organization. *International Statistical Classification of Diseases and Related Health Problems*. 10th revision (ICD-10). Geneva: World Health Organization; 1992.

[14] World Health Organization. *Multiaxial presentation of ICD-10 for use in adult psychiatry*. Cambridge, UK: Cambridge University Press; 1997.

[15] Testa RO, Otero A. Overall report on the Latin American Guide for Psychiatric Diagnosis (GLADP): Symposia and courses during the last 12 months. *Newsletter of the APAL Section on Diagnosis and Classification*, June 2006.

[16] Mezzich JE, Salloum IM. (Invited Guest Editors) Towards innovative international classification and diagnostic systems: ICD-11 and person-centered integrative diagnosis. *Acta Psychiatrica Scandinavica* 2007;116(1): pp. 1–5.

[17] Berganza CE, Mezzich JE, Jorge MR. Latin American Guide for Psychiatric Diagnosis (GLDP). *Psychopathology*, 2002;36: pp. 185–190.

[18] Mezzich JE, Lin KM, Hughes CC. Acute and transient psychotic disorders and culture-bound syndromes. In: Sadock BJ, Sadock VA. (eds.) *Kaplan & Sadock's Comprehensive textbook of psychiatry*. 7th ed. Philadelphia: Lippincott, Williams & Wilkins; 2000. pp. 1264–1276.

[19] Jilek W. Guía Latinoamericana de Diagnóstico Psiquiátrico (GLADP). *Investigación en Salud* 2006;7 p. 63.

[20] Villaseñor SJ, Mezzich JE, Otero A, *et al.* Clinical care, educational and research experience with GLADP: El best given de la guía. *Investigación en Salud* 2006;8 (1) pp. 4–6.

[21] Rojas-Malpica C. Diagnóstico idiográfico en psiquiatría. *Interpsiquis* 2003. Downloaded from *Psiquiatría.com*, at:www.psiquiatría.com/articulos/psisocial/10544/

[22] Alonso I, Otero A. *Cumplimiento de las pautas diagnósticas (CIE - 10) en pacientes del Hospital Psiquiátrico de la Habana* [Fulfilling ICD-10 diagnostic criteria in patients from the Havana Psychiatric Hospital]. Graduation Thesis. University of Havana; 2006.

[23] Saavedra J, *et al. Broad bases for International Classification: Americas Perspectives*. Paper presented at the WPA International Congress in Melbourne, Australia, 28 November - 1 December 2007.

[24] Mezzich JE, Berganza CE, von Cranach M, *et al.* Essentials of the World Psychiatric Association's International Guidelines for Diagnostic Assessment (IGDA). *British Journal of Psychiatry* 2003;182(suppl. 45): pp. s37–s66.

[25] World Health Organization. *The ICD-10 Classification of Mental and Behavioral Disorders: Diagnostic Criteria for Research*. Geneva: World Health Organization; 1993.

CHAPTER 27

Chinese Classification and its Future Perspectives

Yanfang Chen
Professor, Beijing Huilongguang Hospital,
Teaching Hospital of Peking University, Beijing, China
Zhong Chen
Professor, Shandong Mental Health Center,
Teaching Hospital of Shandong University, Jinan, China

27.1 INTRODUCTION: THE EDITION PRINCIPLES OF CCMD-3

The edition principles of CCMD-3 are intended to improve the service for patients, and to meet the needs of contemporary society. In CCMD-3, Chinese psychiatrists seek either to be accordance with ICD-10, or to sustain a nosology with Chinese cultural characteristics [1, 2]. Therefore broad similarities between the ICD-10 and CCMD-3 are obvious. However, based on the prospective field trials, in CCMD-3, there are particular additions (e.g., hysterical psychosis, mental disorders related to culture, and travelling psychosis, etc), deletions (e.g., mixed anxiety and depressive disorder, acute polymorphic psychotic disorder without symptoms of schizophrenia, etc) [1, 2].

In CCMD-3, Code 0 Organic Mental Disorders, regards dementia as only one of the important symptoms associated with brain organic diseases. For example, F01 Vascular Dementia in ICD-10 is named Mental Disorders due to Vascular Disease in CCMD-3; and F02.2 Dementia in Huntington's Disease in ICD-10 is named Mental Disorders due to Huntington's Disease in CCMD-3 [1, 2].

The major mental disorders in CCMD-3 are compiled in the following sequence: descriptive definition; symptom criteria; severity criteria; course criteria: exclusion; and note. For example, for Code 42 Neurosis in CCMD-3:

Descriptive definition: A group of mental disorders with certain factors, without any demonstrable organic basis, usually onset after psychosocial factors and last for a long time. The main manifestations are anxiety, depression, phobia, obsession-compulsion, hypochondriasis, somatoform symptoms, or neurasthenic symptoms, which are disproportional to the patient's actual situation. The patient has insight of the illness, but feels affliction.

(a) **Symptom criteria:** With at least one of the following symptoms:

- phobia;
- obsessive;
- panic attack;
- anxiety;
- hypochondriac symptom;
- somatoform symptom or neurasthenic symptom;
- mixture of above symptoms.

(b) **Severity criteria:** Impairment of social function or inextricable mental agony, which forces the patient to seek medical help.

(c) **Course criteria:** Its condition meeting symptom criteria lasts for at least three months, except for panic disorder.

(d) **Exclusion:** Excluding organic mental disorder, mental disorder due to psychoactive or non-dependent substances, schizophrenia, paranoid psychosis, psychotic disorder, and mood disorder.

Note: It is necessary to point out that various neurotic symptoms can be seen in infection, intoxication, visceral disease, endocrine, or metabolic disease and brain organic disease, which should be called neurosis-like syndrome.

The classification of neurosis is based on the results of the national prospective field trials. It is the main reason why we keep the concept of neurosis, and separate dissociative-convertive disorder from neurosis.

27.2 THE USE OF CCMD-3 IN CHINA [3]

In China, we use CCMD-3 in daily work and research, domestically. If we participate in international collaborative research, we use ICD-10; and for research with American colleagues, we use DSM-IV. The frequency of using CCMD-3 in clinical researches in three major Chinese journals of psychiatry between 2004 and 2007 is 79.1%, 78.1%, 77.0% and 78.0% respectively [Table 27.1].

Table 27.1 Frequency of use of deferent diagnostic criteria in clinical research (in three major Chinese journals of psychiatry 2004–2007*).

Years	ICD-10	CCMD-3	DSM-IV	
2004	14 (7.5%)	148 (79.1%)	25 (13.4%)	187
2005	21 (9.6%)	171 (78.1%)	27 (12.3%)	219
2006	19 (7.8%)	187 (77.0%)	37 (15.2%)	243
2007	14 (9.9%)	110 (78.0%)	17 (12.1%)	141
Total	68 (8.6%)	616 (78.1%)	106 (13.3%)	790

*Chinese Journal of Psychiatry; Shanghai Journal of Psychiatry; Journal of Clinical Psychiatry-Nangjing.

A survey of CCMD-3 or ICD-10 use in China was conducted during the Annual Meeting of the Chinese Society of Psychiatry (CSP) in 2006. The results indicated 94.8% (192 psychiatrists from all over China) used CCMD-3 or ICD-10, and 5.2% used DSM-IV [4].

We hope that the ICD-11 Chinese version will be published after ICD-11 is published in 2011. In the ICD-11 Chinese version, the mental disorders with Chinese cultural characteristics will be included in the appendix.

27.3   RATING TEST FOR HEALTH AND DISEASES (RTHD)

ICD-10 has the Schedules for Clinical Assessment in Neuropsychiatry (SCAN [5]), and DSM-IV has the Structured Clinical Interview for DSM-IIIR Axis I Disorders (SCID-I/P [6]) as their diagnostic instruments. On the basis of previous work, and after 4341 ratings for 1553 patients with 17 different mental disorders, CCMD-3 developed its own diagnostic instrument, RTHD. The seven-axial diagnostic system RTHD can be used not only for CCMD-3, but also for ICD-10, and DSM-4.

RTHD employs a clinical language that is familiar to clinicians from different theoretical backgrounds and, thus, is suitable for clinical work, research projects and epidemiological studies. RTHD contains a glossary of differential diagnoses and a computerized logical decision tree that provides diagnoses on seven axes (RTHD-Logical Verdict System; LVS). Users of RTHD made it clear that they wanted the new instrument to remain compatible with SCAN, SCID and other rating scales so that the RTHD-LVS algorithms could generate diagnoses that could be compared with data from earlier studies [7]. One of the trials of RTHD assessed the suitability of the seven axes of diagnosis for alcohol dependence [8].

Three senior clinicians independently assessed 1553 patients who were originally diagnosed with 17 different mental disorders, using the RTHD according to the diagnostic criteria of CCMD-3. Of these, 79 patients met CCMD-3 (Axis I) criteria for alcohol dependence, and also identified related physical conditions (Axis III); 32 (40.5%) mostly related to dysfunctions or diseases of the liver, spleen, stomach, and brain; and 42 (53.2%) patients with personal changes (Axis II). For bio-psycho-social stressors occurring in the past year (Axis IV), 25 (31.7%): of the 79 patients had had negative life events in the past year. In addition to alcohol abuse, 34 (49.4%) of the subjects were heavy smokers and 2 (2.5%) were abusing benzodiapines. For social functions (Axis V), the assessment of the most severe impairment during the current episode (F50) found that all 79 patients (100%) had poor to grossly inadequate social functioning at some time during the current episode. On Axis VI Global Assessment of Present State (GAPS), all 79 (100%) patients were rated '5 '(no change) at the time of the first evaluation [9]. As mentioned above, Axis VII The Relationship between Axes aims to integrate the information provided in the previous six axes. The results indicate that raters are able reliably to make these judgments.

CASE EXAMPLE: Zhang X, 36, male [CNH 250014.024102]

1. **Complaint:** Drinking for 18 years, alcohol dependence with irritability for eight years, hearing voices and quarrelling with others past week.
2. **Personality traits:** Extroversive

3. **Current history:** Dependent on alcohol since age 31, he currently drinks 250-500g daily. His social functioning has been severely impaired due to alcohol. He has tried to stop drinking many times but failed. He is often drunk and quarrelsome. An ultrasound examination showed liver cirrhosis and an X-ray showed necrosis of the head of the femur. He has been smoking for 15 years more, on average, 20 cigarettes a day.
4. **Mental examination:** He had a strong urge to obtain alcohol, was irritable, had no insight, and had persecutory delusions and auditory hallucinations.

CCMD-3/RTHD:

Axis I: Mental disorder due to use of alcohol (G32 96 Ms)

Psychotic syndrome due to alcohol
Dependence on alcohol
Dependence on tobacco

Axis II: Extroversive trait [P10(3), P10a(5)] and personal change
Axis III: Liver cirrhosis and necrosis of head of femur due to abuse of alcohol
Axis IV Bio-psychosocial Stressors: F10(7) Extreme, F10B(5) Drinking, F10B(7) Smoking
Axis V: 50 the most impairment of social functions (7) grossly inadequate F51 current social functions (6) more poor; F52 premorbidity of social functions (1) Normal
Axis VI Global Assessment of Present State: (6) no change
Axis VII The Relationship between Axes: X4F10 (7) Extreme, F10B (5) drinking—3→X1(3) mental disorders due to alcohol abuse, F10B (7) smoking—2→X1(3); F10B (5) —3→X3(3) physical diseases due to alcohol abuse; X1,X3 (3) —3→X5: F50(7), F51(6). The functional impairment was the outcome of the mental and physical disorders due to alcohol use.

The RTHD was also used to make diagnosis for children/adolescents with mental disorders. For example, the children and adolescents with mental disorders in the DSM-IV Case Book [10] were evaluated. In this book, there are 29 children/adolescents aged between 7 and 17 years old. The percentage of diagnostic consistency between a Chinese psychiatrist using RTHD/DSM-IV and the authors of the Case Book is 96.6% (n=28/29). The only difference between them of a diagnosis of a child case is as follows:

Case 174: Thin Tim

Eight-year-old Tim was referred by a paediatrician, who asked for an emergency evaluation because of a serious weight loss during the past year, for which the paediatrician could find no medical cause. Tim is extremely concerned about his weight and weighs himself daily. He complains that he is too fat, and if he does not lose weight he cuts back on food.

Tim has lost 10 pounds in the past year and still feels that he is too fat, though it is clear that he is underweight. In desperation, his parents have removed the scales from the house; as a result, Tim is keeping a record of the calories that he eats daily. He spends a lot of time on this, checking and rechecking that he has done it just right.

In addition, Tim is described as being obsessed with cleanliness and neatness. Currently he has no friends because he refuses to visit them, feeling that their houses are 'dirty'; he gets upset when another child touches him.

The central feature of the subjective component of obsessive compulsive symptoms is as follows: they are experienced as occurring against conscious resistance, i.e., the ideas and impulses are experienced as entering the mind against conscious resistance. The subject tries to resist them but fails. They are unpleasantly repetitive. They are recognized as part of his/her own thoughts and this causes much distress, since the thoughts may be embarrassing or blasphemous [5].

This child is described as being obsessed with cleanliness and neatness. Currently, he has no friends because he refuses to visit them, feeling that their houses are 'dirty'. But he does not think that his feelings that they are 'dirty' are ideas experienced as entering the mind against conscious resistance. And he has avoidant behaviour that causes him to have no friends. Therefore, we consider the child has specific phobias.

The RTHD involves affirming the whole person of the patient in context, as the centre and goal of clinical care and health promotion at individual, familial, and community levels, because there is no health without both mental health and physical health, and by focusing health efforts on the totality of the person's recovery [11]. Both the mental health and physical health care fields emphasize long-term management until the subject's recovery [12].

REFERENCES

[1] Chinese Society of Psychiatry. *The Chinese Classification and Diagnostic Criteria of Mental Disorders-Version 3* (CCMD-3) (both in Chinese and in English). Jinan, China: Chinese Society of Psychiatry; 2001.

[2] World Health Organization: *International Statistical Classification of Diseases and Related Health Problems* 10th revision. Geneva: World Health Organization, 1994.

[3] American Psychiatric Association. *Diagnostic and Statistical Manual of Mental Disorders*. 4th Edition. (DSM-IV) Washington: American Psychiatric Association; 1994.

[4] Yizhaung Zou . *Classification of mental disorders in China*. WPA regional conference, Shanghai 39, 2007.

[5] World Health Organization: *SCAN (Schedules for Clinical Assessment in Neuropsychiatry)*. Geneva: World Health Organization; 1992.

[6] First MB, Spitzer RL, Gibbon M. *et al. The Structured Clinical Interview for DSM-IIIR Axis I Disorders* (SCID-I/P). New York: Biometrics Research Dept. of New York Psychiatric Institute; 1990.

[7] Chen YF. (ed.) *Rating Test for Health and Diseases (RTHD) and its field trail*. Beijing: Chinese Society of Psychiatry; 1994, pp. 101–142.

[8] Chen YF, Chen Z. (eds.) *Analysis on Seven Axes of Diagnosis for Alcoholic Patients in Mental Test* (English version 1). Peking Union Medical College Press; 2007. Appendix F2; pp. 522–530. (.)

[9] Chinese Medical Association. *The Chinese Criteria of Treatment Effects*. Beijing: Chinese Medical Association; 1958.

[10] Spitzer RL, Gibbon M, Skodol AE, *et al. DSM-IV-TR Case Book*. Washington, DC: American Psychiatric Publishing. Inc.; 2002.

[11] Mezzich JE. Psychiatry and medicine for the person: articulating medicine's science and humanism. *World Psychiatry* 2007;6 (2): pp. 1–4.

[12] Reesal RT, Lam RW. Clinical guidelines for the treatment of depressive disorders. II. Principles of management. *Canadian Journal of Psychiatry* 2001;46(Suppl) 1: pp. 21S–28S.

CHAPTER 28

Multiaxial Schemas for Psychiatric Diagnosis

Claudio E. M. Banzato
Associate Professor of Psychiatry, University of Campinas – UNICAMP, Brazil
Miguel Roberto Jorge
Professor, Department of Psychiatry, Federal University of São Paulo, Brazil; Secretary for Sections, World Psychiatric Association
Marianne Kastrup
Head, Centre Transcultural Psychiatry Psychiatric Clinic, Rigshospitalet, Copenhagen, Denmark

28.1 INTRODUCTION: HISTORICAL BACKGROUND

The first multiaxial system for psychiatric diagnosis was designed by Essen-Möller and Wohlfahrt [1], on the grounds that aetiology and syndrome should be separately classified. But before that, Kretschmer [2] had already argued in favour of a pluridimensional account of the mental disturbances, encompassing three different kinds of causal factors: a characterological, an organic, and a psychosocial one (*Erlebnisfaktor*). Each one of them would contribute somehow to the onset of psychosis and they were likely to be etiologically intertwined. Kretschmer asked why we should then limit ourselves to using only one scale to understand and to measure the mental diseases. Instead, he suggested a multi-tiered approach to diagnosis (*Schichdiagnose*) in which such dimensions should be simultaneously considered [2].

It is interesting to note that Lecomte [3] in France developed a biaxial system separating aetiology and syndrome in the same year Essen-Möller and Wohlfahrt's proposal appeared. Later, a couple of triaxial systems were put forward: in Poland by Bilikiewicz [4]; and in Brazil by Leme Lopez [5]. Besides axes focusing on syndrome and etiopathogenesis, there was a third axis underlying features of personality related to the episode of illness. Furthermore, Leme Lopez argued – in addition to the dynamic pluridimensional, clinical diagnosis, and in order to complement it – in favour of a functional classification, a therapeutical classification (taking into account the place where the patient should be treated) and a medico-legal diagnosis.

Psychiatric Diagnosis: Challenges and Prospects Edited by I.M. Salloum and J.E. Mezzich
© 2009 John Wiley & Sons, Ltd

The biaxial system proposed by Essen-Möller and Wohlfahrt was further developed by another Swedish group [6] who added axes on severity and course of illness to the two axes proposed previously. The same biaxial rationale was also behind the pentaxial approach suggested by Helmchen [7], which included intensity, certainty and time frame axes. Though these developments were not received with great enthusiasm, such an approach was seen as an ingenious contribution to facilitate communication and increase the reliability and validity of psychiatric diagnosis [8].

In general medicine, the pioneer multiaxial initiative seems to be the Standard Nomenclature of Pathology (SNOP) [9]. Within this schema, diseases were to be described in the four following axes: I topography, II morphology, III aetiology and IV symptoms.

The first attempt to incorporate the multiaxial approach into a standard classification system was made by Rutter *et al.* [10], who proposed a triaxial classification of childhood mental disorders. The current child and adolescent psychiatric classification system by WHO places the ICD-10 diagnoses in a multiaxial context, including: Axis I on clinical psychiatric syndromes; Axis II on specific disorders of psychological development; Axis III on intellectual level; Axis IV on general medical conditions; Axis V on associated abnormal psychosocial situations; and Axis VI on global assessment of psychosocial disability [11].

The DSM-III [12] was the first important and widely used classification to adopt a multiaxial format, and further revisions kept it, with a few minor changes, mostly in the rating procedures for axes IV and V. Thus, in DSM-IV, the multiaxial system is still meant to facilitate comprehensive and systematic evaluation of five different domains of information [13]. The DSM-IV-TR [14] multiaxial system contains the following five axes:

Axis I: for clinical disorders and other conditions that may be a focus of clinical attention. All mental disorders, except for personality disorders, should be recorded there.

Axis II: for personality disorders and mental retardation (intellectual disability). Axis II may also be used for noting prominent maladaptive personality features and defence mechanisms.

Axis III: for current general medical conditions potentially relevant to the understanding or management of the individual's mental disorder.

Axis IV: for psychosocial and environmental problems that may affect the diagnosis, treatment and prognosis of the mental disorders coded on axes I and II. The clinician may note as many factors as found relevant, but in general, only factors that were present in the year preceding the current evaluation are recorded. In addition to their relevance in the development of the individual's mental disorder, the factors coded on Axis IV may also be a consequence of the mental disorder or constitute a problem for its treatment or management.

Axis V: measures global assessment of functioning. This is carried out using the Global Assessment of Functioning Scale, a scale from 1 to 100 to rate overall psychopathological status and social and occupational functioning using a single measure or score. In general, the assessment will refer to the current period, but functioning may also be rated for other time periods, e.g. highest level of functioning during the past year.

Later, the ICD-10 presented a multiaxial format for use in adult psychiatry, comprising three different aspects of the psychiatric patient's clinical condition [15]. The ICD-10 multiaxial system uses the following three axes:

Axis I: Clinical Diagnoses: this axis is used to record diagnoses of both mental (including personality) and general medical disorders.

Axis II: Disabilities: this axis covers disabilities resulting from the disorders recorded on Axis I and is accompanied by the WHO Short Disability Assessment Schedule (WHO DAS-S), a semi-structured instrument rating difficulties: a. in maintaining personal care; b. in performance of occupational tasks; c. in functioning in relation to family; and d. in a broader social context due to mental and physical disorders [16].

Axis III: Contextual Factors: this axis is intended for recording the psychosocial, environmental and personal lifestyle factors contributing to the presentation, course or outcome of disorders recorded on Axis I [17]. These factors come from original ICD-10 Z codes, i.e., factors influencing health status and contact with health services.

Another further development building on ICD-10 multiaxial presentation was the World Psychiatric Association's International Guidelines for Diagnostic Assessment (WPA-IGDA), with the main goal of considering the patient in his/her totality and not just as someone with a symptom or disease [18]. The IGDA stresses that the clinician should take into account all key areas of information necessary to describe pathology, dysfunctions and problems as well as assets, and resources of the patient.

As part of the IGDA diagnostic model, there is a Standardized Multiaxial Diagnostic Formulation. This proposal is based on a tetra-axial approach; the first three axes are basically the same as ICD-10's, while the axis IV constitutes an innovation. Axis IV deals with a global assessment of the patient's self-perceived well-being, in terms of physical and emotional status, satisfaction with occupational and interpersonal functioning, with social, emotional, and instrumental supports, and overall personal fulfilment.

28.1.1   Purposes of Multiaxial Systems

The basic aim of a multiaxial format is to evaluate several different domains of information assumed to be of high clinical relevance, and each domain or axis is assessed as quasi-independent of each other [19]. Multiaxial classification seeks to facilitate an understanding of the complexity of mental disorders and psychiatric diagnoses. It takes into account that diagnoses contain various components reflecting different aspects of the psychiatric disease. The multiaxial approach reflects more readily a multifaceted etiopathogenesis [20]. This is important given the fact that a shortcoming of a biological approach has been a frequent disregard for other significant aspects of the patient's situation or condition [21]. In addition, it has been argued that multiaxial diagnosis, by providing a more detailed holistic picture of the patient's condition, would contribute both to improving the validity of psychiatric diagnosis and to creating a better basis for planning a comprehensive treatment and optimizing a longitudinal assessment of a patient's health status [18].

The multiaxial model has been applied both to deal with the illness complexity and to portray the patient's whole condition [22]. The first purpose of the multiaxial approach is thus to articulate the fundamental components of the disorder. The different axes that have been developed in the various diagnostic systems would all contribute to this urge to reflect illness complexity [22]. The second major purpose is to give a comprehensive picture of the patient's totality of the condition [22], accounting for the impact of the disorder on the functioning of the person concerned, and making therapeutic decisions less arbitrary. Here the multiaxial approach may be a particularly useful tool in psychiatric settings where a global and comprehensive clinical assessment of the patient is required in a limited amount of time [23]. Such an approach may also be valuable for educational purposes and in the enhancement of epidemiological research.

28.2   EVALUATING THE CURRENT SYSTEMS

There are several recent reviews of the empirical evidence obtained hitherto with established multiaxial diagnostic schemas [8, 24–26]. In the last three decades, a limited number of articles were published in the literature evaluating DSM and ICD specific axes or their multiaxial schemas as a whole, taking into consideration the overall literature on DSM-IV and ICD-10. A brief summary of the main findings is presented in this section and each system is considered separately below.

28.2.1   Evaluating the DSM Multiaxial System

The DSM multiaxial system as a whole was considered highly (66.7%–84%) useful for clinical care (e.g., Velamoor et al. [27]; Mezzich [28]) and also for training (Tasman [29]). Tasman highlighted its utility in overcoming the rigidity and narrowness of syndromic checklists by enhancing the doctor-patient relationship within a biopsychosocial framework. Some other papers reported its utility for administration [30, 31] and research (e.g., [28]), and also its cultural sensitivity [32, 33]. Nevertheless, some authors have noted that some axes were not systematically used in clinical care – particularly axes IV and V. There are several explanations for this: the fact that the multiaxial approach is considered optional to the classic diagnosis of the main illness, lack of proper training in residency programs, and the perceived need to improve their user-friendliness to help the patient evaluation (e.g., [34–36]).

Concerning the evaluation of personality disorders and mental retardation in a different axis (II) than the main clinical disorder (I), it seems that their identification has substantially increased since the establishment of a multiaxial system [37] though with low reliability [38].

Regarding general medical disorders, the implementation of an individualized axis since DSM-III has contributed to increase their identification and record in clinical charts, both for inpatients [39] and outpatients [40].

Axis IV was differently represented in DSM-III [12] and DSM-IV [13]: while in the former it was related to the evaluation of stressor severity, in the latter it was focused on listing psychosocial problems. Stressor quantification was identified as an important problem for the use of Axis IV evaluation in DSM-III [41, 42], which could possibly be responsible for the moderate to low reliability found for this axis [43, 44]. Though the DSM-IV move away from stressor severity has been perceived as more helpful for clinical care planning, empirical studies are needed to substantiate such impression.

Functioning has received pointed attention lately and, indeed, the DSM-IV [13] included a proposal modification for its current Axis V (the GAF – Global Assessment of Functioning – Scale), excluding symptoms from its scope (in order to avoid overlapping with Axis I and II) and renaming it as SOFAS – Social and Occupational Functioning

Assessment Scale. Hilsenroth *et al.* [45] have found very good reliability for both scales and stated that their findings support the validity of the GAF as a scale to measure global psychopathology and the SOFAS as a measure of problems in social, occupational and interpersonal functioning. But according to Goldman [46], who wrote the editor's introduction to a special section of *Psychiatric Services* on the GAF, the papers featured in that issue showed mixed results regarding its utility.

28.2.2 Evaluating the ICD Multiaxial System

There are few papers aimed at evaluating the ICD-10 multiaxial system. Actually, an international survey published five years after the publication of the ICD Multiaxial Presentation Manual showed that among 202 psychiatrists from 66 countries, only 14% reported having had access to that system [28]. Nevertheless, in some preliminary field trials conducted in Germany and Japan, the perceived usefulness of the ICD-10 multiaxial presentation was considered fairly good [47, 48]. Reliability for each of its three axes was in general good [15]. Michels *et al.* [47] have described data supporting the treatment and prognostic validity of the ICD-10 multiaxial system. Kastrup and Mezzich [24] have suggested adding a measure of quality of life to the ICD-10 multiaxial system.

Recent surveys carried out in Brazil, Japan and New Zealand showed that less than one third of the psychiatrists routinely use all axes of either DSM-IV or ICD-10 in their clinical practice and that, unsurprisingly, the ICD-10 multiaxial system is the least known and used [49, 50].

In summary, both multiaxial systems, but particularly the ICD-10, have not been much used in routine clinical practice and have not been sufficiently empirically evaluated either. It seems that multiaxial systems are more appealing because of their capacity to portray the 'whole figure' of what is going on with the patient and his/her needs, which goes beyond the disorder domain. On the other hand, current axes need to be refined and become more adaptable for everyday practice in different settings. Regular training on multiaxial schemas during residency is essential to broaden their use among psychiatrists, and the inclusion of patient strengths and his/her family and community resources in their scope should be a must in linking them to treatment planning. Some tentative proposals towards such goals are featured in the next section.

28.3 MULTIAXIAL PROPOSALS TOWARDS A PERSON-CENTRED INTEGRATIVE DIAGNOSIS (PID)

As it was stated before, the perceived utility of multiaxial schemes for reaching a comprehensive diagnostic assessment has not been sufficient to grant their everyday use in psychiatric clinical settings [8, 49, 50]. Though multiaxial formulation is usually seen as desirable in psychiatry, it has hardly been considered as an essential resource for effective therapeutic and management decision-making. Indeed, for most psychiatrists, multiaxial diagnosis seems to have a supplementary and optional character; something that is worth doing whenever one can afford the time. Two lines of explanation for such a state of affairs can be thought of (and most likely, they should be combined): first, the available multiaxial schemes fail somehow to capture and reflect clinical reasoning and judgment, and therefore to properly facilitate treatment planning; second, no right balance between comprehensiveness, thrift and practicality has been struck in the current systems. So the question remains: is it possible to design a broad, yet simple diagnostic model? Accordingly, can multiaxial diagnosis be made more usable, helpful to patients and clinician-friendly across the world? These issues are briefly addressed in this last section, within the framework of WPA Institutional Program Psychiatry for the Person (IPPP).

The thrust of the Person-Centred Integrative Diagnosis (PID) envisaged by the WPA IPPP is not just to stress the ultimate centrality of the patient, but also to emphasize the centrality of the clinic. Psychiatry, as any other branch of medicine, is quintessentially a modificatory activity, so diagnosis is supposed to be linked to some sort of rationale for interventions that target certain kinds of human suffering. But in psychiatry, a medical speciality not strictly defined in terms of biological substrata, it should be much clearer that the person is the unity of analysis par excellence.

One working idea, which emerged recently, is to build such a PID model (covering the domains both of ill and positive health) by including only those aspects or factors that are indeed critical for tailoring any individualized treatment plan. The concept of 'clinical validity' – as practical devices, diagnostic tools would be valid to the extent they effectively inform clinical care and have some predictive power – provides the rationale behind it. A rough and very tentative sketch of what such a multiaxial PID model could look like is presented below.

There is a growing worldwide trend that mental health care should be delivered by multidisciplinary teams. Furthermore, the role played by general practitioners in such a task has been acknowledged as a key one as well. Thus, there is a need for classificatory systems to be useable not only by psychiatrists, but also by all those involved in clinical care, which in fact has been highlighted in surveys carried out recently with stakeholders from Brazil, Japan and New Zealand [50]). Accordingly, simplicity and user-friendliness, already valued by psychiatrists (who reported, for instance, to prefer classifications with less than one hundred diagnostic categories [50]), should become even more important for future diagnostic systems.

One plausible option towards improving the clinical validity of psychiatric diagnosis might be to replace current diagnostic criteria by multilevel psychopathological prototypes. Probably, the adoption of an actual and explicit prototypical approach could also concur to some decrease in the number of diagnostic labels, which would represent a welcome simplification of the diagnostic systems. For such a move, either a summary prototype model or an exemplar model could be chosen, or they might both perhaps be used in combination (in the former, a given set of typical features, none of them being necessary, works as a standard of comparison; in the latter, within a series of typical concrete instances, each of them on its own serves as a standard of comparison) [51][1]. Furthermore, diagnostic training should emphasize the process of operating with fuzzy categories, where membership is really a matter of degree and members are arrayed along a continuum of fit [51]. In such a framework, the widespread poor case-category fit seen in clinical practice should not need to be treated as errors provoked by flawed classifications, but instead as an indication of great variability of cases found in the real world. Another anticipated advantage is that prototypical categorization may lend itself readily to concomitant dimensional description, in terms of closeness to prototype or goodness of fit.

Within the WPA IPPP framework, the design of the PID is a work in progress. The aim is to make it simple and yet comprehensive, useful from the very start, though it should allow growth in depth along the course of the diagnostic assessment. In a multilevel diagnostic model, that is, one with different levels of aggregations and description, the clinician should have a clear grasp of where a given process of assessment stands at any time. In the following paragraphs, the domains and axes currently under consideration are briefly presented.

In one axis, a number of psychopathological summary prototypes could be featured along with a few selected dimensions. It should be noticed that a prototypical approach could be used not only for diagnostic categories but also for psychiatric symptoms themselves. Still regarding the domain of ill health, in order to further complement the transversal characterization of the clinical picture (signs and symptoms presentation), dimensional variables that cut across psychopathology (and that must be necessarily taken into account in every diagnostic assessment), such as degree of subjective suffering and disability, could be recorded and linked to the nosological prototypical categories. Closeness to prototype or goodness of fit is yet another dimension that might receive special attention within some contexts (training, for example). Alternatively, such dimensions could stand together in a separate axis.

In another axis, transnosological variables related to development, personality, temperament and character, which are very important for the sake of treatment planning, should be considered. Of course these are very complex domains. What has been suggested is that they could be assessed – however briefly – dimensionally in a standardized way, either by selecting some of the empirically tested instruments or by combining key elements from them, as recently argued by Widiger [52].

Complementing the depiction of the domain of ill health, key contextual factors from the social domain, such as psychosocial stressors, could possibly be featured in a separate axis whenever their relevance for onset, maintenance, or treatment of a condition is presumed. It should also be mentioned that a case has recently been made for the inclusion of a separate risk management axis in our diagnostic systems [53, 54].

Finally, regarding the appraisal of the positive health domain in PID, the general idea is to combine different tools and approaches, using categories, dimensions and narratives. Three broad areas have been identified: the first encompasses self-awareness, resilience, resources and protective factors; the second features the quality of life; and the third involves cultural assessment and formulation. However, no decisions have been made as yet about its formal architecture.

28.4 CONCLUSIONS

The multiaxial approach to psychiatric diagnosis, despite its relatively long history, remains to be fully evaluated. Not many studies have actually been carried out to assess its usefulness for everyday clinical practice and research. The lack of specific and formal training during psychiatric residency is certainly an issue. But some intrinsic reasons probably play a role as well, once the appeal such systems might have at a first glance has been insufficient to grant their widespread use. So it is crucial that new initiatives, such as the undergoing development of the PID, take past experience with multiaxial systems into account, particularly the difficulties faced in having them fully implemented in practice.

NOTE

1. **Summary prototype model**: 'This approach is based on a similarity-matching procedure whereby category membership is determined by the degree of similarity between a particular instance and a standard of comparison, the prototype.' In opposition to classical 'necessary and sufficient' features approach to categorization, the features of a prototype are by no means criterial. **Exemplar (multiple-examples) model**: There are many ways to be a good example of a category, the use of multiple concrete examples is stressed and membership then depends on the existence of a sufficient match to at least one exemplar. [51, pp. 241–242].

REFERENCES

[1] Essen-Möller E, Wohlfahrt S. Suggestions for the amendment of the official Swedish classification of mental disorders. *Acta Psychiatrica Scandinavica* 1947;47(Supp.) pp. 551–555.

[2] Kretschmer E. Über psychogenese Wahnbildung bei traumatischer Hirschwäche. *Z. ges. Neurol. Psychiat* 1919;45: pp. 272–300.

[3] Lecomte M, Daney A, Delage E, Marty P. Essai d'une statistique synoptique de médicine psychiatrique. *Techniques Hospitalières* 1947;18: pp. 5–8.

[4] Bilikiewicz T. Próba układu nozograficznego etioepigenetycznego w psychiatrii.*Neurologia I Neurochirugia Polska* 1951;13: pp. 68–78.

[5] Leme Lopes J. As dimensões do diagnóstico psiquiátrico. Rio de Janeiro: Agir; 1954.

[6] Ottoson JO, Perris C. Multidimensional classification of mental disorders. *Psychological Medicine* 1973;3: pp. 238–243.

[7] Helmchen H. Multiaxial systems of classification. *Acta Psychiatrica Scandinavica* 1980;61: pp. 43–45.

[8] Banzato CEM. Multiaxial diagnosis in psychiatry: review of the literature on DSM and ICD multiaxial schemas. *Jornal Brasileiro de Psiquiatria* 2004;53: pp. 27–34.

[9] College of American Pathologists. *Systematized Nomenclature of Pathology (SNOP)*. Chicago: College of American Pathologists: 1965.

[10] Rutter M, Lebovici S, Eisenberg L, *et al.* A tri-axial classification of mental disorders in childhood. An international study. *Journal of Child Psychology and Psychiatry* 1969;10: pp. 41–61.

[11] World Health Organization (WHO). *Multiaxial Classification of Child and Adolescent Psychiatric Disorders*. Cambridge: Cambridge University Press; 1996.

[12] American Psychiatric Association. *Diagnostic and Statistical Manual of Mental Disorders*. 3rd edition. Washington, D.C.: American Psychiatric Association; 1980.

[13] American Psychiatric Association. *Diagnostic and Statistical Manual of Mental Disorders*. 4th edition. Washington, D.C.: American Psychiatric Association; 1994.

[14] American Psychiatric Association. *Diagnostic and Statistical Manual of Mental Disorders*. 4th edition. Text Revised. Washington, D.C.: American Psychiatric Publishing Inc.; 2000.

[15] World Health Organization (WHO). *Multiaxial Presentation of the ICD-10 for use in Adult Psychiatry*. Cambridge: Cambridge University Press; 1997.

[16] Janca A, Kastrup M, Katschnig H, *et al.* The World Health Organization Short Disability Assessment Schedule (WHO DAS – S): a tool for the assessment of difficulties in selected areas of functioning of patients with mental disorders. *Social Psychiatry and Psychiatric Epidemiology* 1996;31: pp. 349–354.

[17] Janca A, Kastrup M, Katschnig H, *et al.* Contextual aspects of mental disorders: a proposal for axis III of the ICD-10 multiaxial system. *Acta Psychiatrica Scandinavica* 1996;94: pp. 31–36.

[18] Mezzich JE, Berganza CE, von Cranach M, *et al.* (eds.) Essentials of the World Psychiatric Association's International Guidelines for Diagnostic Assessment. *British Journal of Psychiatry* 2003;182(Supp. 45): pp. 37–66.

[19] Williams JBW. The multiaxial system of DSM-III: Where did it come from and where should it go? I. Its origins and critiques. *Archives of General Psychiatry* 1985;42: pp. 175–180.

[20] Mezzich JE. Architecture of clinical information and prediction of service utilization and cost. *Schizophrenia Bulletin* 1991;17: pp. 469–474.

[21] Ditmann V. Modern psychiatric classification in research and clinical practice. *Archives Suisse de Neurologie et de Psychiatrie* 1991;142: pp. 341–353.

[22] Mezzich JE. Multiaxial diagnosis: Purposes and challenges. In: Mezzich JE, *et al.* (eds.) *Psychiatric diagnosis: A world perspective.* New York: Springer; 1994.

[23] Janca A, Kastrup M, Katschnig H, *et al.* The ICD-10 multiaxial system for use in adult psychiatry. *Journal of Nervous and Mental Disease* 1996;184: pp. 191–192.

[24] Kastrup M, Mezzich JE. Quality of life: a dimension in multiaxial classification. *European Archives of Psychiatry and Clinical Neuroscience* 2001;251(Suppl. 2) pp. II.32–II.37.

[25] Mezzich JE, Janca A, Kastrup M. Multiaxial diagnosis in psychiatry. In: Maj M, *et al.* (eds.) *Psychiatric Diagnosis and Classification.* New York: John Wiley & Sons Inc.; 2002. pp. 163–176.

[26] Mezzich JE, Banzato CEM, Cohen P, *et al. Report of the American Psychiatric Association Committee to Evaluate the DSM Multiaxial System.* Presented to the APA Assembly, Atlanta, 21 May 2005.

[27] Velamoor VR, Waring EM, Fisman S, *et al.* DSM-III in Residency Training: Results of a Canadian Survey. *Canadian Journal of Psychiatry* 1989;34: pp. 103–106.

[28] Mezzich JE. International Surveys on the Use of ICD-10 and Related Diagnostic Systems. Psychopathology 2002;35: pp. 72–75.

[29] Tasman A. Lost in the DSM-IV checklist: Empathy, meaning and the doctor-patient relationship. *Academic Psychiatry* 2002;26: pp. 38–44.

[30] Mezzich JE, Sharfstein SS. Severity of illness and diagnostic formulation: Classifying patients for prospective payment systems. *Hospital & Community Psychiatry* 1985;36: pp. 770–772.

[31] Gordon RE, Eisler RL, Gutman EM, Gordon KK. Predicting Prognosis by Means of the DSM-III Multiaxial Diagnosis. *Canadian Journal of Psychiatry* 1991;36: pp. 218–221.

[32] Alarcón RD. Culture and Psychiatric Diagnosis – Impact on DSM-IV and ICD-10. *The Psychiatric Clinics of North America* 1995;18: pp. 449–465.

[33] Mezzich JE, Good BJ. On Culturally Enhancing the DSM-IV Multiaxial Formulation. In: Widiger TA, Frances AJ, Pincus HA. (eds.) *DSM–IV Sourcebook – Volume 3.* Washington, D.C.: American Psychiatric Association; 1997. pp. 983–989.

[34] Jampala VC, Sierles FS, Taylor MA. Consumers' Views of *DSM-III*: Attitudes and Practices of U.S. Psychiatrists and 1984 Graduating Psychiatric Residents. *American Journal of Psychiatry* 1986;143: pp. 148–153.

[35] Bassett AS, Beiser M. DSM-III: Use of the Multiaxial Diagnostic System in Clinical Practice. *Canadian Journal of Psychiatry* 1991;36: pp. 270–274.

[36] Williams JBW. DSM-IV Multiaxial System: Final Overview. In: Widiger TA, Frances AJ, Pincus HA *et al.* (eds.) *DSM-IV Sourcebook – Volume 4.* Washington, D.C.: American Psychiatric Association; 1998. pp. 939–946.

[37] Loranger AW. The Impact of *DSM-III* on Diagnostic Practice in a University Hospital. *Archives of General Psychiatry* 1990;47: pp. 672–675.

[38] Mellsop G, Varghese F, Joshua S, Hicks A. The Reliability of Axis II of DSM-III. *American Journal of Psychiatry* 1982;139: pp. 1360–1361.

[39] Salloum IM, Mezzich JE, Saavedra JE, Kirisci L. Usefulness of DSM-III Axis III in Psychiatric Inpatients: An Actuarial Comparison with the DSM-II Period. *American Journal of Psychiatry* 1994;151: pp. 768–769.

[40] Saavedra JE, Mezzich JE, Salloum IM, Kirisci L. Impact of DSM-III on the Diagnosis of Physical Disorders in Ambulatory Psychiatric Patients. *The Journal of Nervous and Mental Diseases* 1995;183: pp. 711–714.

[41] Zimmerman M, Pfohl B, Stangl D, Coryell W. The Validity of *DSM-III* Axis IV (Severity of Psychosocial Stressors). *American Journal of Psychiatry* 1985;142: pp. 1437–1441.

[42] Skodol AE. Axis IV: A Reliable and Valid Measure of Psychosocial Stressors? *Comprehensive Psychiatry* 1991;32: pp. 503–515.

[43] Rey JM, Plapp JM, Stewart GW, *et al.* Reliability of DSM-III Axis IV. *Archives of General Psychiatry* 1987;44: pp. 96–97.

[44] Rey JM, Stewart GW, Plapp JM, *et al*. DSM-III Axis IV Revisited. *American Journal of Psychiatry* 1988;145: pp. 286–292.

[45] Hilsenroth MJ, Ackerman SJ, Blagys MD, *et al*. Reliability and validity of DSM-IV Axis V. *American Journal of Psychiatry* 2000;157: pp. 1858–1863.

[46] Goldman HH. 'Do you walk to school, or do you carry your lunch?' *Psychiatric Services* 2005;56: p. 419.

[47] Michels R, Siebel U, Freyberger HJ, *et al*. The Multiaxial System of ICD-10: Evaluation of a Preliminary Draft in a Multicentric Field Trial. *Psychopathology* 1996;29: pp. 347–356.

[48] Takada K, Nakane Y. Progress of ICD-10 (F) family in Japan: Research, field trials and publications. *Psychiatry and Clinical Neurosciences* 1998;52(Supp.): pp. S341–S343.

[49] Banzato CEM, Pereira MEC, Santos Jr A. O que os psiquiatras brasileiros esperam das classificações diagnósticas? *Jornal Brasileiro de Psiquiatria* 2007;56: pp. 88–93.

[50] Mellsop GW, Banzato CEM, Shinfuku N, *et al*. An international study of the views of psychiatrists on present and preferred characteristics of classifications of psychiatric disorders. *International Journal of Mental Health* 2007;36(4): pp. 17–25.

[51] Cantor N, Genero C. Psychiatric Diagnosis and Natural Categorization: A Close Analogy. In: Millon T, Klerman GL. (eds.) *Contemporary Directions in Psychopathology*. New York: The Guilford Press: 1986. pp. 233–256.

[52] Widiger TA. Dimensional models of personality disorders. *World Psychiatry* 2007;6: pp. 15–19.

[53] Mellsop GW, Kumar S. An axis for risk assessment in our psychiatric classification. *World Psychiatry* 2008;7(3): pp. 182–184.

[54] Mellsop GW, Banzato CEM. *Proposal for an evidence-based psychiatric classification structure with improved utility*. Submitted, 2008.

CHAPTER 29

The Science of Well-Being and Comprehensive Diagnosis

C. Robert Cloninger

Wallace Renard Professor of Psychiatry, Genetics & Psychology, Washington University School of Medicine, Department of Psychiatry, St Louis, MO, USA

29.1 INTRODUCTION

Contemporary psychiatric practice ignores a crucial fact about human nature. The clinical processes that promote mental health and well-being are not the same as the processes that reduce the symptoms of mental illness. As a result, psychiatrists who focus only on reduction of symptoms and risk of harm are often failing to help their patients to recover a positive quality of life.

The failure to promote self-directedness and other perspectives necessary for well-being is largely a result of psychiatrists' relying on an inadequate approach to psychiatric diagnosis. The diagnostic approach currently represented by the World Health Organization's International Classification of Diseases and the American Psychiatric Association's Diagnostic and Statistical Manual fails to provide an adequate description of the person as a whole human being who is self-aware. Instead, people are reduced to abstract and stigmatizing categories without providing the comprehensive person-centred context necessary to understand their human capacity for recovery and development of well-being.

At the same time that many psychiatrists neglect positive health, advocates of recovery sometimes fail to recognize the reality and psychobiological complexity of mental ill-health. Mental illness is real, not a fiction of the imaginations of authoritarian doctors, and its reality and complexity is shown by the specificity of inheritance and the complexity of the neurobiological mechanisms underlying mental disorders [1]. The traits that predict recovery, such as self-directedness, are partly heritable themselves and interact in complex ways with other genetic and environmental factors that predispose to specific mental disorders. In order to have effective dialogue between psychiatrists and patients, there must be a scientific way to understand the psychobiological mechanisms underlying the development of mental health in ways that are health promoting and not judgmental or stigmatizing.

Psychiatric Diagnosis: Challenges and Prospects Edited by I.M. Salloum and J.E. Mezzich
© 2009 John Wiley & Sons, Ltd

Table 29.1 The World Health Organization's definition
of mental health as well-being.

Mental health is a state of well-being in which a person:
- realizes and uses his or her own abilities;
- can cope with the normal stresses of life;
- can work productively and fruitfully;
- is able to contribute to his or her community.

The science of well-being is a theory-driven and empirically-based field of mental health
that has identified key facts about the psychobiology of well-being that are crucial for
comprehensive diagnosis in psychiatry [1]. Well-being is defined as the state of being well
and happy, and flourishing as an adaptive and self-aware being. Well-being refers to a state
of welfare, health and comfort, which is more than the absence of disease. Since its
inception, the WHO has included well-being in its definition of health: 'health is a state
of complete physical, mental, and social well-being and not merely the absence of disease
or infirmity'. Furthermore, that WHO has recently defined mental health as a state of well-
being, as described in Table 29.1 [2].

The science of well-being has developed from many fields including psychiatric studies
of character development and recovery, from positive psychology, and many related
disciplines ranging from physics and neurobiology to philosophy [1]. Its application to
psychiatric diagnosis provides a rigorous, scientific way for mental health professionals to
be more comprehensive in their assessment and treatment planning in a practical and
efficient manner.

Knowledge of the personalities of people provides the psychobiological context in which
their behaviour and relationships can be adequately understood as a complex, adaptive
process, which is crucial for all diagnosis and treatment. As a result, no psychiatric
assessment is adequate without a description of the patient's personality and its development across the lifespan. The understanding of personality and its disorders is what
distinguishes psychiatry fundamentally from all other branches of medicine. A person is
a self-aware human being, not a machine-like object or an animal that lacks self-awareness.
Personality refers to all the characteristics that distinguish a person from an object.
Therefore, personality refers to all the ways someone shapes and adapts in a unique way
to an ever-changing internal and external environment. Fortunately, it is now possible to
assess personality in a way that provides a comprehensive perspective for diagnosis to
promote mental health as a state of well-being.

29.2 THE ESSENTIALS OF COMPREHENSIVE PERSON-CENTRED DIAGNOSIS

The assessment of a comprehensive person-centred diagnosis can be made during routine
assessment, combining information from mental status and the lifetime psychiatric history.
Integrating this information means that the clinician must recognize and understand the
invariance of the organization of human thought regardless of time scale: mental status
observations spans milliseconds (e.g., a transient smile, fear or anger) to minutes
(e.g., perceptual awareness, fluidity of speech, resourcefulness and speed in problem

solving), whereas the lifetime history spans months (e.g., episodes of depression, gambling, substance abuse) to decades (e.g., repeated divorces, achievements). Human thought is dynamic, with an average of 10 different thoughts per second, involving sudden shifts in attention, emotion and intention, but it varies in ways that can also be observed to develop over the entire lifespan of the same individual. To be able to describe and understand this variability coherently, it is helpful for a clinician to have an integrated model of the structure of human thought and personality.

Human personality has five layers or 'planes of being' [1]. The five layers of personality are concerned with human adaptations in situations that are perceived to be predominantly concerned with reproduction and sexuality ('sexual plane'), practical everyday activities concerned with power and possessions ('material plane'), emotional bonds and social attachments ('emotional plane'), communication and culture ('intellectual plane') and understanding what is beyond individual human existence ('spiritual plane'). The brain systems that make it possible for human beings to adopt these different perspectives have evolved in a hierarchy of discrete steps over time, to allow the survival of progressively more flexible, aware and creative organisms.

With practice, a clinician can learn to identify the layer of personality that is active at any particular moment by recognizing the predominant concern and motivation of the patient by their displayed pattern of emotion and intention, as well as the thoughts and feelings evoked by the patient in others (particularly the clinician) [1]. Specifically, frustration of the emotional drive for reproduction and sexuality elicits anxiety and startle responses, which are regulated by the temperament trait called Harm Avoidance (i.e., anxiety-prone versus risk-taking). Frustration of the material drive for power and possessions elicits anger and defence reactions (fight or flight), which is regulated by the temperament trait called Novelty Seeking (i.e., impulsive-aggressive versus rigid-stoical). Frustration of the emotional drive for succour and attachment produces feelings of rejection and disgust, which is regulated by the temperament trait called Reward Dependence (i.e., approval-seeking versus aloof). Frustration of intellectual goals for communication and creativity is regulated by individual differences in the extinction of intermittently reinforced behaviours, which is measured by the temperament trait called Persistence (i.e., ambitious overachieving versus underachieving). The fifth layer of personality, spirituality, is characterized by growth in self-awareness of the person as a whole, not by basic emotional variables like anxiety, anger, disgust, or ambition. As a result, the fifth layer of personality is regulated entirely by character development, not by a fifth temperament.

Character development does more than regulate the spiritual layer of personality. The development of well-being and the regulation of potential conflicts among emotional drives in self-aware consciousness involves three higher cognitive processes of foresight, judgment, and insight, which correspond to the character traits that should be systematically assessed during mental status examination. Each of these three cognitive functions has modules for adapting to each type of situation or layer of personality, which can be measured reliably by specific facets of character.

The three branches of mental self-government and their components are summarized in Table 29.2, along with the specific subscales of the Temperament and Character Inventory (TCI) designed to measure these functions [3]. Self-directedness in the TCI measures the executive functions of foresight, as shown by a person being self-directed in the sexual plane (i.e., responsible), in the material plane (i.e., purposeful), in the emotional plane (i.e., resilient and self-accepting), in the intellectual plane (i.e., resourceful), and in the

Table 29.2 Descriptions of three higher cognitive processes of foresight, judgment and insight that regulate the emotional drives relevant to each of the five layers of human personality, which are defined by the predominant focus of the person's perspective in a situation. Within each layer of personality, maturation involves increasing each of the three character dimensions. Integration of the whole person requires working through these functions in each of the layers of personality. TCI subscales predicted to measure these processes are indicated in parentheses. (Adapted from Cloninger [[1], pp. 219–225]).

Cognitive function (character dimension)	Characteristics of the sexual layer	Characteristics of the material layer	Characteristics of the emotional layer	Characteristics of the intellectual layer	Characteristics of the spiritual layer
Foresight (self-directedness)	Responsible vs Irresponsible (SD1)	Purposeful vs Aimless (SD2)	Resilient vs Moody (SD4)	Resourceful vs Inadequate (SD3)	Spontaneous vs Predetermined (SD5)
Judgment (cooperativeness)	Tolerant vs Prejudiced (CO1)	Forgiving vs Revengeful (CO4)	Empathic vs Inconsiderate (CO2)	Helpful vs Unhelpful (CO3)	Principled vs Opportunistic (CO5)
Insight (self-transcendence)	Self-forgetful vs Alienated (prelogical enaction-categorizing) (ST1)	Idealistic vs Materialistic (concrete-abstract logic)	Transpersonal vs Avoiding (non-verbal emotive imagery) (ST2)	Creative vs Conventional (vocal-archetypal symbols)	Spiritual vs Skeptical (preverbal holistic schemas) (ST3)

spiritual plane (i.e., spontaneous so that habits and intentions are congruent). On mental status exam, a person may be emotionally resilient in response to stress, impartial and realistic in their thinking, high in self-esteem, and far-sighted in their planning if they are highly self-directed, or they may be emotionally vulnerable, biased and unrealistic in their thinking, low in self-esteem, and short-sighted in planning. Remember that rating this one characteristic (foresight expressed as self-directedness) reveals more than any other feature of the mental status, the level of a person's maturity, their vulnerability to psychopathology, and their prognosis for recovery with a positive quality of life. Self-directedness is the expression of a life guided by a sense of hope that allows a realistic acceptance of reality as a path to understand the wonders and mysteries of life, even if they appear inconsistent with past expectations. Self-directedness is not a fixed trait – it can be temporarily reduced during stress, trauma, intoxication or psychosis, and it can be enhanced by psychotherapy or life experiences such as opportunities to gain in self-directedness by one's accomplishments from responsible work. Everyone can grow in self-directedness under appropriate therapeutic conditions, such as reduced stress, non-violence and sobriety, especially when encouraged by the hope and compassion of others.

Cooperativeness measures the legislative function of judgment, which involves making rules that allow us to get along with one another in a reasonable and flexible manner in each plane of our life. Cooperativeness can be recognized in the sexual plane as tolerance instead of prejudice, in the material plane as forgiveness instead of vengefulness, in the emotional plane as empathy instead of self-centredness, in the intellectual plane as helpfulness instead of hostility, and in the spiritual plane as a sense of principle and fairness instead of opportunism. In brief, good judgment is shown by a person's flexibility and ability to get along with others with values guided by compassion and principle. Poor judgment is shown by prejudice, lack of impulse control, insecure or hostile attachments, difficulty with teamwork, and opportunism. Comparison of a person's interaction during mental status examination with their life history is important to understand the range of cooperativeness they have demonstrated at different times during their life. For example, a person who is usually cooperative may temporarily become inflexible and hostile under stress or in the aftermath of violent trauma. Alternatively, a person who has been uncooperative in the past, may develop better judgment. A person may also have a blind spot in their awareness that elicits uncooperativeness in a recurrent but specific type of situation, but allows good judgment in most other situations.

Self-transcendence measures the judicial function or depth of insight that allows us to know intuitively when our legislative rules apply in a particular situation. The depth of a person's insight is shown in the sexual plane by a person's capacity to be absorbed in what they like to do, rather than feeling victimized, thinking pre-logically, and being repressive when dealing with situations that they don't like. Insight is shown in the material plane by problem solving that is logical and practical. In the emotional plane, insight is shown by awareness of one's transpersonal connections with nature and other people, which leads to a sense of abundance, cheerful exuberance and being gracious. In the intellectual plane, insight is shown by creativity, fluid intelligence and oceanic feelings. In the spiritual plane, insight is shown by a sense of connectedness to what is divine or beyond human existence, expressed as feelings of well-being, spiritual awareness and wisdom. In general, poor insight is shown by shallowness of awareness or magical ideation, whereas good insight is shown by wisdom, creativity and depth of understanding. In most people, the depth of insight is indicated by the frequency of peak experiences of transpersonal union, inseparable connectedness with nature, or oceanic feelings. However, reports of such peak experiences are sometimes the product of magical thinking in people who are very low in self-directedness.

29.3   THE SPIRAL PATH TO WELL-BEING

The full three-dimensional structure of personality can be visualized as a three-dimensional spiral with five planes, and increasing in height, width, and depth from the sexual to the spiritual plane. The height of the spiral indicates a person's foresight, as measured by their level of TCI Self-Directedness. The width of the spiral indicates a person's broadness of social concern and flexibility of judgment, as measured by their level of TCI Cooperativeness. The depth of the spiral indicates a person's depth or shallowness of insight, as measured by their level of TCI Self-Transcendence. Essentially, a person's thoughts can shift rapidly throughout their possible range, spiralling down with increasing negative emotions and other indicators of ill-health when stressed (e.g., preoccupied with fears, threats or desires) or spiralling up with increasing positive emotions and other indicators of well-being when calm and secure (e.g., feeling hopeful, kind and aware).

The job of a psychiatrist is to help their patient's thoughts spiral upward toward well-being. A psychiatrist is often presented with a patient in a state of distress in which their thoughts have fallen to a low point in the range. The first step in treatment is to create conditions that allow the patient's thoughts to ascend in the spiral of self-aware consciousness through validation, encouragement, medication and mental exercises that allow a person to regain their more hopeful, kind and coherent perspective toward life. Later work can help to understand and reduce their vulnerabilities for relapse and recurrence. A number of specific mental and physical exercises have been developed to promote the development of well-being (see https://psychobiology.wustl.edu).

The effective clinician must make a comprehensive diagnosis that looks beyond presenting symptoms to understand and treat the underlying processes that produce symptoms. Such a comprehensive understanding is not possible with categorical diagnoses or multidimensional systems designed to compare and judge one person against another. Nevertheless, it is possible to use information about clinical syndromes to help identify the underlying processes that are most likely. Table 29.3 lists the personality traits that are most consistently associated with different clinical disorders and states of mental health. This is not meant to be an exhaustive listing of all the personality correlates of different mental disorders, but only the traits that are so strongly related to different disorders that a clinician can use the information in the differential diagnostic process. For example, high Harm Avoidance is commonly associated with most forms of psychopathology, but it has a particularly strong relationship as a cause of mood and anxiety disorders. Therefore, high Harm Avoidance should be suspected as a predisposing trait in mood and anxiety disorders. The presence of Harm Avoidance can be quickly evaluated by inquiring about child and adolescent traits like being a worrier, a pessimist or shy. Likewise, high Novelty Seeking should be suspected if a person is alcoholic, drug abuser, gambler or bulimic. Novelty Seeking can be quickly evaluated by inquiring about a person having a quick temper in their youth, being impulsive, extravagant or disorganized, instead of slow-tempered and liking order and structure in what they do.

Table 29.3 Personality traits* that are highly likely to be high (+) or low (-) in different mental disorders and states of mental health and well-being

Mental disorder	HA	NS	RD	PS	SD	CO	ST
Schizophrenia	+		−		−	−	+
Mood disorder							
− depression	+				−		
− bipolar	+	+		−			+
Anxiety disorder							
− GAD, panic	+						
− OCD	+	−					
− social anxiety	+		+				
Eating disorder							
− anorexia	+			+			
− bulimea	+	+					
Personality disorder							
− OCPD	+	−		+	−	−	
− Cluster A			−		−	−	+
− Cluster B		+			−	−	
− Cluster C	+				−	−	
Mental order							
Recovered life quality					+		
Well sib of depressive					+		
Well sib of schizophrenic					+	+	
Resilience	−	+	+	+	+	+	+

*The personality traits are symbolized as HA (Harm Avoidance), NS (Novelty Seeking), RD (Reward Dependence), PS (Persistence), SD (Self-Directedness), CO (Cooperativeness) and ST (Self-Transcendence).

29.4 PERSON-CENTRED TARGETS FOR RESILIENCE AND RECOVERY OF WELL-BEING

Mature character development confers well-being and resilience to psychopathology, as summarized in Table 29.3. For example, TCI Self-Directedness predicts indicators of recovery of well-being in schizophrenia, including a sense of coherence, internal locus of control, self-mastery, self-esteem and life satisfaction [4]. In addition, mature character developments, such as high Self-Directedness and Cooperativeness, protects the sibs of people with major depression or schizophrenia from developing mental disorder themselves [5, 6]. Thus, the assessment of temperament traits, which are value-neutral, and character traits, whose development can facilitate recovery and well-being, provides a comprehensive perspective for person-centred diagnosis that is encouraging and not stigmatizing.

REFERENCES

[1] Cloninger CR. *Feeling Good: The Science of Well Being*. New York: Oxford University Press; 2004.
[2] Hermann H, Saxena S, Moodie R. (eds.) *Promoting Mental Health: Concepts, Emerging Evidence, Practice*. Geneva: World Health Organization; 2004.

[3] Cloninger CR, Svrakic DM, Przybeck TR. A psychobiological model of temperament and character. *Archives of General Psychiatry*1993;50: pp. 975–990.

[4] Eklund M, Hansson L, Bengtsson-Tops A. The influence of temperament and character on functioning and aspects of psychological health among people with schizophrenia. *European Psychiatry* 2004;19: pp. 34–41.

[5] Farmer A, Mahmood A, Redman K, Harris T, Sadler S, McGuffin P. A sib-pair study of the Temperament and Character Inventory in major depression. *Archives of General Psychiatry* 2003;60(5): pp. 490–496.

[6] Smith MJ, Cloninger CR, Harms MP, Csernansky, JG. *Temperament and character as schizophrenia-related endophenotypes in non-psychotic siblings.* Submitted for publication, 2008.

CHAPTER 30

Towards a Person-Centred Integrative Diagnosis

Juan E. Mezzich

*Professor of Psychiatry and Director,
International Center for Mental Health and Division of Psychiatric Epidemiology,
Mount Sinai School of Medicine, New York University, NY, USA;
Past President of the World Psychiatric Association*

Ihsan M. Salloum

*Professor of Psychiatry and Director,
Division of Alcohol and Substance Abuse: Treatment and Research, University of
Miami Miller School of Medicine, FL, USA;
Section on Classification, Diagnostic Assessment and
Nomenclature, World Psychiatric Association*

30.1 INTRODUCTION

The World Psychiatric Association has established an initiative on Psychiatry for the Person, in response to historical concerns and aspirations, and current policy statements and clinical developments in the health field. As part of this initiative, and in order to facilitate its implementation, a Person-Centred Integrative Diagnostic model (PID) is being designed. This chapter presents the background for these evolving concepts and presents the steps that are being taken for the design of the theoretical model, including health domains, descriptive tools and evaluators.

30.2 HISTORICAL AND CONCEPTUAL BASES

The broad conceptualization of health can be noted in the traditions of major ancient civilizations. For example, Chinese and Ayurvedic medical traditions promote a broad concept of health and a highly personalized approach to care and health promotion [1].

Psychiatric Diagnosis: Challenges and Prospects Edited by I.M. Salloum and J.E. Mezzich
© 2009 John Wiley & Sons, Ltd

Ancient Greek philosophers and physicians, such as Socrates, Plato and Hippocrates, also advocated holism in medicine [2]. Socrates stated that 'if the whole is not well it is impossible for the part to be well' [3]. Those early historical perspectives are echoed in today's world and serve as substantiation of a range of key health action such as prevention and health promotion [4].

In a widely quoted statement [5], the WHO's Director General proclaimed, 'there is no health without mental health', and several major international policies have cogently argued for paying greater attention to the totality of the person in clinical care and the integration of health and social services [6, 7].

A number of recent clinical developments are consistent with the above perspectives. The **recovery** movement [8, 9], which started in the rehabilitation field and was promoted by patient/user groups and like-minded clinicians, attempts to go beyond symptoms removal and functional improvement, to advance a flourishing of the whole person and quality of life. Also relevant is the **need-adaptive assessment and treatment approach** designed and studied by Irjo Alanen and colleagues in Finland. Furthermore, the **values-based practice** advocated by Fulford *et al.* [10] and the multilevel **philosophy of science schemas** presented by Schaffner [11, 12] are at the core of a renaissance of applied philosophical research in psychiatry.

30.3   WPA'S INSTITUTIONAL PROGRAMME ON PSYCHIATRY FOR THE PERSON

In 2005, the WPA's General Assembly established an Institutional Program of Psychiatry for the Person (IPPP) in response to the above historical perspectives and recent developments. The IPPP proposes the whole person in context, as the centre and goal of clinical care and public health. In this sense, it endorses Ortega y Gasset's dictum: 'I am I and my circumstance'.

This initiative is aimed at promoting a psychiatry of the person (of his/her whole health, covering both ill and positive aspects), a psychiatry by the person (with psychiatrists and health professionals extending themselves as total human beings and not merely as healing technicians), a psychiatry for the person (promoting the fulfilment of the person's health aspirations and life project, and not merely disease management), and a psychiatry with the person (working respectfully and in an empowering manner with the person who consults).

This initiative seems to represent a conceptual shift in psychiatry and, potentially, in medicine at large [13]. It is already attracting wide attention throughout WPA and other major international medical and health organizations, as evidenced in recent major conferences in London (October 2007), Paris (February 2008) and Geneva (May 2008).

The IPPP has four components, including conceptual bases, clinical diagnosis, clinical care and public health. The first component involves the reviewing of the historical, philosophical, ethical, biological, psychological, social, cultural-spiritual, and arts and literature perspectives of person-centred psychiatry [14]. The diagnostic component includes two major tasks: collaborating with the WHO for the development of the best possible classification of mental disorders and health conditions at large, and developing a Person-Centred Integrative Diagnosis (PID) [15]. The latter includes a theoretical model and its implementation in terms of a practical guide or manual. The clinical care component is focusing attention on the development of a set of guidelines on person-centred clinical care, and on the design of the curricula for person-centred training for psychiatrists and other health care professionals. The public health component is examining the role of service users as persons in mental health care training and research and designing person-centred approaches in community settings and for health promotion.

30.4 CONCEPTUAL BASES FOR PERSON-CENTRED INTEGRATIVE DIAGNOSIS

In reference to diagnosis in medicine at large, Feinstein [16] has noted that diagnosis articulates how clinicians observe, think, remember and act. In this sense, diagnosis is crucial for both clinical care and public health.

The etymological meanings of diagnosis include identification of a disorder (from the Greek *dia)* and understanding a clinical condition and situation (from *diagignoskein)*. Of relevance, the eminent philosopher of medicine Pedro Lain-Entralgo [17] has argued that identification of a disorder can be regarded as **nosological diagnosis** and the differentiation of one disorder from another as **differential diagnosis**. He reserved the fuller meaning of diagnosis to understanding what is going on in the mind and body of the person presenting for care. This more comprehensive meaning of diagnosis seems highly relevant for person-centred diagnosis.

Another important analysis involves the distinction between diagnosis as a formulation and diagnosis as a process (involving interaction among clinician, patient and family). The importance of the latter was highlighted by the conference chair at the final conclusions session of the WPA Thematic Conference on Diagnosis in Psychiatry held in Vienna, 19–22 June 2003. A further elaboration of this process is reflected in the *Trialogs* among patient, families and health professionals as documented by Amering [18].

30.5 PRECEDENCE AND RESOURCES

As we approach the development of improved diagnostic models, we should note that WPA has an established track record of contributions to the central issue of international diagnosis in psychiatry [19, 20]. Also relevant is the publication of WPA's International Guidelines for Diagnostic Assessment (IGDA) [21]. At the core of the IGDA is a diagnostic model articulating standardized multiaxial and idiographic personalized components. There has been wide acceptance of this model, as illustrated by the Latin American Guide for Psychiatric Diagnosis [22] and the use of this model in different countries in Latin America. Consequently, the IGDA diagnostic model is a significant reference point for the development of envisioned future diagnostic models.

Key participants in the development of the PID model and guide are members of the IPPP diagnostic component. Other relevant resources are WPA scientific sections (particularly the section on Classification, Diagnostic Assessment and Nomenclature), as well as member societies and their participation in a global network of national classification and diagnosis groups. Also available for consultation are the members of the IPPP Advisory Council. Specific efforts will be made to engage patients who are representative at various points in the developmental process.

Work procedures will include communication through the Internet and teleconferences, as well as face-to-face meetings. An Internet platform will be established to facilitate information exchanges and storage.

30.6 BASIC THEORETICAL MODEL OF PERSON-CENTRED INTEGRATIVE DIAGNOSIS (PID)

The construction of the new PID diagnostic model or schema requires attention to the following points.

First are the informational domains to be covered. The current draft organizes these domains into ill health and positive health [23, 24, 25]. The first level corresponds to ill health and its burden in the ill health column; and well-being in the positive health column. Here, the first sublevel corresponds to clinical disorders, both mental and general health, in the ill health column; and recovery (health restoration and growth) in the positive health column. The second sublevel corresponds to disabilities (regarding self-care, occupational functioning, functioning with family and participation in community activities) in the ill health column; and functioning in the positive heath column. The second level covers risk factors in the ill health column. This includes inner risk factors such as genetic vulnerability, and external risk factors such as stressors. It also covers protective factors in the positive health column, which include inner protective factors such as resilience, and external protective factors such as social support. The third level covers experience of illness (e.g. suffering, values and cultural experience of illness and care) in the ill health column, and experience of health (e.g. quality of life, values and cultural formulation of identity and context) in the positive health column (see Figure 30.1, which represents schematics of the PID domains).

Second, are the descriptive tools to be employed. This includes categories, particularly of a probabilistic type. The second descriptive tools are dimensions, which offer the

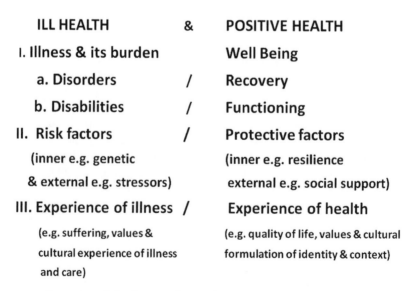

ILL HEALTH   &   **POSITIVE HEALTH**

I. **Illness & its burden**   **Well Being**

   a. **Disorders**   /   **Recovery**

   b. **Disabilities**   /   **Functioning**

II. **Risk factors**   /   **Protective factors**

   (inner e.g. genetic   (inner e.g. resilience

   & external e.g. stressors)   external e.g. social support)

III. **Experience of illness** /   **Experience of health**

   (e.g. suffering, values &   (e.g. quality of life, values & cultural

   cultural experience of illness   formulation of identity & context)

   and care)

Figure 30.1   Domains of the Person-Centred Integrative Diagnosis (PID).

opportunity to measure particular domains in a more quantitative manner. This greater use of the information available also affords categorical assignment above a threshold level. The third descriptive tool involves narrative. This offers the possibility of a deeper and richer description of a relevant domain.

Third, are the evaluators involved in the diagnostic process. These can include the clinicians as the conventional scientific experts, the patient as the main protagonist as informational source and centre of ethical clinical care, and other important participants such as family, carers and pertinent community representatives (e.g., teachers for child diagnosis).

30.7   NEXT STEPS IN PID DEVELOPMENT

Further development of the PID will involve the construction of a practical guide and application manual. This PID guide or manual will involve the translation and specification of the theoretical model into a set of procedures for practical use, according to the following phases.

First, a draft PID guide will be prepared, including its structure, schemas and procedures. It will also identify the instruments to be used, and it will describe the procedures to be employed for the assessment of the domains of the PID.

Next, the draft PID will be evaluated through field trials across different realities and settings. They will appraise the feasibility, reliability and validity of the guide.

Based on the results of the evaluation process discussed above, and on expert discussions and input from health stakeholders, a final version of the PID guide will be produced.

Eventually, the PID Guide will be translated into prominent world languages and training aids will be developed.

30.8   CONCLUSIONS

Psychiatry for the Person is a current major World Psychiatric Association (WPA) initiative. One of its endeavours is the development of Person-Centred Integrative Diagnosis (PID). This diagnostic model articulates science and humanism to obtain a diagnosis of the person (of the totality of the person's health, both ill and positive aspects), by the person (with clinicians extending themselves as full human beings), for the person (assisting the fulfilment of the person's health aspirations and life project), and with the person (in respectful and empowering relationship with the person who consults). This broader and deeper notion of diagnosis goes beyond the more restricted concepts of nosological and differential diagnoses. The proposed Person-Centred Integrative Diagnostic model, involving both a formulation and a process, employs all relevant descriptive tools (categorization, dimensions, and narratives), in a multi-level structure, engages the interactive participation of clinicians, patients, and families, and intends to provide the informational basis for person-centred integration of health care.

REFERENCES

[1] Patwardhan B, Warude D, Pushpangadan P, Bhatt N. Ayurveda and traditional Chinese medicine: a comparative overview. *Evidence-based Complementary and Alternative Medicine* 2005;2: pp. 465–473.

[2] Christodoulou GN. (ed.) *Psychosomatic Medicine*. New York: Plenum Press; 1987.

[3] Plato. *Charmidis Dialogue, 156 E*. Athens: Papyros; 1975.

[4] Herrman H, Saxena S, Moodie R. *Promoting Mental Health: Concepts, Emerging Evidence, Practice*. Geneva: WHO; 2005.

[5] World Health Organization. WHO's New Global Strategies for Mental Health. *Factsheet* 217; 1999.

[6] U.S. Presidential Commission on Mental Health. *Achieving the Promise: Transforming Mental Health Care in America. Final Report*. DHHS Pub N: SMA-03-3832. Rockville, Maryland: Department of Health and Human Services; 2003.

[7] World Health Organization European Ministerial Conference on Mental Health. *Mental Health Action Plan for Europe: Facing the Challenges, Building Solutions*. Helsinki, Finland, 12–15 January 2005. EUR/04/5047810/7.

[8] Anthony W. Recovery from mental illness. The guiding vision of the mental health service systems in the 1990s. *Psychosocial Rehabilitation Journal* 1993;16: pp. 11–23.

[9] Amering M, Schmolke M. *Recovery – Das Ende der Unheilbarkeit. Bonn: Psychiatrie-Verlag*; 2007.

[10] Fulford KWM, Dickenson D, Murray TH. (eds.) *Healthcare Ethics and Human Values: An Introductory Text with Readings and Case Studies*. Malden: Blackwell; 2002.

[11] Schaffner KF. Discovery and explanation in biology and medicine. In: Hull DL (ed.) *Science and its Conceptual Foundations*. Chicago: University of Chicago Press; 1993.

[12] Schaffner KF. The validity of psychiatric diagnosis: Etiopathogenic and clinical approaches. In: Salloum IM, Mezzich JE. *Psychiatric Diagnosis: Context and Prospects*. Chichester: Wiley-Blackwell. In press.

[13] Mezzich JE. Psychiatry for the Person: articulating medicine's science and humanism. *World Psychiatry* 2007;6(2): pp. 1–3.

[14] Christodoulou GN, Fullford B, Mezzich JE. Conceptual bases of Psychiatry for the Person. *International Psychiatry*. In press.

[15] Mezzich JE, Salloum IM. Towards innovative international classification and diagnostic systems: ICD-11 and person-centered integrative diagnosis. *Acta Psychiatrica Scandinavica* 2007;116: pp. 1–5.

[16] Feinstein AR. *Clinical judgment*. Huntington, NY: Robert E. Krieger; 1967.

[17] Lain-Entralgo P. *El Diagnostico Medico: Historia y Teoria*. Barcelona: Salvat; 1982.

[18] Amering M. *Trialog on Psychiatric Diagnosis. WPA Classification Section Newsletter*, August 2003. www.wpanet.org

[19] Mezzich JE, Ustun TB. International Classification and Diagnosis: Critical Experience and Future Directions. *Psychopathology* 2002;35: Special Issue, 55–202.

[20] Banzato CEM, Mezzich JE, Berganza CE. (eds.) Philosophical and Methodological Foundations of Psychiatric Diagnosis. *Psychopathology* 2005;38: Special Issue, Jul–Aug.

[21] World Psychiatric Association. Essentials of the World Psychiatric Association's International Guidelines for Diagnostic Assessment (IGDA). *British Journal of Psychiatry* 2003;182(Supp. 45): pp. s37–s66.

[22] APAL. *Guia Latinoamericana de Diagnostico Psiquiatrico (GLADP)* (*Latin American Guide of Psychiatric Diagnosis*). Mexico: Editorial de la Universidad de Guadalajara; 2004.

[23] Cloninger CR. *Feeling Good: The Science of Well-Being*. New York: Oxford University Press; 2004.

[24] Cox J, Campbell A, Fulford KWM. *Medicine of the Person*. London: Kingsley Publishers; 2007.

[25] Mezzich JE. Positive health: Conceptual place, dimensions and implications. *Psychopathology* 2005;38: pp. 177–179.

Index

Psychiatric Diagnosis: Challenges and Prospects   Edited by I.M. Salloum and J.E. Mezzich
© 2009 John Wiley & Sons, Ltd